Lecture Notes in Electrical Engineering

Volume 426

About this Series

"Lecture Notes in Electrical Engineering (LNEE)" is a book series which reports the latest research and developments in Electrical Engineering, namely:

- Communication, Networks, and Information Theory
- Computer Engineering
- Signal, Image, Speech and Information Processing
- Circuits and Systems
- Bioengineering

LNEE publishes authored monographs and contributed volumes which present cutting edge research information as well as new perspectives on classical fields, while maintaining Springer's high standards of academic excellence. Also considered for publication are lecture materials, proceedings, and other related materials of exceptionally high quality and interest. The subject matter should be original and timely, reporting the latest research and developments in all areas of electrical engineering.

The audience for the books in LNEE consists of advanced level students, researchers, and industry professionals working at the forefront of their fields. Much like Springer's other Lecture Notes series, LNEE will be distributed through Springer's print and electronic publishing channels.

More information about this series at http://www.springer.com/series/7818

Filippo Cavallo · Vincenzo Marletta
Andrea Monteriù · Pietro Siciliano
Editors

Ambient Assisted Living

Italian Forum 2016

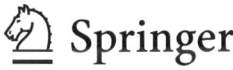 Springer

Editors
Filippo Cavallo
Scuola Superiore Sant'Anna
Pontedera
Italy

Vincenzo Marletta
DIEEI
Università degli Studi di Catania
Catania
Italy

Andrea Monteriù
Università Politecnica delle Marche
Ancona
Italy

Pietro Siciliano
IMM-CNR
Lecce
Italy

ISSN 1876-1100   ISSN 1876-1119 (electronic)
Lecture Notes in Electrical Engineering
ISBN 978-3-319-85362-8   ISBN 978-3-319-54283-6 (eBook)
DOI 10.1007/978-3-319-54283-6

Printed on acid-free paper

This Springer imprint is published by Springer Nature
The registered company is Springer International Publishing AG
The registered company address is: Gewerbestrasse 11, 6330 Cham, Switzerland

Preface

Active and Assisted Living (AAL) has been recognized for its crucial role in determining the quality of life in the future of our society. This principle has been confirmed by such institutions as the European Commission, an organization that clearly sees AAL as the "fundamental block" in addressing the challenges of demographic changes, sustaining people in productive and healthy work, keeping people at home healthy, independent and integrated, and improving the delivery of care where and when needed. These are very demanding challenges for which AAL can guarantee products and services that improve the quality of life for people in all phases of life, combining new technologies and social environments. Recent advances in a number of research areas have helped the vision of AAL to become a reality and have allowed integration of new AAL technologies into human lives in a way that will benefit all.

All these aspects were explored during the Seventh Italian Forum on Active and Assisted Living (ForItAAL), in June 2016, Pisa, Italy. It is one of the most important annual showcase events for researchers, professionals, developers, policy makers, producers, service providers, carriers, and end user organizations working in the different fields of AAL, who want to present and disseminate their results, skills, prototypes, products, and services.

This book presents the refereed proceedings of the Forum and reviews the status of researches, technologies, and recent achievements on AAL. Different points of view, from research to practice, cover interdisciplinary topics, combine different knowledge, expertise, needs, and expectations, and thus offer a unique opportunity to all those directly or indirectly interested and involved in the field of AAL.

Moreover, the book discusses the promises and possibilities of growth in AAL. It lays out paths to meet future challenges and will provide crucial guidance in the development of practical and efficient AAL systems for our current and future society.

Pontedera, Italy   Filippo Cavallo
Catania, Italy   Vincenzo Marletta
Ancona, Italy   Andrea Monteriù
Lecce, Italy   Pietro Siciliano

Organization Committee

General Chair

Filippo Cavallo, Istituto di BioRobotica—Scuola Superiore Sant'Anna

Honorary Chairs

Pietro Siciliano, IMM—Consiglio Nazionale delle Ricerche
Paolo Dario, Istituto di BioRobotica—Scuola Superiore Sant'Anna

Scientific Committee

Bruno Andò, DIEEI—Università di Catania
Roberta Bevilacqua (Istituto Nazionale Riposo e Cura Anziani, Ancona)
Manuele Bonaccorsi (Istituto di BioRobotica—Scuola Superiore Sant'Anna)
Niccolò Casiddu (Scuola Politecnica—Università degli Studi di Genova)
Amedeo Cesta (ISTC—Consiglio Nazionale delle Ricerche)
Paolo Ciampolini (Università di Parma)
Gabriella Cortellessa (ISTC—Consiglio Nazionale delle Ricerche)
Assunta D'Innocenzo (Abitare Anziani)
Leopoldina Fortunati (Università di Udine)
Michele Germani (DIISM—Università Politecnica delle Marche)
Alessandro Leone (IMM—Consiglio Nazionale delle Ricerche)
Sauro Longhi (DII—Universita' Politecnica delle Marche)
Massimiliano Malavasi (Ausilioteca Bologna)
Vincenzo Marletta (DIEEI—Università di Catania)
Andrea Monteriù (DII—Università Politecnica delle Marche)

Massimo Pistoia (E-result srl)
Lorena Rossi (Istituto Nazionale Riposo e Cura Anziani, Ancona)
Lorenzo Scalise (DIISM—Università Politecnica delle Marche)

Organizing Committee

Federica Radici (Istituto di BioRobotica—Scuola Superiore Sant'Anna)
Damiano Giuntini (TechnoDeal srl)
Teresa Pagliai (TechnoDeal srl)
Laura Fiorini (Istituto di BioRobotica—Scuola Superiore Sant'Anna)
Giorgia Acerbi (Istituto di BioRobotica—Scuola Superiore Sant'Anna)
Raffaele Esposito (Istituto di BioRobotica—Scuola Superiore Sant'Anna)
Alessandra Moschetti (Istituto di BioRobotica—Scuola Superiore Sant'Anna)
Raffaele Limosani (Istituto di BioRobotica—Scuola Superiore Sant'Anna)
Grazia Pastucci (Istituto di BioRobotica—Scuola Superiore Sant'Anna)

Contents

Part I
Care Models and Algorithms

The Mo.Di.Pro Experimental Project at the Galliera Hospital: I.C.T., Robots and Care of the Environment for the Rehabilitation of Patients Before Discharge

Niccolò Casiddu and Claudia Porfirione

Abstract The project Mo.Di.Pro, which stands for "Assisted Discharge modal" is a pilot study to test and validate an innovative form of hospitalisation which provides domestic assistance following treatment in the acute stage, during which, for a vast number of patients (mainly elderly) their discharge is delayed due to reasons independent from purely sanitary needs. The model proposes a domestic environment with sanitary assistance and monitoring with a discreet staff presence, in order to gradually prepare patients to return to their household after being discharged. This goal was pursued by designing and realising hi-tech, semi-hospital accommodation prototypes with domestic characteristics. They integrate the domestic environment with current technology in monitoring, telepresence, and teleassistance, thus reducing the need for continuous assistance from the medical staff. This contributed to increased safety and autonomy for patients.

Keywords Protected discharge · Telemedicine · Rehabilitation · Tech support

1 Introduction

The study involves the collaboration between the Hospital Board of Galliera and the University of Genoa, (DSA—Architectural Science Department, DIBRIS—Department of Computer Science, Bioengineering, Robotics and Systems Engineering) for the construction of a shelter facility of domiciliary nature adjacent

N. Casiddu (✉) · C. Porfirione
Architectural Science Department—Design Area, University of Genoa,
Stradone S. Agostino 37, 16123 Genoa, Italy
e-mail: casiddu@arch.unige.it

C. Porfirione
e-mail: claudia.porfirione@arch.unige

© Springer International Publishing AG 2017
F. Cavallo et al. (eds.), *Ambient Assisted Living*, Lecture Notes
in Electrical Engineering 426, DOI 10.1007/978-3-319-54283-6_1

to the hospital allowing scheduled visits by doctors and immediate intervention in health emergencies, at a lower cost to the current hospital costs (approx. 1000 €/day) and to assist the return to a home environment more gradually and effectively.

Accordingly the study activity has concerned, first of all, the design and construction of prototype semi-hospital housing of domiciliary nature and with high-tech equipment and subsequently the design of interface systems for the monitoring and control of activities during the model testing.

1.1 *Objectives*

The aim of the study, which started in January 2015, is to develop a model of "protected discharge" in premises with high technological and architectural content for elderly patients, clinically dischargeable but not able to return home, for social care issues. It is an experimental pilot study, coordinated by Dr. Gian Andrea Rollandi (Scientific Coordinator, E.O. Ospedali Galliera).

The experimental activity includes the involvement of 30 subjects chosen among patients in hospital discharge, discharged and sent for monitoring in the area of temporary in-hospital residence for a period of approximately 5–2 days.

The primary objective of the study is to evaluate the feasibility in terms of protected discharge, with the help of appropriate monitoring of the main vital/clinical signs using the automated system, in the context of specifically dedicated discharge premises of domiciliary type. Accordingly, the primary endpoint is represented by the hospitalisation days of patients enrolled in an experimental model. The achievement of this objective will be identified by the number of hospitalisation days.

The secondary objectives, since this is a pilot study, are varied and include a series of evaluations, with exploratory intent, which will be used to better define the objectives of any subsequent stage of experimentation. They are mainly identified in assessing the hospitalisation costs, life quality for patients and their caregivers, the degree of cognitive and physical frailty, assistive devices and remote connection.

2 Materials and Methods

Recent data show that a predictable percentage of around 8% of patients admitted to hospitals prolongs stay in hospital despite being clinically dischargeable and with no need to carry out diagnosis and/or in-hospital therapy [1]. This involves, on the one hand, an unsuitable occupation of hospital beds with an increase in the number of hospitalisation days and hospital health expenditure and, on the other hand, hardship for patients with increased risk of creating conditions of disability and iatrogenic diseases by "prolonged hospitalisation", well documented mainly in more compromised and older subjects [2, 3].

The reasons for the continued stay in hospital may include [4, 5]:

1. degree of disability and frailty of the patient with heavy care burden once returned to his/her domestic environment (distance from the hospital, assistance availability, etc.);
2. prolonged waiting for activation of home care processes;
3. prolonged waiting for supplying aids/devices at home;
4. unwillingness on the part of family members/caregivers to receive the patient at home;
5. bed unavailability in protected residential structures (RSA) or rehabilitation facilities.

The conditions of the study result from the analysis of the times and course of hospitalisation: the average time of hospitalisation of patients with non-surgical pathologies is slightly longer (at the Galliera hospital, the average is 15 days) and while, normally, most of the diagnoses and the most important therapies are conducted in the first week of admission, usually, in the last days before the discharge, the medical assistance to patients decreases to almost zero.

In this respect one of the most important elements to consider is the time gap between the time a patient is deemed clinically dischargeable and the time this patient is actually discharged. This time gap is due mainly to social welfare problems related to the difficulties for families to receive a member who is less self-sufficient and in need of more care and time of insertion in the RSA (nursing residence) in several respects (rehabilitation, clinical stabilisation, relief and more).

On this basis a shelter structure, adjacent to the hospital, is planned to be built, so that scheduled visits and immediate action of doctors is easily enabled in the event of a health emergency, provided with all the architectural and premise features to be perceived as a receptive domestic/lodging facility that enables a significant reduction in the daily management cost (the current average cost of hospitalisation is nearly 1000 €/day).

The stay is planned in larger rooms, with home like furnishings and with a different discipline from the perspective of the relatives' access, in order to "accompany" more gradually and effectively both patients and relatives back to their home environment.

The goal of the experiment aims at identifying design (architectural and technological) solutions, to assist the rehabilitation of hospitalised patients before their final discharge [6].

So the choice has been made to experiment with new project proposals and to generate an "ecosystem" with materials, furniture, accessories and technology platforms already available in the market, implementing the functions for achieving predetermined objectives: for example to monitor the domestic space, to facilitate opportunities for communication and user participation in every aspect of daily life, etc.

2.1 Accommodation Design

The objective of the first testing phase aims at creating and studying the functionality of (architectural and technological) design solutions, to enhance autonomy, independence and mobility of the dischargeable patient [7]. The study is based on the principle that, going through a transition period in an environment of mainly domestic reception features, these persons can regain the ability to live actively and independently at home.

Architectural (distribution, material, structural and formal) choices in the study are conceived according to criteria designed to guarantee maximum safety, comfort and ease of use (for guests, their families and professionals) and to optimise the procedure and timing for operation and maintenance of the premises in relation to the expected hygiene standards. The project aims at verifying solutions for those needs [8].

New project proposals will be experimented and a "domestic ecosystem" will be generated with materials, furniture, accessories and technology platforms already available on the market, implementing functions for achieving present objectives: for example, to monitor domestic space, to facilitate opportunities for user communication and participation in every aspect of daily life, etc.

Starting from the identification of needs and the users' needs, the work aims to identify solutions and products that allow the integration of architectural environment with systems of monitoring, control and assistance (with particular attention to the protection of privacy), involving different technological areas such as: telecommunications, computer science, microsystems, robotics, new materials, according to the AAL (Ambient Assisted Living) approach [9].

The study applied to the project was conducted on two interdependent levels:

- Definition of finishing materials, furnishings and accessories, colour harmonies, textures, etc. designed according to ergonomics, usability, accessibility and security (passive technological design);
- Choice of technologies, devices and systems that are integrated into the domestic ecosystem, both in current use and to be developed specifically to provide environmental control and personal monitoring and offer assistance, care and companionship (active technological design).

The integration of "passive" solutions (e.g. resilient floor surfaces, to reduce damage in the event of a fall or impact, shape and arrangement of furnishings, position of control devices etc.) and "active" hi-tech systems (integrated sensor panels for the control of posture and warning in the event of recognition of a fall) makes it possible to implement smart environments, which are still designed to be perceived as domestic and in which the comfort and safety of the guest and family members is guaranteed and at the same time monitoring and care facility is optimised [10].

2.1.1 Bedroom

The spaces intended for curative periods and at night, being of a private nature, are defined by the use of cool colours, designed to separate clearly the public spaces from the private ones [11, 12]. Colour has been used as signage and orientation to accentuate the differentiation between the different spaces of the accommodation and the transition from one to another [13]. The light fixtures are predominantly composed of domestic purpose lights (such as floor lamps and lampshades over nightstands). In particular, the lighting during the night, for the safety of our guests, is guaranteed by a LED step light for orientation, automatically operated by getting out of bed.

The furnishings have light wood finishes, more similar to the home than the hospital environment [14]. The bed nets are of orthopaedic type with variable inclination (Fig. 1).

2.1.2 Bathroom

In toilets, scaled so they are easily adaptable to the use of a wheel chair, the installation is expected of acrylic stone shower trays flush with the sanitary floor and equipped with full access, while maintaining the typical characteristics of the home environment. Specific measures have been developed to prevent the risk of falling due to tripping or slipping and of impact or injury (Fig. 2).

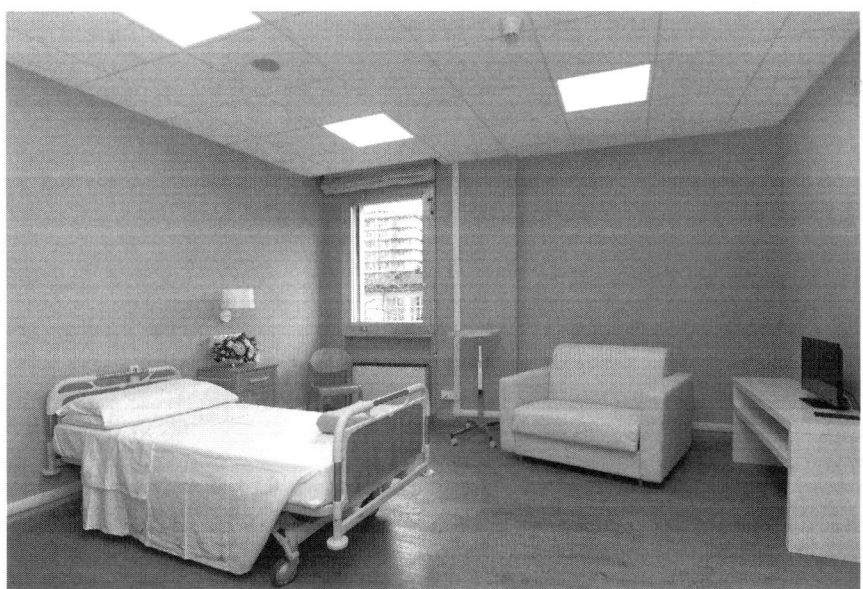

Fig. 1 Single room

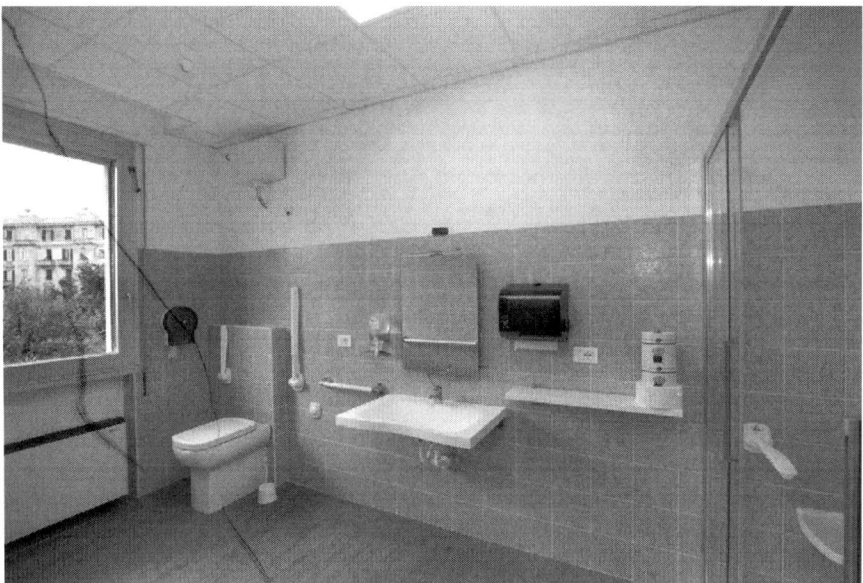

Fig. 2 Single bathroom

2.1.3 Corridor

In the corridor (partially adjacent to the living room), as throughout the accommodation, the floors were completely coated in 2 mm thick PVC with a wood effect, with hot-welded joints, to ensure perfect homogeneity of the environments and also their cleanliness [15] (Fig. 3).

2.1.4 Living Area

Warm colours characterise the bright living room [16]. The kitchenette is equipped with refrigerator, electric hob with induction heating for heating food, microwave oven, sink with mixer tap and mobile storage facilities with easy handling (e.g., handles easily reached and recognisable by colour and shape) [17]. Fittings and components are safe, pleasant and characterised by a high level of performance (i.e., without materials which are excessively cold to the touch). A "Design for All" principles-based design has guaranteed the best approach possible to all worktops [18].

The lights, kitchen ceiling light points, the floor of the living room and the light fixtures on the ceiling of the corridor are linked to the presence detection system (Figs. 4 and 5).

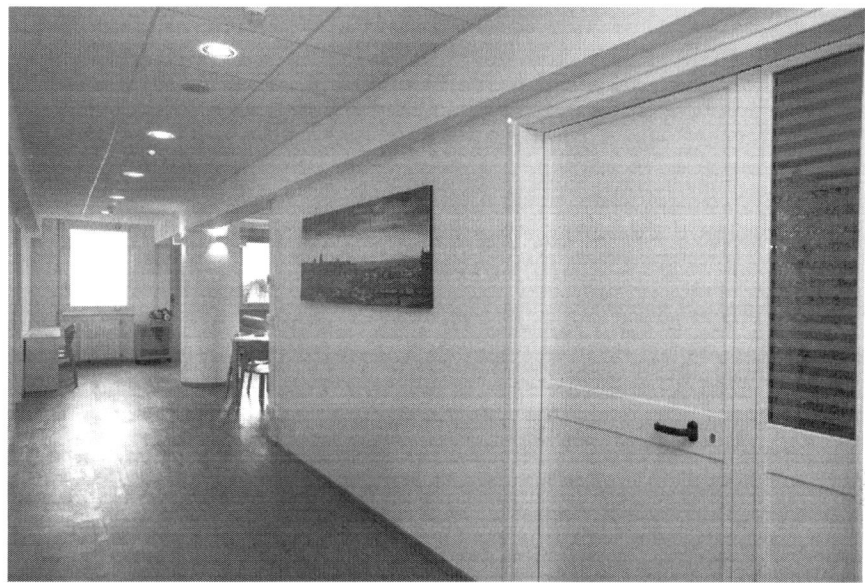

Fig. 3 The wide corridor from the entrance leads to the living area

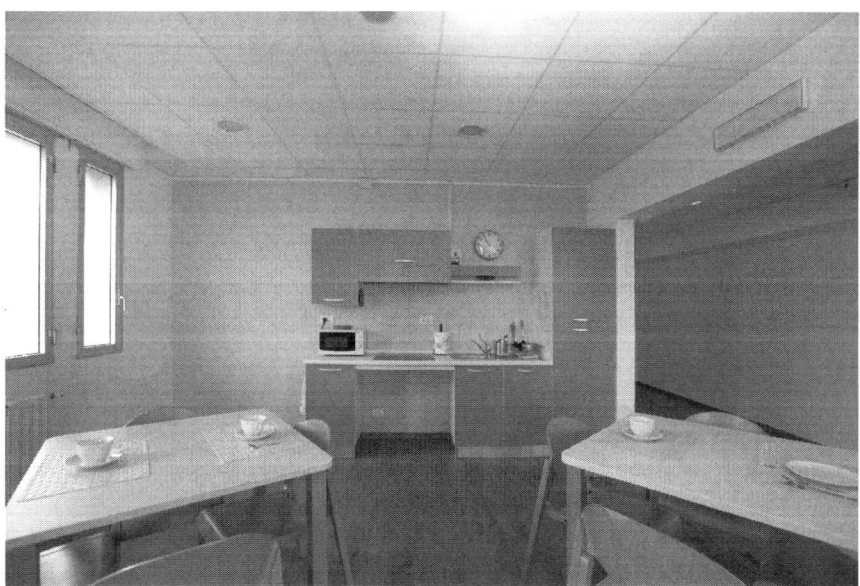

Fig. 4 Kitchen

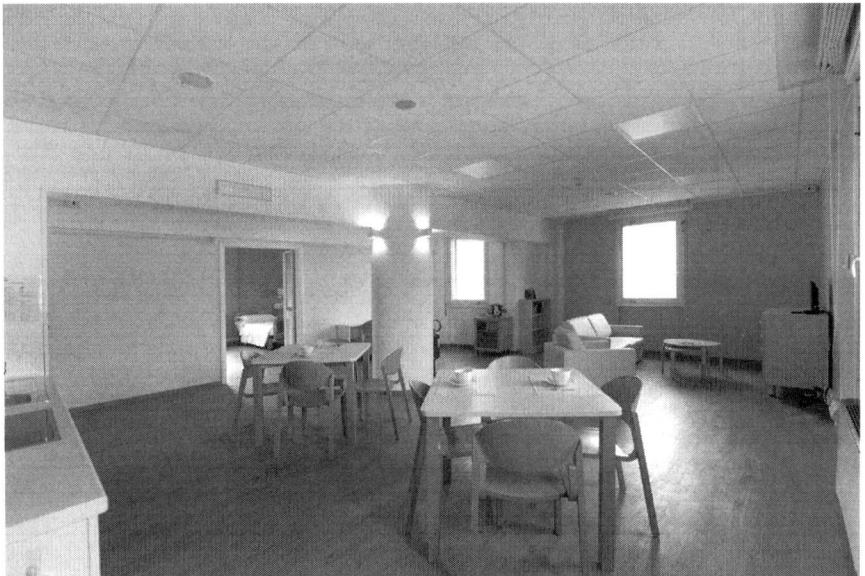

Fig. 5 Living area

2.1.5 Gym

Dominated by the colour yellow, it has retained the lighting from the ceiling [19]. Usable for rehabilitation activities under the guidance of the responsible staff member, it has a space dedicated to the technical IT compartment.

2.2 Monitoring of Parameters

During the stay in the semi-hospital residence certain data will be monitored which is collected using worn devices and properly coordinated environmental devices.

The intention is to monitor a series of vital signs using non-invasive wearable devices that give the subject enrolled complete freedom of movement and that perform analyses on the data captured (through the implementation of mathematical methods and statistical analyses) [20].

In particular, we intend to observe the following vital signs: temperature, blood pressure, heart rate and oxygen saturation, breathing rate and body weight.

In addition to monitoring vital parameters, there will also be monitoring of the following laboratory parameters when necessary: glycaemia, INR, cholesterol.

The analysis of sleep and movement, the risk of falling (fluctuations and swings, as well as changing the centre of gravity) and ADL (Activity of Daily Living) are

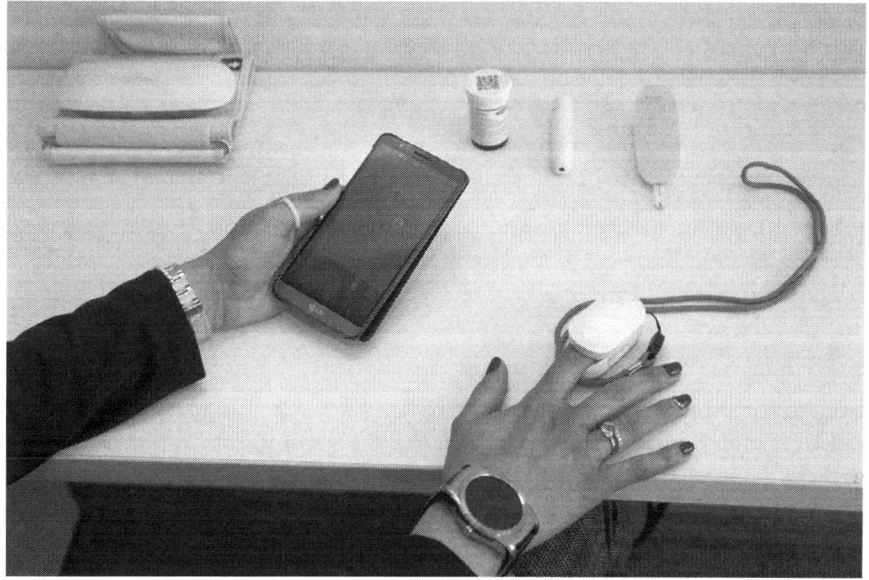

Fig. 6 Some of the monitoring equipment supplied to the facility

monitored. Sleep quality, understood as the number of nocturnal awakenings, is monitored as an indicator of the overall health of the patient (Fig. 6).

The intention is to monitor the amount of time the patient spends sitting, the time and speed of walking and physical activity: this monitoring activity (motion analysis) both includes the use of wearable sensors and is deployed in the environment.

Using wearable inertial sensors it is possible to estimate the number of steps taken and track/trace the person's posture, while through two cameras, properly positioned, it is possible to obtain synchronised video streams and spatial and temporal information on users (e.g. spatio-temporal sequences of activities: statistics on time spent at a given point, statistics on how often the patient moves around the room and what are the points where he most commonly goes, information related to time slots).

It is also expected that, inside the rooms, monitoring will be performed through wearable devices, positioning systems and RFID tags. To give some examples:

1. force sensors that detect the status (free/occupied) of chairs, armchairs, sofas, beds;
2. sensors to detect the presence of persons in the apartment;
3. tags placed on key items that will recognise a specific type of activity through interaction with them.

In addition to the proposed set-ups, it is intended to also to offer the testing and subsequent marketing of devices currently in the engineering phase (Fig. 7).

CLASSE	MISURA	ESISTENZA
Parametri vitali	Temperatura corporea	SI
	Pressione Arteriosa	SI
	Frequenza cardiaca	SI
	Frequenza respiro	SI
	Saturazione ossigeno	SI
	Peso corporeo	SI
Esami di Laboratorio	Glicemia	SI
	INR	SI
	Disidratazione	NO
Sonno	Sonno	NO
Rischio di caduta		SI
Movimento		SI
ADL		NO

Fig. 7 List of parameters to be observed and the relevant devices available on the market

2.3   Ethics: Informed Consent

The study protocol is in compliance with the principles established by the 18th World Medical Assembly in Helsinki, 1964 and subsequent amendments/additions as well as Good Clinical Practice.

The nature of the study, its purpose, the procedures, the expected duration and the potential risks and benefits should be explained to each patient. Each patient must be informed that the participation in the study is voluntary and that he/she may withdraw at any time. Withdrawal of consent will not affect its subsequent clinical treatment or relationship with the doctor.

Informed consent will be drafted by the coordinating centre by means of a written statement, using non-technical language. The patient will have to demonstrate that he/she understands the information contained in the consent, by signing and dating it; also the copy of the document must be provided. No patient will be enrolled in the study without having obtained his/her prior informed consent. An original copy of the signed written informed consent of the patient must be kept by the enrolling centre in a dedicated section of the study documentation.

3   Results and Discussion

No data is currently available in the literature on the methodology of management intervention tested in this study and in a similar context (hospital): no sufficient data is therefore available from previous experimental experiences on which to base the foundations to build valid hypothesis testing.

It follows that no formal sample calculation has been performed. The study is therefore intended as a pilot type with exploratory intent, with the main objective being to assess the feasibility of a managerial change in hospital discharge standard procedures. The standard assumable sample of about 30 subjects to be enrolled in a time of approximately 3 months (10 persons/month) has been therefore established on the basis of practical considerations considering eligible cases that normally involve the hospital. This sample will be sufficient, however, to consider first the technical feasibility of the project, but may also be useful in testing, on an exploratory basis, the initial assumptions of efficacy (maintenance of fragility indices, popularity testing, reducing hospitalisation time and operating costs) and to lay the groundwork for possible future studies, even with larger randomised drawing on case studies and specifications.

Descriptive statistics used for continuous parameters shall be mean, standard deviation, median, quartiles, minimum and maximum; the discrete parameters will be absolute frequency and relative frequency. The normality of deployments will be tested and, if necessary, the necessary transformations to normality will be applied.

Any statistical tests used with purely exploratory intent will be the Fisher exact test and chi-square for comparison between proportions; mainly nonparametric tests (given the limited sample size) will be used in the case of comparison between continuous variables.

3.1   *Experimentation with Telepresence Robots*

The purpose of the trial made by the group of researchers of the DSA (Architectural Science Department) in the semi-hospital facility is the evaluation of operating modes for using tele-presence robots in assisting elderly patients.

Fig. 8 Padbot, telepresence robot

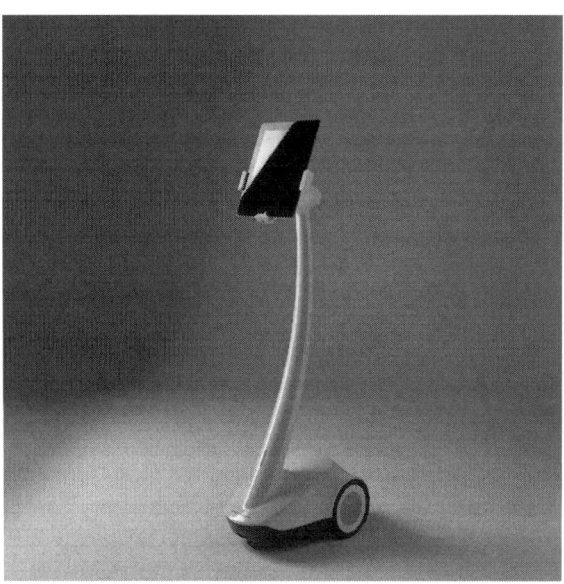

Evaluation by users, service personnel and customers, will cover the robot interface, which is the component of the product that allows the user to actually take action. For this purpose two Padbots will be used in the treatment rooms, a telepresence robot developed by Inbot Technology Ltd, a company based in Guangzhou [21]. Padbot allows users to move and communicate remotely with actions-reactions in real-time voice and video, in a simple and natural manner. The launch campaign suggests using them in the work and private environments, particularly in long distance relationships, since they can amplify the degree of satisfaction with telepresence communication (Fig. 8).

This tele-presence robot consists of a body about 90 cm allowing it to move freely on wheels within the department. The head consists of a tablet—which can be an iPad or Android tablet—which makes it possible to connect remotely with a 4G connection or wi-fi. This telerobot is equipped with sensors antifall and anticollision enabling it not to collide with potential obstacles that can be found in the environment in which it moves, and it can be controlled remotely via the appropriate smartphone app (iOS or Android). The robot has an independent operating time of 8 h and when it has lost its charge goes independently to its charging base to recharge, and it also has Bluetooth and speakers. From a design point of view, Padbot is characterised by soft and sinuous lines that resemble a white goose, a quality that makes it particularly elegant, pleasant and friendly [22].

The two rooms of the department will be equipped with a Padbot operated by service personnel of the department or by a physician who can remotely connect to the patient.

If authorised by the patients, the system can be activated even with family members, so that they can get from the outside, on their mobile devices, in connection with patients within the department.

The conduct of these operations will be assessed through appropriate cards and interviews, for the purposes of analysing the problems encountered in the use of robots, both by patients and by service personnel and assessing the object's usability as well as the user's related perception [23].

3.1.1 Specific Procedures

The trial will cover in particular the assessment of certain procedures for calling for assistance staff, which are usually outside the department. Two scenarios will be analysed:

- local (patient);
- Remote (doctor or family);

The scenarios identified will configure three different types of communication-interaction with the robot:

1. Video chat without Padbot (between 2 SmartPhone/Tablet type terminals)
2. Video chat via Padbot activated by the local device (between 2 terminals).
3. Video chat via Padbot by two terminals.

The development is expected of specific secondary procedures aimed at improving the existing functionalities or their specific implementation in areas of interest for research. The following is a list of the main ones:

- development of an application or a specific computer software;
- increase of the quality of communication by wi-fi;
- increased level of video call alert on the SmartPhone/Tablet (currently the automatic answer works only when the Padbot App is active);
- development of the ability to send images or other multimedia files;
- development of the ability to send text messages or images during a video call (like Skype).

The evaluation of the procedures will involve medical and welfare staff in filling out a questionnaire concerning the efficiency of the communication and usability of the robotic system.

A parallel evaluation of quality will be performed through interviews conducted for guests by the researchers of the DSA, via video call with Padbot, at agreed times.

4   Conclusion

This project, initiated in January 2015, has already led to the creation of a model of "protected discharge" of high technological and architectural content.

The experimental activity, launched in April 2016, is affecting successfully the first subjects chosen among patients in hospital discharge (for approximately 5–2 days).

The trial is intended to test the feasibility of positive rehabilitation of patients being discharged, to familiarise them with the use of self-monitoring technologies for communication and data transmission, and it is functional to be able to transfer the rehabilitation situation to situations at home so as to enable a functional relationship of assistance which continues over time, in order to improve quality of life, safety and autonomy and reduce recidivism in recovery, such as often happens in patients, especially the elderly and frail, after discharge [24].

Acknowledgements The research activity carried out was launched in January 2015, in a collaboration between the Hospital Board of Galliera (contact: Dr. Gian Andrea Rollandi) and the two departments of Genoa University: DSA—Science Department for Architecture (contact: Prof. Niccolò Casiddu) and DIBRIS—Department of Computer Science, Bioengineering, Robotics and Systems Engineering (contact: Prof. Alessandro Verri). Technical sponsor: Malvestio s.p.a and Ponte Giulio S.p.A.

References

1. Lenzi J, Mongardi M, Rucci P (2014) Sociodemographic, clinical and organisational factors associated with delayed hospital discharges: a cross-sectional study. BMC Health Serv Res 14:28–36
2. Volpato S, Onder G, Cavalieri M (2007) Characteristics of nondisabled older patients developing new disability associated with medical illnesses and hospitalization. J Generel Intern Med 22:668–674
3. Bo M, Fonte G, Pivaro F (2015) Prevalence of and factors associated with prolonged length of stay in older hospitalized medical patients
4. Challis D, Hughes J, Xie C, Jolley D (2014) An examination of factors influencing delayed discharge of older people from hospital. Int J Geriatr Psychiatry 29:160–168
5. Percorsi di dimissioni ospedaliere protette nelle Regioni italiane. Le buone prassi. Project (VS/2011/0052)—supported by the European Union Programme for Employment and Social Solidarity—PROGRESS (2007–2013)
6. Clarkson PJ, Keates S (2003) Inclusive design: design for the whole population. University of Cambridge, Springer
7. Pullin G (2009) Design meets disability. MIT Press, Cambridge, Mass
8. Briganti F (2009) Corpo, tecnologie e disabilità. Le tecnologie integrative, invasive ed estensive. Napoli, Edizioni Manna
9. Wichert R, Eberhardt B (2012) Ambient assisted living. Springer, Londra
10. Pierce D (2012) The accessible home: designing for all ages and abilities. Taunton Press, Newtown
11. Gazzola A (2011) Uno sguardo diverso: la percezione sociale dello spazio naturale e costruito. Franco Angeli, Milano
12. Santagostino P (2006) Il colore in casa. Urra, Milano

13. Fagnoni R (2006) A colori. Alinea, Milano
14. Perkins LB, Hoglund JD (2013) Building type basics for senior lining. Wiley, Hoboken
15. Rossi S (2008) I rivestimenti: la pelle del design. Alinea, Firenze
16. Ridolfi F (2000) Casa e colore. Mondadori, Milano
17. Bleicher S (2011) Contemporary color, theory & use. Cengage Learning, USA
18. Accolla A (2009) Design for All: il progetto per l'individuo reale. Franco Angeli, Milano
19. Romanello I (2002) Il colore: espressione e funzione. Hoepli, Milano
20. Bennett KB, Flach JM (2011) Display and interface design: subtle science, exact art. CRC Press, Londra
21. http://www.padbot.co [18 gennaio 2016].
22. Spadolini MB (2000) Progettazione amichevole. Rima, Milano
23. Moggridge B (2007) Designing interaction. The Mit Press, Cambridge
24. Rosenfeld J, Chapman W (2011) Unassisted living: ageless homes for later life. Monacelli Press, New York

Theoretical Model for Remote Heartbeat Detection Using Radiofrequency Waves

V. Di Mattia, G. Manfredi, M. Baldini, V. Petrini, L. Scalise, P. Russo, A. De Leo and G. Cerri

Abstract Recently there is an increasing demand for contactless and unobtrusive techniques able to ensure a complete, comfortable and unobtrusive monitoring of human vital signs even in critical situations, such as burn victims and newly born infants, or when a long time monitoring is needed. This paper describes a preliminary theoretical investigation about the possibility of using an electromagnetic approach, already successfully tested for respiration monitoring, to detect the heart activity of a human subject in indoor environments. In particular, the electromagnetic model presented has been implemented to investigate the physical mechanism of interaction between the heart movement and an electromagnetic wave impinging on the human chest and to find out what is possible to observe from the outside without any electrodes.

V. Di Mattia (✉) · G. Manfredi · M. Baldini · V. Petrini ·
P. Russo · A. De Leo · G. Cerri
Dip. Ing. dell'Informazione, Univ. Politecnica delle Marche, Ancona, Italy
e-mail: v.dimattia@univpm.it

G. Manfredi
e-mail: g.manfredi@univpm.it

M. Baldini
e-mail: baldinim89@gmail.com

V. Petrini
e-mail: v.petrini@univpm.it

P. Russo
e-mail: paola.russo@univpm.it

A. De Leo
e-mail: a.deleo@univpm.it

G. Cerri
e-mail: g.cerri@univpm.it

L. Scalise
Dip. Ing. Industriale e Scienze Matematiche,
Univ. Politecnica delle Marche, Ancona, Italy
e-mail: l.scalise@univpm.it

© Springer International Publishing AG 2017
F. Cavallo et al. (eds.), *Ambient Assisted Living*, Lecture Notes
in Electrical Engineering 426, DOI 10.1007/978-3-319-54283-6_2

Keywords Electromagnetic sensor · Heartbeat detection · Remote sensing

1 Introduction

The heartbeat is an important vital sign which indicates the health and the physiological vital status of a subject and represents a predictive parameter for many pathologies. The early diagnosis of the heart disease is a more and more significant goal considering that, according to the World Health Organization (WHO), the cardiovascular disease is one of the leading causes of death and the proportion of deaths related to cardiovascular disease is increased by 5.7% globally between 1990 and 2013 [1].

The electrocardiography (ECG) is the *gold standard* among monitoring cardiac techniques and it measures the bioelectrical signal generated by the myocardial cells involved in cardiac activity. The mechanisms of contraction involved generate an electrical potential difference, which propagates to all the surrounding tissues and can be measured by several electrodes placed on the body surface. In some cases, such as burn victims or newly born infants or when a long time monitoring is needed, the fixed electrodes represent a contraindication (discomfort, skin irritation, subject confined) with a consequent need for a noncontact measurement method [2].

In this context, the electromagnetic (EM) technology can provide a useful approach to remotely monitoring humans' vital signs. Previous studies [3, 4] demonstrated the feasibility of using EM fields to monitor the respiration activity of human subjects in indoor environments, highlighting some important advantages as the possibility of non-contact measurements at significant distances (even 2 or 3 m), and most importantly, through tissues (bed sheets, blankets, clothes), because common fabrics are generally transparent to EM waves. These aspects may represent a clear advantage for both the monitoring of non-collaborative or burnt patients and the remote monitoring for Ambient Assisted Living applications. In fact, an EM system may be easily installed inside hospital rooms or even at home without the need to have a direct collaboration of the subject, the intervention of medical personnel nor of the subject and without privacy issues. The next step of this research field is to investigate the possibility of using a similar EM technology to detect without contact the cardiac activity. A preliminary theoretical study about the feasibility of such an approach will described in this paper.

The normal heart rate in adult subjects ranges from 1 to 3 Hz, corresponding to 60–100 beats per minute (bpm) but in some cardiac arrhythmia disease, it can significantly change. During ventricular tachycardia, the heart rate can increase over 200 bpm; it can also decrease below 60 bpm during bradycardia. These changes influence the respiration rate, which increases above 1–2 Hz in emergency cases, while the normal respiration rate varies between 0.1 and 0.3 Hz (12–20 breaths per min), demonstrating that is often important to consider the frequency components of both the heart and the respiration rates. It is equally true that the two signals are hardly distinguishable from each other. In fact, the breathing activity produces a chest displacement ranges from 4 to 12 mm, which is summed to the exiguous skin movement caused by the heart activity, which ranges from 0.2 to 1 mm.

A lot of experimental researches have already been conducted on non-invasive monitoring of heart rate. Some examples are: a 2.4 GHz Doppler radar on chip used to detect the heart rate with an accuracy up to 80% [5]; a wavelet transform performed to detect the heart rate at various distances from the radar [6] and an investigation about the effect of the frequency on the detection accuracy [7]. On the contrary there is a lack of theoretical studies able to give a physical explanation of the relation between the heart movement and the EM signal reflected by the human chest and observed from the outside without any electrodes. Actually the values relative to the impedance, the attenuation, the speed and the thickness of various tissues crossed by the EM field while travelling through the human thorax from the skin to the heart can be found in [8, 9], allowing predict some parameters related to the EM signal reflected by the human chest. Starting from these and other studies related to the dielectric properties of biological tissues of a human chest [10], the idea has been to review and modify the multilayer model presented in [11] to better understand the physical mechanism of interaction between an EM wave and the human chest and its consequences on the reflected wave, in order to define some guidelines for the realization of an EM non-contact monitoring system.

The paper is divided as follows: Sect. 2 describes the EM model implemented and its application to the detection of the cardiac activity; Sect. 3 presents a comparison between the results obtained using the models and those calculated by analytical formulation and by experimental measurements; at the end, Sect. 4 resumes the goals and the most important results of the research activity presented and proposes some hints for future developments.

2 The Electromagnetic Multilayer Model

Starting from the positive results achieved in terms of respiration monitoring by means of an EM sensor [3, 4], the next step has been to investigate the feasibility of monitoring the cardiac activity without contact and with a similar technology. In particular, it has been taken into account the use of a Doppler continuous wave radar technology. The research activity started with a preliminary study to understand which is the physical quantity related to the heart movement that can be significantly detected from the outside and without contact with the human body. In fact, while the respiration activity causes a chest displacement of about few centimeters (depending on the breath depth) visible even to the naked eye, the movement of the cardiac muscle is hard to detect because it is placed under several layers (chest, lungs…) and causes a skin displacement of maximum 1 mm. For this reason, the first step has been the development of an EM multilayer model to simulate the interaction between an EM wave and the heart movement. This allows to understand if the EM wave is able to penetrate all the tissues to directly detect the reflection caused by the cardiac movement, or whether it is necessary to detect the reflection caused by the superficial thoracic movement due to the cardiac activity. In fact, it is commonly known that the phenomena of depolarization and polarization are responsible for the contractions movements of the cardiac muscle, that are variations of shape and volume of the heart. Such movements do not remain organ-confined but they propagate through the adjacent tissues and the ribs, thus causing a skin vibration slightly perceptible from the outside. Moreover, the extent of this external movement caused by the heartbeat varies depending on the conditions of the monitored subject, considerably decreasing for patients in conditions of obesity or over fifty years and by the position taken by the subject. The size of the skin vibration caused by the heartbeat can be assumed between 0.2 and 1 mm and to this exiguous displacement is summed the much higher chest movement caused by the breathing activity. Therefore, not only a small spatial resolution is required, but even a suitable signal processing to distinguish the two signals. Table 1 resumes the average amount of the variables related to the two phenomena.

2.1 Multilayer Model Implementation

An EM wave transmitted at a sufficient distance from the subject to monitor, that means assuming the target is in the far field zone with respect to the transmitter, can be considered as a plane wave. At this point there are two main factors that influence the characterization of the reflected wave: the morphology of the human body and the dielectric properties of the tissues crossed by the wave. It is understandable that taking into account the complex morphology of the body would mean also considering the variability of these characteristics not only from one person to another, but also depending on the position of the same subject. On the contrary, the dielectric properties of the tissues crossed by the incident wave with slightly approximations are quite comparable among subjects. Therefore, it is reasonable to consider that an EM model will be an approximation of the real scenario but sufficient to estimate the amount of reflection and attenuation of an EM wave that travels through the different tissues of the body.

The propagation of an EM wave through biological tissue is mainly governed by the dielectric constant, the conductivity, the source configuration and geometric factors that describe the structure of the tissues themselves. These parameters also determine the amount of power density absorbed by a given tissue. When the radius of curvature of a surface is larger than both the wavelength and the beam width of

Table 1 Comparison between the fundamental features of respiration and heart activities

	Respiration activity	Heart activity
Rate (breaths/beats per minute)	6–40	40–180
Frequency (Hz)	0.1–0.6	0.6–3
Chest displacement (mm)	4–12	0.2–1

the incident radiation, it is possible to use planar tissue models to estimate the absorbed power density and its distribution within the body. In the view of this hypothesis, the one-dimensional layered model proposed in [11] to study the dependency of dielectric proprieties of biological tissues on the frequency, has been chosen as the starting point for the implementation of a more complete model. In fact, among the models present in literature, it is the most satisfactory to represent the geometry and the dielectric characteristic of the human chest. Actually, to the end of our study, it has been reviewed and extended in order to consider also the contribution of the cardiac muscle. In fact, the original model includes Skin, SAT, Muscle, Bone Lungs, where SAT (Subcutaneous Adipose Tissue) represents the subcutaneous fat and contains various types of fat tissue. Figure 1 shows a schematic representation of the proposed EM model, where a layer for heart has been added between the bone and lungs layers. Table 2 reports the range relative to the thicknesses of the tissues used in the model and relative to the frontal chest area of a male adult subject, aged between twenty and sixty years, normo-weight [11]. The values chosen for the simulation are the maximum, the minimum and the averages values of the ranges indicated in Table 2. The dielectric properties of these tissues are taken from [12].

Thanks to this simple EM model it has been possible to investigate at various frequencies, the behavior of the reflection coefficient at the air-skin interface. Such reflection coefficient provides a quantitative indication of the reflected wave useful to estimate the intensity of the actual EM signal to be detected by a Doppler radar system.

The layered model described in Fig. 1 has been analyzed as a transmission line with losses, see Fig. 2, considering that the impedance of the nth layer can be written as:

$$Z_n = \eta_n \frac{Z_{n+1} + \eta_n tanh\gamma_n d_n}{\eta_n + Z_{n+1} tanh\gamma_n d_n} \tag{1}$$

where η_n, γ_n and d_n respectively represent the characteristic impedance, the propagation constant and the dimension of the n-th layer. Therefore, by applying recursively the transmission line model, it is possible to calculate the reflection coefficient at the air-skin interface as:

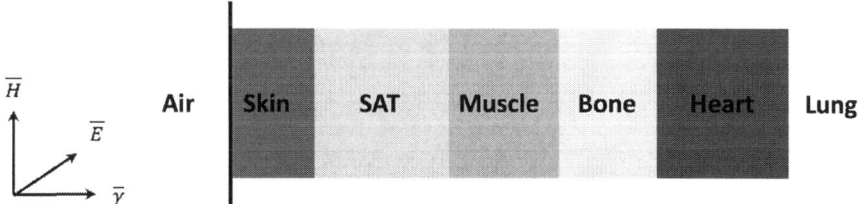

Fig. 1 The multilayer EM model proposed to study the interaction between an EM wave and human chest

Tissue	Thickness (mm)
Skin	0.8–2.6
SAT	1.4–23.2
Muscle	0.0–30.0
Bone	5.6–6.6

Table 2 Thickness of biological tissues [11] adopted in the multilayer model

$$\Gamma_{\text{air}-\text{skin}} = \frac{Z_{in\_skin} - \eta_0}{Z_{in\_skin} + \eta_0} \qquad (2)$$

where η_0 is the free space characteristic impedance and Z_{in_skin} is the input impedance of the EM model depicted in Fig. 2.

The model has been used to estimate the value of the reflection coefficient at the air-skin interface at different working frequencies (from 236 MHz up to 10 GHz) in two different scenarios: (a) thickness variation of 1 cm of the layer corresponding to the heart; (b) 1 mm skin surface displacement caused by the heartbeat movement.

In the following the two different scenarios and the results obtained with the multilayer EM model will be described in details.

2.1.1 Scenario (a): Heart-Layer Movement

In the first scenario, the reflection coefficient at the air-skin interface has been evaluated at various frequencies, firstly in the rest condition and then when the longitudinal dimension of heart-layer is increased of 1 cm, representative of the heart contraction, leaving the thickness of the other layers unchanged with respect to the rest condition. Therefore the variations of module and phase of the reflection coefficient have been calculated for each frequency in the range 236 MHz–10 GHz as the difference between the values obtained with the two configurations. Figure 3 depicts only the phase variation, that is more significant than the module variation,

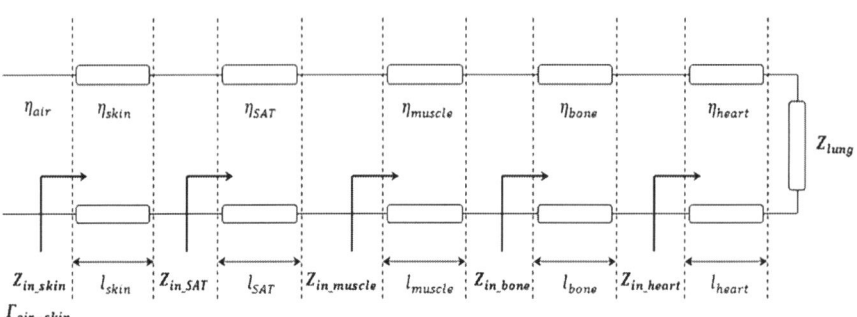

Fig. 2 Multilayer EM model of human chest represented as a transmission line

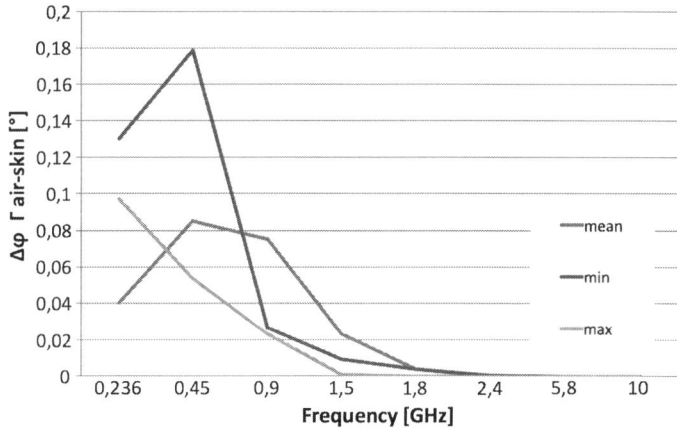

Fig. 3 Phase variation of the reflected EM wave due to 1 cm heart layer displacement (the *lines of different colors* refers to tissue layer thickness parameterization) (Color figure online)

of the reflected wave evaluated all over the frequency range of interest and relative to three different EM models, obtained considering the minimum, the mean and the maximum thickness of the layers according to the variability range reported in Table 2.

Three main evidences can be highlighted:

- Variations of both the module and the phase of the reflected wave are very small and hardly detectable by a standard EM monitoring system. Anyway, the highest values are obtained at about 400 MHz since moving up in the frequency the attenuation phenomena become predominant and the EM wave is not able to arrive at the last layer and come back with a significant intensity. Therefore only the low frequency EM waves reach the heart layer, but their wavelengths are much larger than the displacement to detect (about 1 cm) and consequently the phase variation caused in the reflected wave is exiguous.
- At the high frequencies the EM wave is not able to penetrate through all the tissues because the attenuation phenomena become predominant, so its penetration depth significantly decreases and the EM field remains confined in the first layers. Therefore no variation of phase caused by the dimension changes of the heart layer can be appreciated, as clearly shown in Fig. 3.
- Considering that an incident EM wave is mostly reflected at the first interface air-skin, when the longitudinal dimensions of layers are changed the curves slightly differ from each other: the values of phase variations increase when considering the minimum layer thicknesses of the range defined in [11] but the different between curves reduces with frequency.

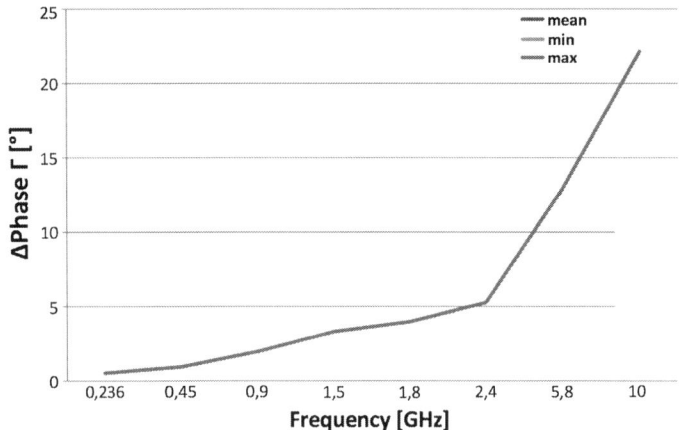

Fig. 4 Phase variation of the reflected EM wave due to 1 mm chest wall displacement (the *lines of different colors* refers to tissue layer thickness parameterization)

2.1.2 Scenario (b): Chest-Layer Movement

The second scenario is related to the outside chest displacement that is the secondary effect (skin vibration) created by the heartbeat movement. In the multilayer model this phenomenon is reproduced by varying the antenna—skin distance.

Figure 4 shows the variation of phase caused by the skin displacement with respect to the rest condition (even in this scenario the simulation have been repeated considering the minimum, the mean and the maximum values of tissue thickness, according to [11]).

Three main evidences can be highlighted:

– the displacement of 1 mm is too small to be detected by low-frequency waves. In fact Fig. 4 shows that the phase shift becomes greater as the frequency increases, because by reducing the wavelength the resolution increases allowing detect smaller displacements.
– the movement of the skin surface, albeit is an order of magnitude lower than the heart-layer displacement considered in the previous scenario, causes a significant phase modulation of high frequency waves reflected by the outside layer, thanks to the small wavelength.
– As in the previous scenario, the longitudinal dimensions of tissues slightly influence the phase variation of the reflected wave. Anyway in Fig. 4 the three lines seems to overlap, because the difference is extremely smaller than the phase variation obtained at high frequencies.

3   Validation of the Model

In order to validate the EM multilayer model presented in the previous section, the results obtained have been compared with theoretical and experimental values. In particular, the theoretical values have been calculated according to:

$$\Delta\varphi = \frac{4\pi \cdot \Delta x}{\lambda} \qquad (3)$$

which defines the phase variation as a function of the displacement Δx and the wavelength λ of the incident EM field.

As concerns the experimental values they have been obtained reproducing as faithfully as possible the simulated scenario. The set up consists of a wide band commercial horn antenna and a Vector Network Analyzer to transmit and receive a continuous wave at the frequencies in the range of interest. The measurements campaign has been carried out inside an anechoic angle set in our laboratory, even if there are not particular requirements concerning the surrounding environment. In fact, for each test, a reference signal is subtracted via software to the measured signal, so as to delete the contribution of the static clutter and enhance the one due to moving parts, as the target's chest. This expedient allows conduct the measure in whatever outdoor or indoor environments, as hospitals or houses, without any issues caused by surrounding reflective surfaces.

This first campaign of measurement (8 tests, each 40s long) involved a male subject in a state of good health. He wore normal clothes, and he has been asked to maintain the default location for the test (sitting in front of the antenna, at a distance of 1 m) avoiding suddenly movements all over the duration of the measure. For all the tests carried out, the respiratory act of the subject is to be considered normal.

Table 3 summarizes the values obtained for a chest displacement of 1 mm at 236 MHz and 10 GHz, radiating a power level of 0 dBm. Looking at the values it is clear that the very good agreement between simulated and calculated results. The slight difference with the measured values is quite reasonable and it is probably due to the real scenario in which the measure has been carried out and to the measurement uncertainty. Therefore, once defined the displacement and the frequency, the simulated values are to be considered as an upper limit, that is, as the maximum values obtainable.

Table 3 Comparison between simulated, calculated and measured values of phase variation

Frequency (GHz)	$\Delta\varphi$ simulated (EM model)	$\Delta\varphi$ calculated (Eq. 3)	$\Delta\varphi$ measured
0.236	0.26°	0.56°	0.25°
10	23.99°	23.98°	18°

4 Conclusions

A preliminary study about the use of EM technology to remotely monitor the cardiac activity has been presented. The research activity started with the implementation of a simple but efficient model able both to explain the physical mechanism of the interaction between an EM wave and the human chest and to define some guidelines for a future realization of an EM non-contact monitoring system.

To this end, a multilayer model of the human chest, including different materials as skin, fat, bone, lungs and heart, has been reviewed for this specific application. Then the multilayer model has been analyzed as a transmission line in order to define the reflection coefficient at the air-skin interface and to investigate the variations of its module and phase depending on the variation of the length of the heart layer (displacement of about 1 cm) or of the skin layer (secondary effect of heart beat causing an outside displacement of about 1 mm).

The preliminary study carried out, whose results have been compared with theoretical and experimental values, allowed to deeply understand how an EM continuous wave interacts with the human chest and what are the actual mechanisms that can be observed depending on the working frequency. In detail, using low frequencies of about few hundreds of MHz it is possible to penetrate all the tissue of the human chest up to the heart and directly observe the movement of the cardiac muscle. Unfortunately, because of the strong attenuation of the EM wave through biological tissues and the large values of its wavelength with respect to the displacement to observe, the variations of the reflection coefficient are too exiguous and very hard to be detected using a standard EM system. On the contrary using high frequencies, the attenuation mechanisms are so significant that the EM wave is not able to penetrate all the tissues and it remains confined within the first layers, meaning that it is not possible to directly detect the movement of the cardiac muscle, but due to the small wavelength, the EM wave is able to resolve the 1 mm skin displacement, which causes a phase variation of about 20 degree at 10 GHz. Moreover, the small penetration depth avoids the interaction with any type of electronic devices eventually implanted inside the human chest, as pacemakers.

It is worth noting that further studies could be carried out in order to investigate what happen at higher frequencies, although 10 GHz seems to be a good trade off between resolution, simplicity and cost of realization. Moreover according to what has been done in regards to the respiration monitoring [3, 4], it could be convenient to investigate the use of a frequency sweep technique rather than a single continuous wave paving the way for a future integration of the two monitoring systems.

References

1. GBD (2013) Mortality and Causes of Death Collaborators. Global, regional and national age-sex specific all-cause and cause-specific mortality for 240 causes of death, 1990–2013: a systematic analysis for the global burden of disease study 2013, 17 Dec 2014. Lancet 385 (9963):117–171
2. Li C, Cumings J, Lam J, Graves E, Wu W (2009) Radar remote monitoring of vital signs. IEEE Microw Mag 10(1):47–56
3. Petrini V, Di Mattia V, De Leo A, Russo P, Mariani Primiani V, Manfredi G, Cerri G, Scalise L (2015) Domestic monitoring of respiration and movement by an electromagnetic sensor. In: Andò B, Siciliano F, Monteriù A (eds) Ambient assisted living. Springer, Berlin, pp 133–142
4. Scalise L, Petrini V, Di Mattia V, Russo P, De Leo A, Manfredi G, Cerri G (2015) Multiparameter electromagnetic sensor for AAL indoor measurement of the respiration rate and position of a subject. In: 2015 IEEE international instrumentation and measurement technology conference (I2MTC), pp 664–669, 11–14 May 2015
5. Droitcou AD, Boric-Lubecke O, Lubecke VM, Lin J, Kovacs GTA (2004) Range correlation and I/Q performance benefits in single chip silicon doppler radars for noncontact cardiopulmonary monitoring. IEEE Trans Microwave Theory Tech 52(3):838–848
6. Tariq A, Ghfouri-Shiraz H (2011) Vital sign detection using Doppler radar and continuous wavelet transform. In: Proceedings of the 5th European conference on antennas and propagation (EUCAP), pp 285–288, 11–15 Apr 2011
7. Serra A, Nepa P, Manara G, Corsini G, Volakis JL (2010) A single on-body antenna as a sensor for cardiopulmonary monitoring. IEEE Antennas Propag Lett 9:930–933
8. Chang YJ (2016) The NPAC visible human viewer. Syracuse University, NY. Available at http://zatoka.icm.edu.pl/vh/paper/index.htm. Accessed Feb 2016
9. Gabriel C (1996) Compilation of the dielectric properties of body tissues at RF and microwave frequencies. Physics Department, King's College London, London WCR2lS, UK, Armstrong Laboratory (AFMC), Occupational Environmental Health Directorate, Radiofrequency Radiation Division, Report: AOE-TR-1996–0037
10. Staderini EM (2002) UWB radars in medicine. IEEE Aerosp Electron Syst Mag 17(1):13–18
11. Christ A, Klingenbock A, Samaras T, Goiceanu C, Kuster N (2006) The dependence of electromagnetic far-field absorption on body tissue composition in the frequency range from 300 MHz to 6 GHz. IEEE Trans Microw Theory Tech 54(5):2188–2195
12. Andreuccetti D, Fossi R, Petrucci C (1997) An internet resource for the calculation of the dielectric properties of body tissues in the frequency range 10 Hz–100 GHz. Available at http://niremf.ifac.cnr.it/tissprop/. Accessed Feb 2016

A Wearable System for Stress Detection Through Physiological Data Analysis

Giorgia Acerbi, Erika Rovini, Stefano Betti, Antonio Tirri,
Judit Flóra Rónai, Antonella Sirianni, Jacopo Agrimi,
Lorenzo Eusebi and Filippo Cavallo

Abstract In the last years the impact of stress on the society has been increased, resulting in 77% of people that regularly experiences physical symptoms caused by stress with a negative impact on their personal and professional life, especially in aging working population. This paper aims to demonstrate the feasibility of detection and monitoring of stress, inducted by mental stress tests, through the analysis of physiological data collected by wearable sensors. In fact, the physiological features extracted from heart rate variability and galvanic skin response

Giorgia Acerbi, Erika Rovini, Stefano Betti Equal contribution to the work.

G. Acerbi (✉) · E. Rovini · S. Betti · F. Cavallo
The BioRobotics Institute, Scuola Superiore Sant'Anna,
Viale Rinaldo Piaggio, 34, 56025 Pontedera, PI, Italy
e-mail: g.acerbi@sssup.it

E. Rovini
e-mail: e.rovini@sssup.it

S. Betti
e-mail: s.betti@sssup.it

F. Cavallo
e-mail: f.cavallo@sssup.it

A. Tirri · J.F. Rónai · A. Sirianni
Telecom Italia | TIM WHITE Joint Open Lab, Via Cardinale Pietro Maffi,
27, Pisa, Italy
e-mail: antonio.tirri@telecomitalia.it

J.F. Rónai
e-mail: juditflora.ronai@telecomitalia.it

J. Agrimi
Life Science Institute, Scuola Superiore Sant'Anna,
Piazza Martiri Della Libertà, 33, 56127 Pisa, PI, Italy
e-mail: j.agrimi@sssup.it

L. Eusebi
Telecom Italia | TIM S-Cube Joint Open Lab, Via Camillo Golgi, 42, Milan, Italy
e-mail: lorenzo.eusebi@telecomitalia.it

© Springer International Publishing AG 2017   31
F. Cavallo et al. (eds.), *Ambient Assisted Living*, Lecture Notes
in Electrical Engineering 426, DOI 10.1007/978-3-319-54283-6_3

showed significant differences between stressed and not stressed people. Starting from the physiological data, the work provides also a cluster analysis based on Principal Components (PCs) able to showed a visual discrimination of stressed and relaxed groups. The developed system would support active ageing, monitoring and managing the level of stress in ageing workers and allowing them to reduce the burden of stress related to the workload on the basis of personalized interventions.

Keywords Stress monitoring · Stress induction test · Heart rate variability · Galvanic skin response · Feature extraction · Psychometric instruments · Clusterization algorithms

1   Introduction

Stress is a physiological response to the mental, emotional, or physical challenge and it can be defined as the reaction of a person to the environmental requests or influences [1]. Stress conditions can cause physical and emotional exhaustion that leads to symptoms such as headaches, stomach complaints and difficulties in sleeping. A study conducted by the American Institute of Stress (Statistic Brain Research Institute, NY) has shown as in 2015 the 48% of people feels that their stress condition has increased over the past five years. 77% of people regularly experiences physical symptoms caused by stress with a negative impact on their personal and professional life [2]. The influence of stress and its consequences on society concerns also the economic aspect. According to the recent EU-funded project 2013, the cost to Europe of work-related stress and depression was estimated to be 617 billion annually. The total amount includes loss of productivity, health care costs and social welfare costs [3]. The early detection of stress can positively affect personal wellbeing and society affluence.

Traditionally, the level of personal stress has been established using some psychometric instruments and scales [4], which are subjective. Subsequently the correlation between the variation of the physiological signals and stress was investigated in order to make the measurement more objective.

1.1   Physiological Signals and Stress Concept

Physiological phenomena are extremely correlated with stress and anxiety, such as heart rate variability and galvanic skin response. Human stress response can be described through Psychoneuroimmunology that tries to link together the physiological systems involved in the stress response: the nervous system, the endocrine system and the immune system [5].

Several studies have shown that stress has an impact on the Autonomic Nervous System (ANS) [6]. The ANS provides a rapidly responding mechanism to control a wide range of functions and organs, including heart, skin resistance, digestive tract, lungs, bladder and blood vessels [7]. The ANS has two components, the sympathetic nervous system (SNS) and the parasympathetic nervous system (PNS). In particular, the response "fight-or-flight" is associated with SNS, through the release of adrenaline and noradrenaline [5], while PNS is involved in relaxation process. Stress response is structured into 3 main stages: immediate effects of stress involve the SNS, with releasing of adrenaline and noradrenaline in 2–3 s; intermediate effects are characterized by 20–30 s time activity, in which adrenal medulla releases epinephrine and norepinephrine.

That is why alteration of physiological signals and variables can be related to a change of stress condition such as cardiac activity [8], electrodermal activity (EDA) [9, 10], electro-myographic activity [11], breathing (Rottenberg et al. [12], skin temperature [13], electrical brain activity [14], eye blink [15]. In particular SNS and PNS regulate the EDA, the heart rate variability (HRV) and the brain waves that are commonly used in literature to investigate the levels of stress during different tasks [16].

1.1.1 Electrodermal Activity

Psycho physiological measures have been recently used in HRI studies, in which, in addition to HRV, Galvanic Skin Response (GSR) has been used. The neural mechanism and pathways involved in the central control of electrodermal activity are numerous and complex. EDA is related to the level of arousal elicited by an extended range of psychological and emotional states with either positive or negative valence. Different studies investigating anxiety, anger, fear and also joy experiences report increased EDA [17, 18]. It is also an indicator of the cognitive load, stress and arousal [9, 10], because of the variation of the skin electrical resistance in response to various emotional stimuli. When a subject is under mental stress, sweat gland activity is activated and increases skin conductance (SC). Since the sweat glands are also controlled by the SNS, SC acts as an indicator for sympathetic activation due to the stress reaction [1].

GSR has already been used in previous works in combination with other physiological parameters. For example, SC has been combined with electro cardiac activity, electromyographic activity and respiration activity in order to monitor drivers' behaviours through open roads [19]. In particular, the parameters provided were the number of stressors in a given temporal window, the sum of the amplitude of all the stressors counted in that temporal window, the sum of the response durations and the sum of the areas under the peaks counted as stressors. Finally, the integration of GSR, HRV and accelerometer data has been implemented in the work of Sun et al. [1], with the aim to differentiate between physical activity and mental stress. In particular, electrodermal activity has been analysed through three main parameters: the number of the stressor, the related amplitude and the sum of the duration of the responses.

1.1.2 Electro Cardiac Activity

There are two types of neuro-modulatory receptors in cardiac cells: one is for acetylcholine (SNS) and the other is norepinephrine (PNS). These receptors interact with inhibitory or excitatory proteins, which, through chemical exchanges, can modify the Calcium concentration in the heart cells membrane and inhibit or stimulate heart rate (HR) and the strength of contraction [20]. HR describes the cardiac activity when the ANS attempts to tackle with the human body demands depending on the stimuli received. Concretely, ANS reacts against a stressing stimulus provoking an increase in blood volume within the veins, so rest of the body can react properly, increasing the number of heartbeats [8]. In confirmation of this aspects, over recent years clinical researches have shown that one of the most important indicators of stress is HRV. It is the variation in the time interval between one heartbeat and the next one. To study the effect of SNS and PNS activities, starting from ECG signal, it is necessary to analyse the HRV signal both in time and frequency domains. Generally cardiac parameters as mean of Inter-Beat Interval (IBI), HR, signal power in low frequency (LF) and high frequency (HF) bands are used to analyse stress. The HRV analysis has already been used in different studies to detect stress in various condition as mental task [21], high workload [22], car driving [19] and other common daily tasks.

1.2 The Aim of the Study

This paper presents an experimental methodology to collect and analyse physiological data to detect the stress status of the user. The methodology has been applied in a test for the Trans.Safe (The AmbienT Response to Avoid Negative Stress and enhance SAFEty) European research project which has the aim to detect stress levels, through the monitoring and interpretation of physiological signals.

EDA and HRV were the physiological signals measured during the tests since they are two of the most important indicators of stress (see Sects. 1.1.1 and 1.1.2) and they can be revealed through portable and non-invasive devices. Thus, the stress detection activity carried out in this experimentation has been performed through a combination of two wearable sensors, Shimmer GSR Sensor and Zephyr BioHarness™.

A new experimental protocol for the collection of physiological data in different conditions has been defined. It consisted of alternated stages of rest and stress induction phases combined with the administration of psychometric instruments. Then, the data collected was properly processed and analysed in order to investigated the significance of the physiological features in distinguishing stress and relax conditions.

Since the main goal of this study is the monitoring of stress using a ultra-low invasiveness system, it is reasonable to think that improving the comfort, the user could wear the system for a long time, both during work or daily activities.

In the future a such system, using a real time classifier, could act as a portable system control, like medical devices as cardiac holter or pressure monitoring devices (24 h). Furthermore it could also be useful for the user in order to predict the rise of stress and act to reduce it. The feedback for stress presence and any suggestion or intervention to decrease it would allow benefits for the user's health and a reduction in health care costs for stress-related illnesses.

2 Materials and Methods

In this section the sensor devices used for the acquisition of physiological signals, the experimental protocol developed and adopted and the methodology chosen for data analysis are described in detail.

2.1 Instrumentation

The choice of the wearable sensor devices to be included into the test has been performed according to two criteria: accuracy of measurements and unobtrusiveness of the sensors. There are several devices on the market that claim the measurement of cardiac and electro-dermal activity in a unobtrusive way. Unfortunately, not all these devices are accurate enough for a reliable assessment of stress conditions. In order to find a reasonable trade-off, we selected two devices: Zephyr BioHarness™3 and Shimmer GSR Sensor (Fig. 1).

Zephyr BioHarness™3 (BH3) [23] is a Bluetooth chest belt capable of retrieving signals derived from the ECG such Heart Rate and R-R Intervals. The ECG signal is sampled at 250 Hz. Moreover, the BH3 is able to collect other signals such as breathing rate, posture information and skin temperature. For the data analysis and the development of the stress detection algorithm the Inter-Beat-Interval data provided by the device has been used. The GSR Module developed by Shimmer [24] is a wearable sensor composed by two special finger electrodes and a main unit that streams data related to the galvanic skin response with a sample frequency of 51.2 Hz using a Bluetooth connection.

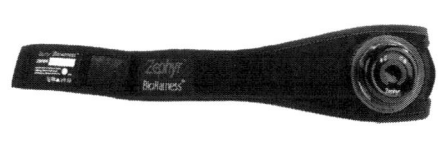
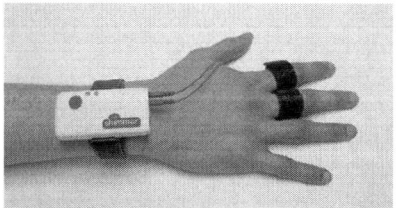

Fig. 1 Zephyr BioHarness™3 on the *left* and Shimmer GSR Sensor on the *right*

2.2 Participants

Twelve voluntary students (3 men, 9 women) with a mean age of 26.0 years old (SD = 4.8 years, range = 21–30 years old) participated on purpose in this study. All the participants did not meet the exclusion criteria that consisted in neurological disorders that made unable the subjects to complete the mental tasks proposed or cardiac diseases that could deface the physiological response in electro cardiac activity.

Participants completed the experimental session in the Scuola Superiore Sant'Anna (Pisa, Italy) and in the Telecom Italia WHITE Joint Open Lab (Pisa, Italy). Written informed consent was obtained from all the participants before starting the tests.

2.3 Experimental Protocol

The experimental protocol was intended to put the subjects in a state of emotional and cognitive stress, in order to measure the variations of their physiological parameters induced by stress.

The experimentation consisted in three phases: a baseline, a stress induction and a recovery stage. During baseline the subjects relaxed in a separate room, for 10 min, without using mobile phone, without music or external sounds, without stimuli and without closing their eyes. This phase was indispensable in order to acquire the personal baseline of each subject, since physiological parameters show a wide inter-subjects variability. At the end of baseline recording, the psychologist administered psychometric instruments to the participants to obtain a subjective perception about the level of stress, anxiety and drowsiness. Then the subjects performed the stress phase, during about 15–20 min, completing a series of extremely demanding cognitive tests handed out by the psychologist in order to induce the stress. People were not aware that this phase was part of the experiment: the psychologist indeed pretended to be sent by University to detect the intelligence quotient (IQ) for a poll. The investigator assumed a very aggressive behaviour towards the subject, behaving rude and correcting the person even when the he accomplished the task properly. Furthermore, the user performed the required tasks by listening a noisy sound in background that simulates high intensity traffic jam. At the end of this phase, the subjects filled out the psychometric instruments again. Afterwards a recovery period of 10 min was performed, in the same conditions as in the baseline phase.

During the whole experimental session (baseline, stress and recovery phases), the tested subjects wore the kit of wearable sensors described in Sect. 2.1, in order to record electro cardiac and electrodermal activities.

2.3.1 Tests for Stress Induction

The aim of this experimental protocol was to arouse stress in tested subjects that would produce major changes in the level of physiological signals. For this reason, in the experimental protocol the stress induction phase consisted of two paths: (i) the use of validated neuropsychological tests that caused a great cognitive effort; (ii) the creation of a stressful social situation that would put the subject under pressure causing a strong emotional reaction.

The five different following tasks (Fig. 2), were executed by the tested subjects:

- **Digit Span:** it is a common measure of short-term memory to evaluate working memory's number storage capacity. In the test of Reverse Digit Span a list of random numbers was read out loud to the person who had to immediately repeat it in a backward order.
- **Stroop Color Test:** it is a common test to measure selective and divided attention, cognitive flexibility and processing speed [25]. This test is a demonstration of interference in the reaction time of a task in which the subject was asked to read out loud and as fast as possible either the written word or the ink color.

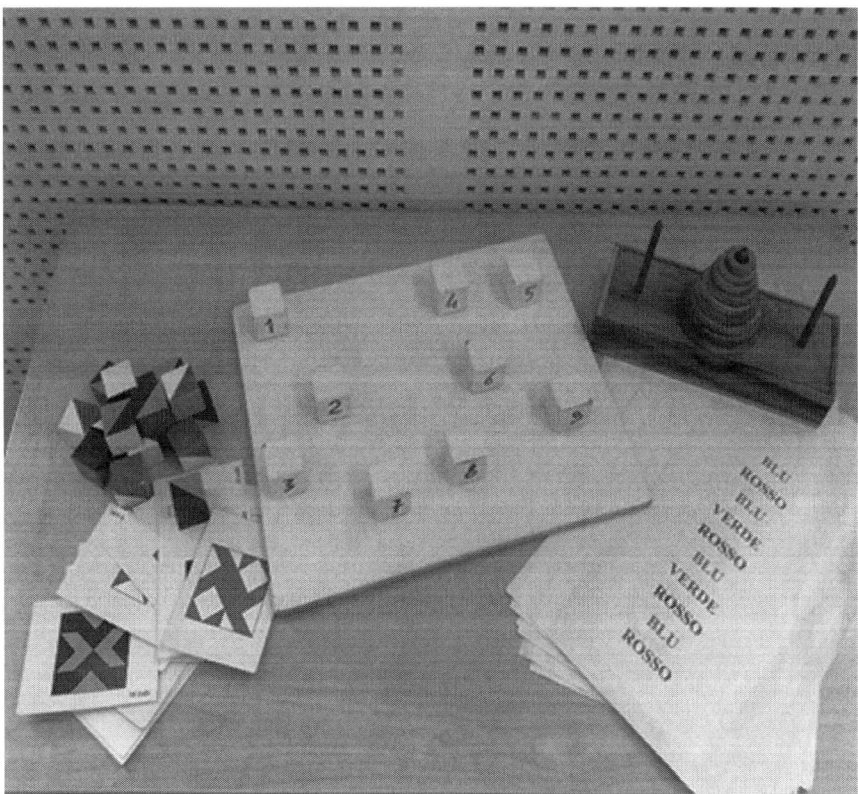

Fig. 2 Stress induction test set administered during the experimental session

- **Corsi Reverse:** The Corsi block-tapping test is a psychological test that assesses visual-spatial short term memory. The experiment is done typically by using a wooden base where nine identical spatially separated blocks are present. In the Reverse Corsi Test [26] the experimenter indicated a sequence of blocks by tapping them and the subject was requested to reproduce the spatial succession of boxes in the reverse way.
- **Kohs Block Design Test:** this is a performance test designed to be an IQ test and to measure visual-spatial skills [27]. The subject was asked to replicate the patterns displayed on a series of test cards by using colored cubes (each side has a single color or two colors divided by a diagonal line).
- **Tower of Hanoi:** this is a mathematical game, common to test problem solving and executive capacity of the subject [28]. It is composed by three rods and a number of disks of different sizes which can slide onto any rod. The subject had to move the entire stack to another rod, following simple rules: only one disk could be moved at a time; only the upper disk from one of the stacks could be moved and placed on top of another stack; no disk could be placed on top of a smaller disk.

2.3.2 Psychometric Instruments

In order to measure the emotional state and the level of stress of the subjects, the following psychometric instruments were administered before and after stress induction phase:

- **State-Trait Anxiety Inventory (STAI):** this scale is one of the most frequently, reliable and sensitive used measures of anxiety in applied psychology research. In this study the short-form of the STAI scale was used, consisting of only six items (STAI-6) since the objective was to establish the level of stress and anxiety produced during the stress phase [29]. Higher STAI scores suggest higher levels of anxiety.
- **Karolinska Sleepiness Scale (KSS):** it is one of the most common sleepiness state tests and it is a 9-point Likert scale based on a self-reported assessment of the person's level of drowsiness at the moment [30]. The subject had to choose his level of sleepiness from 1 = "very alert" to 9 = "very sleepy". KSS was originally developed to constitute a one-dimensional scale of sleepiness and was validated against alpha and theta electroencephalographic activity [31].
- **Shortened State Stress Questionnaire (SSSQ):** The 24-item SSSQ [32], based on the 90 Question Dundee Stress State Questionnaire (DSSQ), provides a rapid, reliable, self-report assessment of the three primary stress dimensions: distress, task engagement and worry [33].

2.4 Data Analysis

The physiological data acquired during the whole experimentation have been offline analysed using Matlab® R2012a.

The acquired data have been examined for baseline phase (10 min of recording), stress phase (ranging from 15 to 20 min, depending from the attitude and behaviour of the tested subject). Thus, for each phase, we obtained a dataset composed by a set of GSR features for each participant and another dataset consisting of features extracted from HRV signal. All these data were analysed in order to investigate variations in physiological parameters that could be attributed to stress statutes of the tested subjects.

2.4.1 Galvanic Skin Response (GSR)

The EDA has been recorded using Shimmer GSR sensor which provides as output the galvanic resistance, that has been converted into galvanic skin conductance. In the features extraction algorithm, the signal has been analyzed with temporal windows of 2 min, after a filtering process, using a moving average filter. The features extraction algorithm is based on startle detection that can lead to a set of computable features. The method used is referred to the scoring multiples response method of Boucsein [34], that establishes a local baseline at the level of the onset of the second response and measures the distance from that baseline to the following peak. The detection algorithm identifies all the occurrences of when the first derivative exceeded to a certain threshold. It was empirically determined as 0.005 µS. Given the variability of GSR signal among subjects, this threshold is not absolute but it has found to be adequate for the 12 subjects analyzed. Furthermore, to ensure to not consider subsequent startles, a minimum distance has been chosen as in (Shumm et al. [35], considering that a startle event is expected to last about 1–3 s. Once the response was detected, the zero-crossing of the derivative preceding and following the response were identified as the onset and end of the startle [36]. Starting from the startle detection, the following parameters have been calculated (Table 1):

2.4.2 Electro Cardiac Activity

Electro cardiac activity has been recorded using the chest belt Zephyr BioHarness™ BH3. The device provides as output the raw ECG signal and the HRV data that specifies the temporal distance between a beat and the following one. Starting from Inter-Beat-Interval (IBI), the algorithm to extract the main features has been developed. The IBI signal has been modified identifying and correcting ectopic rhythm, which is an irregular heart rhythm due to a premature heartbeat. The analysis of cardiac signal has been structured investigating both the time domain

Table 1 Features extracted from GSR signal calculated within a temporal window

Feature Name	Description
Num_Startle	Number of the stressors
Sum_Amplitude	Sum of the amplitude of the stressors
Sum_RiseTime	Sum of the rise duration of the stressors
Sum_RecTime	Sum of the decrease duration of the stressors
Rise_Rate	Mean value of the rise duration of the stressors
Decay_Rate	Mean value of the decrease duration of the stressors
Area_GSR	Mean of the area under each stressor
Mean_GSR	Mean value of GSR signal
Std_GSR	Standard deviation of GSR signal

Table 2 Features extracted from HRV signal in the temporal domain

Feature name	Description
IBI_mean	Mean of inter-beat-interval corresponding to R-to-R interval
SDNN	Standard deviation of all Normal RR intervals (NN intervals)
HR_mean	Mean of heart rate
SDHR	Standard deviation of the heart rate
RMSSD	Square root of the mean of the squared differences between adjacent normal RR intervals
pNN50	Percentage of differences between adjacent normal RR intervals exceeding 50 ms
#ECT	Number of ectopic intervals (abnormal RR intervals)
%ECT	Percentage of ectopic intervals on the total number of RR intervals

and the frequency domain. Regarding the time domain, the following parameters have been selected and computed (see Table 2)

By identifying and correcting ectopic rhythm, a Normal-to-Normal (NN) interval sequence appropriate for HRV analysis is obtained. Since the NN interval sequence is an irregularly sampled time sequence, for spectral analysis it had to be therefore converted to an equidistantly sampled sequence [37]. After a smoothing of the signal, the NN interval sequence has been resampled at 4 Hz. For the analysis in frequency domain, the following parameters have been computed (see Table 3):

2.4.3 Data Processing and Statistical Analysis

After extracting features from physiological signals, Kolmogorov-Smirnov test was applied in order to verify the normal distribution of data. A non-parametric statistical analysis was used because the test showed data were not normally

Table 3 Features extracted from HRV signal in the frequency domain

Feature name	Description
Peak VLF	Frequency peak in very low frequency (VLF) range (0.04–0.15 Hz)
Area VLF	Signal power by Power Spectral Density (PSD) in VLF
%VLF	Percentage of signal power in the VLF respect to the total signal power
Peak LF	Frequency peak in low frequency (LF) range (0.04–0.15 Hz)
Area LF	Signal power by PSD in LF
%LF	Percentage of signal power in the LF respect to the total signal power
Peak HF	Frequency peak in high frequency (HF) range (0.15–0.4 Hz)
Area HF	Signal power by PSD in HF
%HF	Percentage of signal power in the HF respect to the total signal power
LF/HF	Ratio between LF and HF powers

distributed. Then, Kruskal-Wallis (KW) test was used for comparing data acquired in baseline phase and those recorded during stress phase in order to verify a significant difference (p-value < 0.05) on the basis of the extracted parameters. Furthermore the linear correlation between the significant parameters was calculated using the Pearson's coefficient. If the value of correlation between two features was at least rho $= 0.8$, the less significant one was deleted. Then, the remaining features were used for Principal Component Analysis (PCA) in order to identify how the groups investigated, related to different phases of the experimental protocol, could be visualized and separated in the space of the principal components (PCs). Finally, the most important PCs, that included more than 80% of the overall variance of data, were taken into account in order to train and test a Support Vector Machine (SVM) classifier which had to be able to correctly classify a subject as stressed or not-stressed.

Regarding the analysis of the psychometric instruments, a T-test has been conducted in order to assess if significant differences between after and before the stress induction phase could be revealed.

Finally, a linear regression analysis has been implemented with the aim to look for a correlation between the results obtained by the psychometric instruments administered and the physiological parameters measured.

3 Results and Discussion

In this section the results obtained from both the analysis of physiological data and the psychometric instruments are reported and widely discussed, examining the most important features extracted, the evaluation of the psychometric instruments and the algorithm for data classification.

3.1 Physiological Parameters Assessment

Features extracted by physiological parameters are reported in Tables 4 and 5 both
for baseline phase and stress phase as mean values and standard deviations.
Furthermore p-values, calculated with KW test for non parametric data, are also

Table 4 Features extracted from GSR signal: mean values ± standard deviations and
significance

Parameters	Baseline			Stress			p-value
Num_Startle (#)	15.97	±	4.71	17.95	±	3.06	0.119
Sum_amplitude (µS)	11.18	±	12.40	11.18	±	6.79	0.453
Sum_RiseTime (s)	32.25	±	6.94	41.25	±	5.61	0.004*
Sum_RecTime (s)	61.96	±	8.73	64.81	±	2.52	0.488
Rise_Rate (µS/s)	3.61	±	0.90	3.08	±	0.39	0.141
Decay_Rate (µS/s)	9.36	±	4.32	5.59	±	1.21	0.003*
Area_GSR (s·µS)	2.55	±	1.95	2.11	±	1.16	0.773
Mean_GSR (µS)	11.56	±	5.34	16.83	±	5.99	0.028*
Std_GSR (µS)	1.62	±	1.33	1.30	±	0.73	0.862

*Significant difference between groups ($p < 0.05$)

Table 5 Features extracted from HRV signal: mean values ± standard deviations and
significance

Parameters	Baseline			Stress			p-value
IBI_mean (s)	0.788	±	0.126	0.642	±	0.096	0.005*
SDNN (s)	0.065	±	0.021	0.071	±	0.025	0.544
HR_mean (bpm)	78.45	±	12.38	95.54	±	13.69	0.005*
SDHR (bpm)	6.43	±	1.15	10.48	±	3.88	0.001*
RMSSD (s)	0.04	±	0.02	0.03	±	0.01	0.018*
pNN50 (%)	22.89	±	19.44	7.35	±	4.98	0.043*
#ECT (#)	11.42	±	14.57	25.33	±	24.18	0.182
%ECT (%)	1.30	±	1.77	1.29	±	1.31	0.885
Peak VLF (Hz)	0.033	±	0.014	0.011	±	0.017	0.005*
Area VLF (s^2)	195.03	±	253.25	185.88	±	106.16	0.326
%VLF (%)	16.93	±	9.87	28.85	±	9.41	0.009*
Peak LF (Hz)	0.077	±	0.019	0.053	±	0.022	0.016*
Area LF (s^2)	509.75	±	364.71	317.93	±	147.23	0.184
%LF (%)	55.07	±	16.94	51.15	±	9.45	0.194
Peak HF (Hz)	0.219	±	0.078	0.203	±	0.096	0.486
Area HF (s^2)	284.78	±	276.02	120.66	±	59.22	0.106
%HF (%)	27.99	±	20.94	20.01	±	8.88	0.525
LF/HF	3.53	±	2.79	3.27	±	2.28	0.908

*Significant difference between groups ($p < 0.05$)

disclosed because they represent if there are significant differences between the two investigated groups.

Significant differences are observed in some parameters, both for features extracted by electro dermal and electro cardiac activities, representing a concrete variation in physiological response to a psychological stress induction.

In particular for the first signal, Sum_RiseTime, Decay_Rate and Mean_GSR are the significant parameters. For the second signal IBI_mean, HR_mean, SDHR, RMSSD and pNN50 are the significant features in the temporal domain, whereas Peak VLF, %VLF and Peak LF are the ones in the frequency domain.

Discussing significant parameters derived by electrodermal activity, Sum_RiseTime is a parameter that gives an indication of how the global GSR level is varying as time progresses. If the sympathetic branch of the ANS is highly aroused, then sweat gland activity also increases. This fact leads to an increase of skin conductance, that can be then a measure of emotional and sympathetic responses. A significant variation of this parameter from baseline to stress phase can be explained as an increase of arousal level of the subject, probably due to an increment of stress level during the execution of the stressor tasks. A significant variation has been observed from baseline phase to stress phase for other two parameters: Decay_Rate and Mean_GSR. Regarding the mean value of GSR, it reflects the variation of the signals in terms of arousal, cognitive load and stress in general. So, an increase of cognitive load corresponds to an increase of the mean value of the signal, related to a bigger sweat gland activity that modifies SC. Finally a considerable variation in decay rate, which represents an indirect measure of the relaxation pattern experienced by the subject [38] could mean that when the arousal level is high, the GSR needs more time to assume values similar to baseline ones. So it is reasonable to have a variation of the time needed to obtain a relaxation, during a stress phase, respect to the baseline.

Regarding electro cardiac activity variations in the mean values of IBI and HR from baseline to stress phase are absolutely congruent with an increase of stress level: the number of beats in a minute increases, with a related reduction of the time between a heartbeat and the following one. According to Orsila et al. [22] in which RMSSD parameter changed its values among different phases of the experimental session described, this parameter presents a variation from baseline to stress phase. The lower value in the stress stage may suggests the subjects' perceived stress was effectively higher during this phase of the protocol. The difference between baseline and stress conditions in pNN50 was expected, as in [21]. It is probably due to the short term variability, which is lower with a cognitive task than during rest. Also SDHR changes between the phases, being a measure for long term variability. Analysing frequency domain parameters, it is known that sympathetic and parasympathetic activities are reflected into LF and HF power, so a variation in one of the parameters linked to these frequency contributions is justified. The activation of SNS is indeed reflected in the variation of peak LF, peak VLF and %VLF.

3.2 Psychometric Instruments Evaluation

A comparison between the scores of the state tests administered before and after stress induction has been performed (Table 6) using the T-test. The KSS scores did not show significant differences between before and after stress induction phase, whereas the STAI-6 scores showed statistically significant differences between the two phases ($p < 0.05$) indicating a recognisable level of anxiety in the tested subjects. The SSSQ scores also showed significance differences between pre and post stress induction tests ($p < 0.01$) In particular, a highly statistically significant result ($p < 0.01$) emerged from a subscale of SSSQ called "distress" that is the most important factor of SSSQ measuring the negative effect of the situation [32]. A statistically significant result related to the variation of this subscale could mean that the stress induction phase effectively provided a negative effect on participants.

3.3 Correlation Between Physiological Parameters and Psychometric Instruments

From the analysis of both physiological data and psychometric instruments it has been possible to notice a significant difference among the baseline phase and the stress one, indicating that these are valuable instruments to appreciate the arousal of anxiety and stress. The further step has been to assess the correlation between physiological features obtained from electro cardiac and electro dermal activities and questionnaires, in order to establish if it was possible to classify the stress level using psychometric instruments as reference. Unfortunately, the correlation between these two instruments was not high. The p-values calculated and disclosed in Table 7, did not show a significant correlation between physiological data and psychometric instruments.

Among the psychometric scales used, KSS scale is the most correlated, showing a significant p-value. It is indicated to assess the level of sleepiness of the subject. The correlation with the variation of physiological data could explain that the stress

Table 6 Questionnaires results: mean values $\pm$ standard deviations and t-test significance

Scale	Baseline			Stress			p-value
KSS	3.8	$\pm$	1.3	3.3	$\pm$	0.6	0.089
STAI-6	10.9	$\pm$	2.2	13.7	$\pm$	4.1	0.031*
SSSQ	93.4	$\pm$	19.5	117.6	$\pm$	34.2	0.001*
Distress	19.9	$\pm$	10.9	39.5	$\pm$	20.1	0.001*
Task management	36.5	$\pm$	4.1	35.8	$\pm$	6.1	0.639
Worry	37.0	$\pm$	12.9	42.3	$\pm$	19.5	0.174

*Significant difference at T-test between groups ($p < 0.05$)

Table 7 Correlation between psychometric instruments and physiological data

Scale	R^2	p-value
KSS	0.77	0.019*
STAI-6	0.53	0.373
SSSQ	0.55	0.312
Distress	0.53	0.357
Task Management	0.40	0.695
Worry	0.57	0.278

*Significant statistical values ($p < 0.05$)

induction phase provided a reduction of sleepiness, increasing the level of alarm and attention. The lack of significant correlation with the other scales has been probably due to the fact that, generally, self-reports provide valuable information but there could be problems with validity. Users of experimental studies often may not answer exactly how they are feeling. Rather, they answer questions as they feel others would answer them, or in a way they think the researcher wants them to answer. Furthermore, the psychometric responses could be dependent on participants' mood and state of mind on the day of the study [39, 40].

In this study it has been chosen to use physiological measures because, as primary advantage, the participants can not consciously manipulate the activities of their ANS [41–43]. Additionally, physiological measures offer a non-invasive method that can be used to determine the stress levels and reactions of participants interacting with technology [43, 44]. Even if psychometric instruments did not provide a remarkable correlation with physiological response, it is possible to assert that physiological measures provide an indication about the variation in stress level of the tested subjects.

3.4 Data Classification

According to the aim of the paper, a classifier was implemented in order to identify the status of the subjects on the basis of the measured physiological signals. Basically, the classifier should be able to distinguish if a person is stressed or not.

For this purpose, the datasets acquired both in baseline and stress phases were used and, in particular, the parameters resulted significant at the KW test in distinguishing between the two phases have been taken into account (see Sect. 3.1).

The linear correlation between the significant parameters was calculated using the Pearson's coefficient and results were reported in Table 8.

If the value of correlation between two features was at least 0.80, the less significant one was deleted.

Thus, a reduced number of eight parameters has been selected and used for Principal Component Analysis (PCA) that allowed to visualize the separation between subjects in baseline and stress phases in the space of the PCs as shown in Fig. 3.

Table 8 Pearson's coefficient of correlation between significant features

Feature name	IBI_mean	HR_mean	SDHR	RMSSD	pNN50	peakVLF	%VLF	peakLF	Sum_RiseTime	Decay_Rate	Mean_GSR
IBI_mean	1.00	-0.98	-0.55	0.77	0.73	0.34	-0.29	0.28	-0.29	0.56	-0.38
HR_mean	-0.98	1.00	0.62	-0.73	-0.68	-0.35	0.31	-0.30	0.29	-0.50	0.34
SDHR	-0.55	0.62	1.00	-0.22	-0.22	-0.53	0.56	-0.50	0.44	-0.32	0.17
RMSSD	0.77	-0.73	-0.22	1.00	0.96	0.16	-0.23	0.10	-0.20	0.53	-0.27
pNN50	0.73	-0.68	-0.22	0.96	1.00	0.15	-0.28	0.07	-0.22	0.55	-0.35
peakVLF	0.34	-0.35	-0.53	0.16	0.15	1.00	-0.75	0.95	-0.36	0.37	-0.37
%VLF	-0.29	0.31	0.56	-0.23	-0.28	-0.75	1.00	-0.77	0.33	-0.38	0.39
peakLF	0.28	-0.30	-0.50	0.10	0.07	0.95	-0.77	1.00	-0.35	0.39	-0.33
Sum_RiseTime	-0.29	0.29	0.44	-0.20	-0.22	-0.36	0.33	-0.35	1.00	-0.76	0.30
Decay_Rate	0.56	-0.50	-0.32	0.53	0.55	0.37	-0.38	0.39	-0.76	1.00	-0.49
Mean_GSR	-0.38	0.34	0.17	-0.27	-0.35	-0.37	0.39	-0.33	0.30	-0.49	1.00

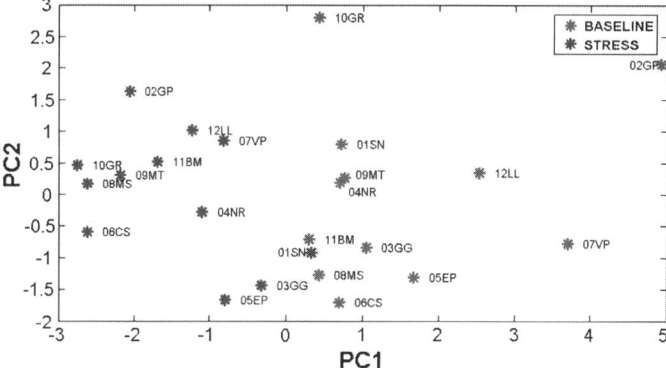

Fig. 3 PCA synthesizes the differences in physiological parameters between baseline (*blue markers*) and stress phase (*red markers*). The first four PCs contains the 87.8% of the overall variance (Color figure online)

4 Conclusion

The presented work described features extraction and processing techniques used for HRV and GSR signals. In particular, the aim was to demonstrate the possibility to monitor stress condition through physiological signals variations. Among the physiological features extracted, significant differences have been observed in some parameters, both for electrodermal activity and electro cardiac activity. This fact can be conferred to a concrete variation in physiological response due to a psychological stress induction. The PCA analysis has shown the capability of the system in distinguishing stressed and not stressed clusters. Then, it is possible to conclude that through physiological features it could be feasible to establish if a subject is stressed or not. The significant difference between the scores obtained by the subjects before and after the stress induction in both the STAI-6 questionnaire and SSSQ questionnaire confirms that the stress protocol designed reaches the goal of inducing a cognitive and emotional arousal. The evidence of the efficacy of the protocol is even more evidenced by the results of the distress subscale which seems very effective in evaluating the situational stress experienced by the subject.

Since physiological signals are influenced by a high level of variability among subjects, it is important to collect even small variations of signals in order to calculate the related features. For this purpose it is needed to take into account both the quality and accuracy of the devices used and the precision of the algorithms implemented.

Regarding psychometric instruments, there was not a remarkable correlation between physiological variations and scores obtained from the questionnaires. The only significant p-value obtained was related to the KSS scale, focused on the level of sleepiness, that probably changed among the different phases of the test, with a reduction in the stress induction phase.

In future, the extraction features will be improved and classification algorithms could be implemented in order to obtain a real time system, able to detect stress levels of the user. The system will suggest also interventions such as physical exercises in order to reduce the stress level. This will support active ageing, allowing also to elderly to work until the retirement, under controlled conditions that could reduce the burden of stress related to the workload on the basis of personalised interventions.

Acknowledgments This work was supported by research funding provided by Trans.Safe (AmbienT Response to Avoid Negative Stress and enhance SAFEty, www.transsafe.eu) project—6th call of the Ambient Assisted Living Joint Programme (AAL JP) with the topic "ICT-based Solutions for Supporting Occupation in Life of Older Adults"

References

1. Sun FT, Kuo C, Cheng HT, Buthpitiya S, Collins P, Griss M (2010) Activity-aware mental stress detection using physiological sensors. In Mobile computing, applications, and services. Springer, Berlin, Heidelberg, pp 211–230
2. Statistic Brain (2015) Stress statistic. Retrieved from http://www.statisticbrain.com/stress-statistics
3. EU-OSHA (2016) European agency for safety and health at work. Retrieved from https://osha.europa.eu/en/tools-and-publications/publications/literature_reviews/calculating-the-cost-of-work-related-stress-and-psychosocial-risks
4. Ulstein I, Wyller TB, Engedal K (2007) High score on the relative stress scale, a marker of possible psychiatric disorder in family carers of patients with dementia. Int J Geriatr Psychiatry 22(3):195–202
5. Seaward BL (1999) Managing stress: principles and strategies for health and wellbeing. Jones & Bartlett Pub, USA
6. Watkins LL, Grossman P, Krishnan R, Blumenthal JA (1999) Anxiety reduces baroreflex cardiac control in older adults with major depression. Psychosom Med 61(3):334–340
7. Tsigos C, Chrousos GP (1994) Physiology of the hypothalamic-pituitary-adrenal axis in health and dysregulation in psychiatric and autoimmune disorders. Endocrinol Metab Clin North Am 23(3):451–466
8. de Santos Sierra A, Ávila CS, Pozo GBD, Casanova JG (2011, October). Stress detection by means of stress physiological template. In: Nature and biologically inspired computing (NaBIC), 2011 Third World Congress on IEEE, pp 131–136
9. Haapalainen E, Kim S, Forlizzi JF, Dey AK. (2010, September) Psycho-physiological measures for assessing cognitive load. In: Proceedings of the 12th ACM international conference on Ubiquitous computing, ACM, p 301–310
10. Park B (2009) Psychophysiology as a tool for HCI research: promises and pitfalls. In: Human-computer interaction. New Trends, Springer, Berlin, Heidelberg, pp 141–148
11. Lundberg U, Kadefors R, Melin B, Palmerud G, Hassmén P, Engström M, Dohns IE (1994) Psychophysiological stress and EMG activity of the trapezius muscle. Int J Behav Med 1(4):354–370
12. Rottenberg J, Wilhelm FH, Gross JJ, Gotlib IH (2002) Respiratory sinus arrhythmia as a predictor of outcome in major depressive disorder. J Affect Disord 71(1):265–272
13. Karthikeyan P, Murugappan M, Yaacob S (2012) Descriptive analysis of skin temperature variability of sympathetic nervous system activity in stress. J Phys Ther Sci 24(12):1341–1344

14. Lim CKA, Chia WC (2015) Analysis of single-electrode eeg rhythms using MATLAB to elicit correlation with cognitive stress. Int J Comput Theory Eng 7(2):149
15. Haak M, Bos S, Panic S, Rothkrantz LJM (2009) Detecting stress using eye blinks and brain activity from EEG signals. In: Proceeding of the 1st driver car interaction and interface (DCII 2008), p 35–60
16. Sharma N, Gedeon T (2012) Objective measures, sensors and computational techniques for stress recognition and classification: a survey. Comput Methods Programs Biomed 108 (3):1287–1301
17. Ritz T, Steptoe A, DeWilde S, Costa M (2000) Emotions and stress increase respiratory resistance in asthma. Psychosom Med 62(3):401–412
18. Stemmler G, Heldmann M, Pauls CA, Scherer T (2001) Constraints for emotion specificity in fear and anger: the context counts. Psychophysiology 38(02):275–291
19. Healey JA, Picard RW (2005) Detecting stress during real-world driving tasks using physiological sensors. Intell Transp Syst IEEE Trans on 6(2):156–166
20. Clifford GD (2002) Signal processing methods for heart rate variability. Doctoral dissertation, Department of Engineering Science, University of Oxford
21. Taelman J, Vandeput S, Spaepen A, Van Huffel S (2009). Influence of mental stress on heart rate and heart rate variability. In: 4th European conference of the international federation for medical and biological engineering. Springer, Berlin, Heidelberg, pp 1366–1369
22. Orsila R, Virtanen M, Luukkaala T, Tarvainen M, Karjalainen P, Viik J, Nygård CH (2008) Perceived mental stress and reactions in heart rate variability—a pilot study among employees of an electronics company. International Journal of Occupational Safety and Ergonomics, 14 (3), 275–283
23. Medtronic (2015). Zephyr™ performance system. Retrieved from http://www.zephyranywhere.com/products/bioharness-3
24. Shimmer (2016) Shimmer3 GSR + Unit. Retrieved from http://www.shimmersensing.com/shop/shimmer3-wireless-gsr-sensor
25. Lansbergen MM, Kenemans JL, van Engeland H (2007) Stroop interference and attention-deficit/hyperactivity disorder: a review and meta-analysis. Neuropsychology. 21 (2):251–262
26. Gillett R (2007) Assessment of working memory performance in self-ordered selection, Cortex. 43(8):1047–1056
27. Barbeau A (1980) Lecithin in Parkinson's disease. J Neural Transm Suppl 16:187–93
28. Miyake A, Emerson MJ, Friedman NP (2000) Assessment of executive functions in clinical settings: problems and recommendations. Semin Speech Lang 21(2):169–183
29. Marteau TM, Bekker H (1992) The development of a six-item short-form of the state scale of the Spielberger state—trait anxiety inventory (STAI). Br J Clin Psychol 31(3):301–306
30. Åkerstedt T, Gillberg M (1990) Subjective and objective sleepiness in the active individual. Int J Neurosci 52(1–2):29–37
31. Kaida K, Takahashi M, Åkerstedt T, Nakata A, Otsuka Y, Haratani T, Fukasawa K (2006) Validation of the Karolinska sleepiness scale against performance and EEG variables. Clin Neurophysiol 117(7):1574–1581
32. Helton WS (2004, September) Validation of a short stress state questionnaire. In: Proceedings of the Human Factors and Ergonomics Society Annual Meeting, Vol 48, No. 11, SAGE Publications, California, pp 1238–1242
33. Pfaff MS (2012) Negative affect reduces team awareness the effects of mood and stress on computer-mediated team communication. Hum Factors J Hum Factors Ergon Soc 54(4): 560–571
34. Boucsein W (2012) Electrodermal activity. Springer Science & Business Media
35. Schumm J, Bachlin M, Setz C, Arnrich B, Roggen D, Troster G (2008, January) Effect of movements on the electrodermal response after a startle event. In: Pervasive Computing Technologies for Healthcare, 2008. PervasiveHealth 2008. Second International Conference on IEEE, pp. 315–318

36. Healey J, Picard R (2000) SmartCar: detecting driver stress. In: Pattern Recognition, 2000. Proceedings of 15th International Conference on IEEE, Vol 4, pp 218–221
37. Mali B, Zulj S, Magjarevic R, Miklavcic D, Jarm T (2014) Matlab-based tool for ECG and HRV analysis. Biomed Signal Process Control 10:108–116
38. Singh RR, Conjeti S, Banerjee R (2012, February) Biosignal based on-road stress monitoring for automotive drivers. In: Communications (NCC), 2012 National Conference on IEEE, pp 1–5
39. Burke J, Christensen L (2004) Educational research: quantitative, qualitative, and mixed approaches. Boston: Pearson Education, Inc. Campbell KT, Forge E, Taylor L (2006). The effects of principal centers on professional isolation of school principals. Sch Leadersh Rev Summer/Fall, 2(1), 1–15
40. Elmes D, Kantowitz B, Roediger III H (2011) Research methods in psychology. Nelson Education, Canada
41. Kidd CD, Breazeal C (2005, April) Human-robot interaction experiments: lessons learned. In: Proceeding of AISB, Vol 5, pp 141–142
42. McCreadie C, Tinker A (2005) The acceptability of assistive technology to older people. Ageing soc 25(01):91–110
43. Picard RW, Vyzas E, Healey J (2001) Toward machine emotional intelligence: analysis of affective physiological state. Pattern Anal Mach Intell IEEE Trans On 23(10):1175–1191
44. Liu C, Rani P, Sarkar N (2006, October) Affective state recognition and adaptation in human-robot interaction: a design approach. In: Intelligent robots and systems, 2006 IEEE/RSJ International Conference on IEEE, pp 3099–3106

Complete Specifications of ICT Services in an AAL Environment

**Laura Burzagli, Paolo Baronti, Marco Billi,
Pier Luigi Emiliani and Fabio Gori**

Abstract Problems concerning services in an AAL kitchen environment are discussed. The complexity of their accurate specification is outlined. An example of implementation is described.

Keywords AAL · Service · Kitchen · Food · Well being

1 Introduction

Despite the amount of resources made available for research and development in AAL (Ambient Assisted Living) and, in particular, for supporting people in activities connected to feeding (kitchen), at the moment the impact on the market of smart home appliances and their integration in a connected system is relatively little. According to the experience of the authors, after many years of activity in projects dealing with the kitchen environment, for example in the AAL Project FOOD [1] and in the Italian project D4ALL [2], the main reason is that what is offered to the potential consumers is probably not perceived by the users as very relevant with respect to their real needs.

L. Burzagli (✉) · P. Baronti · M. Billi · P.L. Emiliani · F. Gori
CNR IFAC, Via Madonna Del Piano 10, 50019 Sesto Fiorentino, Firenze, Italy
e-mail: l.burzagli@ifac.cnr.it

P. Baronti
e-mail: p.baronti@ifac.cnr.it

M. Billi
e-mail: m.billi@ifac.cnr.it

P.L. Emiliani
e-mail: p.l.emiliani@ifac.cnr.it

F. Gori
e-mail: f.gori@ifac.cnr.it

© Springer International Publishing AG 2017   51
F. Cavallo et al. (eds.), *Ambient Assisted Living*, Lecture Notes
in Electrical Engineering 426, DOI 10.1007/978-3-319-54283-6_4

In AAL, services are defined as a support to the activities carried on by people in their daily living at home. What is offered now, apart health care applications that however are not new, is only technology that can perform a specific task, such as standing up or falling detection, or fancy displays on home appliances to have information about their status or connections through the network e.g. to download recipes. On the contrary, what is necessary is that the home system is able to support activities that meet complex and composite needs, such as planning a person's diet, as part of a suite of services that seamlessly address all activities connected to feeding.

This situation is due to many reasons. Out of them, two are considered here. The first, discussed in detail in the paper, is that it is not possible to identify user needs to be satisfied with home-based services, if an accurate analysis in not carried out of the activities of people in their living environments, for example for feeding, and how they perform them. The details of these activities must be carefully identified to produce potentially useful services and then, in interaction with individual users, to find out what are, if any, residual difficulties they may experience to fulfil their goals and/or to use the services themselves, in order to introduce suitable adaptations and/or additional support (e.g. at the level of interaction).

The need of individuals of having specific adaptations of services themselves and/or additional supports is the second reasons for an insufficient uptake of the home technology. As a matter of fact, in the transition from AmI (see the ISTAG documents [3]), i.e. Ambient Intelligence, to AAL, i.e. Ambient Assisted Living, the word "intelligence" has been forgotten. Available systems are not intelligent enough to be really useful, i.e. to be able to adapt themselves to the requirements of the single user.

2   Position of the Problem

As a matter of fact, a lot of activity has been devoted to the adaptation capabilities necessary to match the service features to the different users' profiles, thus overcoming personal limitations, due to lack of user abilities and different contexts. Several studies are already available on static and dynamic adaptation, often cited as adaptivity and adaptability [4, 5]. However, from this perspective, a central role is assumed by the accessibility and the usability of the interface and to this concern laws, standards and guidelines are available [6]. Less activity has been carried out with respect to the adaptation of the functionalities of equipment and corresponding services.

Considering, for example, feeding, all basic necessary activities have been carefully identified in the WHO-ICF document [7]. However, the experience gained in the above cited projects, shows that the design of services in an assisted living environment requires an additional level of analysis. The definition of the main functionalities of the services, of the interface with the user and of its adaptation approach, is not sufficient. Most services, according to users' evaluation reports, do not reach the hoped satisfaction and acceptability level, mainly because they address trivial tasks or functionalities at a too general level.

With reference to the ICF classification, this means that the granularity of the classification of the activities is not sufficient to describe in the details how, for example, people construct a shopping list by collecting and harmonizing information about what they want to eat, what they have available at home, how frequently they are shopping and so on. The design process, as presently carried out, is relevant for the identification of the technical infrastructure, which is often the main concern of many efforts in research and development in the AAL environment, and the adaptation aspects of the human system interface, where a GUI implementation is generally assumed. The necessary complexity and completeness of the service, to be defined before any identification of adaptations of its functionalities to specific user needs or preferences, is often not sufficiently analyzed. The result may be a lack of real impact on the activity to be carried out by the user and therefore a difficulty at the market level.

Actually, the functionalities of services must be developed from the start at a level of detail able to cover most of the aspects concerning the considered human activity (see Fig. 1). Otherwise, a service may be based on a powerful technical infrastructure and have an adapted user interface, without being really effective. The service provides advantages to the user only if it follows the activity normally carried out by her. This is why a service must not only be based on the identification of the necessary information flow. It must be compatible with and adhere to the user's habits. The service should be as much complete and coherent as possible even if complex. Part of the adaptation effort should be devoted to hide the complexity of the service to the user, when necessary.

Fig. 1 Service components

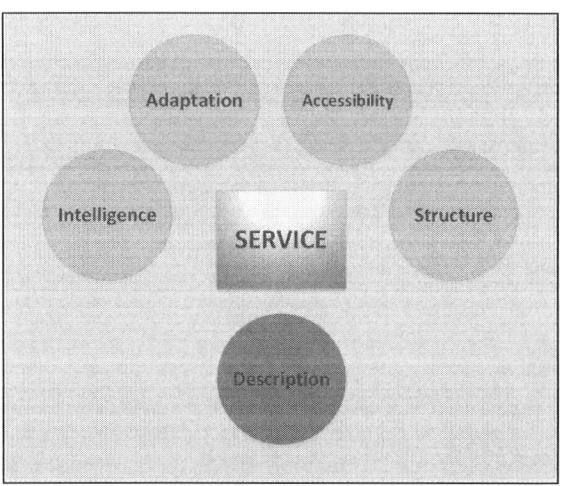

3 Design Approach

Aspect related to a satisfactory description of an AAL service has been studied within a specific context in the D4ALL project, whose main objective is to create a platform for interoperability of ambient equipment and services and their adaptation to individual users. The platform is supposed to help in designing and implementing an inclusive and sustainable domestic environment adaptable and adaptive to the individual users both at the level of human-system interface and of the integration and cooperation of service functionalities. As a demonstration environment, the kitchen was selected. In order to start the process of service development, all offered services are grouped in four basic categories (macro-functions): Cookbook—dietary process (recipes), Diary—food preparation, Pantry—food management, and control of appliances. These categories collect most of the service related to the ICF domestic life activities [7], in particular activity d620 (Acquisition of goods and services) and d630 (preparing meals), because they collect the vast majority of services related to food preparation.

For each of the above basic categories, the component tasks and possible interconnections among them have been identified, trying to take into account, as much as possible, the real sets of operations that the user normally performs in her daily life activities. This approach tries to capture the fact that very often people do not perform single activities, but complex aggregations different activities.

3.1 Cookbook

This macro-function is at the level of interaction with general purpose information accessible from the service and available in principle to all interested users. It is not personalized. It contains recipes accessible through different selection criteria, e.g. the name of the recipe, the presence of an ingredient, the type of dish (e.g. pasta or dessert). For each recipe a list of necessary ingredients can be extracted and information about the availability in the pantry retrieved. Therefore, the cookbook function is connected with the pantry function.

3.2 Diary

This macro-function is available for every user registered with a specific profile. It represents the personal level of interaction with the cookbook. The diary contains the personal notes related with a recipe, including, for example, general comments or specific modifications of ingredients and their doses. This may include a list of already used recipes, a list of recipes under preparation and, consequently, the shopping list. The shopping list can be directly derived from the list of ingredients of the recipes in preparation (components and quantity can be modified) or produced modifying an older shopping list or a list of normally bought items.

3.3 Pantry

This macro-function is in charge of the operations related to the acquisition and storage of food. It is divided in three storage spaces: a space at ambient temperature, a refrigerated space and a deep-frozen space. A search function is available that is able to produce a list of what is available with an indication of where in the pantry the element is available and the expiration date. At the moment, it is assumed that the pantry content is explicitly updated by the user after shopping and according to the use of the different items. However, it is foreseen that, due to the widespread use of new technological developments, as for example RFID tags, in the future the pantry content will be automatically updated. The list of items to be added to the pantry is a combination of elements coming from the recipes under preparation and elements explicitly introduced by the user according to her habits, the information about the conservation status and the expiry dates of the single items.

3.4 Appliances

This macro-function is in charge of the interaction with the home appliances. It gives information about their present status and control on all their functionalities. During the cooking activities it is possible to control the right execution of the recipe (e.g. temperature of the oven).

4 A Case Study—The Example of a Shopping List Service

In order to understand the design process, reference can be made to a specific service, namely a service supporting the preparation of the shopping list. The first step in planning the service is obviously the study of how to replace the paper support with an electronic support, which can guarantee flexibility in use and accessibility by different categories of users, since they can take advantage of multimodal interaction. Then, the selection of the shopping-list components can be based on predefined tables of commonly used items presented as text or as a collection of icons, so favoring people with mild cognitive problems. However, a careful analysis shows that, in order to define the service, it is not sufficient to study the content of the list itself, but also how it is produced. Indeed, a person, when going to the market with the shopping list, has already carried out several activities that must be supported by the service.

Even an informal investigation of these activities gives an idea of the complexity of the necessary service and of the "intelligence" that should be introduced in it to be really useful and probably worth to consider the migration to an assisted environment. This investigation can be carried out with reference to a few short scenarios (sketchy descriptions of rea life situations). These scenarios are not assumed as design tools or supposed to be exhaustive of all possible situations, but are presented only as an attempt of showing the level of complexity which is requested in order to implement a service able to handle the larger number of aspects possible. They come from an evaluation of service requirements carried out by experienced users, in order not to cover every aspects of the service, but to improve their adherence to human activity.

1. Scenario 1: The user invited friends for lunch. Therefore, she selected some recipes, corrected the doses of ingredients according to the number of guests, and probably inserted some changes. For example, she replaced butter with oil, as her doctor suggested. She also introduced bookmarks on the kitchen book to come back fast to the pages of the selected recipes. She also checked the availability of ingredients, some of which she must use, since close to the best-before date. Shopping is also correlated to the food supply she likes to have at home. She checks the fridge, the freezer and the cupboard, since, for example, she generally uses fresh milk, but stores also some packages of long-life milk.

2. Scenario 2: The user decides to go for her weekly shopping. First, she has to check her food supplies, taking also into account the different best-before dates and, for example, the available vegetables in the fridge and in the freezer. She needs to assess what she needs during the week, taking also in account that some packages have already been partially emptied. Moreover, she wants to take into account the dietary suggestions of the doctor.

3. Scenario 3: The user is planning a dinner with her friends, but, at the same time, has also to take care of the weekly shopping. She has a list written the previous day, placed with a magnet on the fridge door. Now, she has to add new ingredients, after having found what product already available at home she can use.

4. Scenario 4: The user comes back from the market with all the items of the list, with the addition of other goods chosen while shopping, e.g. selected for their special price. Therefore, the list of what is available in the kitchen must be outdated.

The presented scenarios do not refer to different user's profiles, but to different situations. An effective service, in addition to be adapted to the different users' profiles, which include physical, cognitive, sensorial and motor abilities, must take into account the above described contexts of use. Therefore, it requires the development of functionalities more complex than editing text or listing icons, even if accessible.

5 Technical Implementation

For the D4All project, an App(lication) on a mobile device with an accessible interface that implements the four macro-functions described above has been implemented. As a multiplatform environment, Cordova [8] is used and the solution is being tested on an Android device with O.S. Android 5.x and 6.01.

For the recipe-book, on the vertical left menu bar the App includes the list of recipes divided in five different courses: starters, first dishes, main dishes, side-dishes, desserts. As can be seen in the right part of Fig. 2, a list of ingredients is present, together with the quantity and an icon describing its availability in the pantry. An emoticon (happy—green, straight face—orange, sad—red) represents in a graphic form (color plus symbol) the presence, uncertainty and absence of the ingredient in the pantry.

Moreover, a picture with four basic comments about the recipe is provided: number of people, level of difficulties, cooking time, preparation. The number of people can be changed, and the system automatically adjusts the quantity of each ingredients and according to the availability, changes the availability icons. A "recipe in process" is foreseen, which implies the shopping of the necessary ingredients and the support for the real cooking.

The Diary macro-function (Fig. 3) includes a list of the used recipes (with the date of use), a list of recipes in preparation and the shopping list. The shopping list

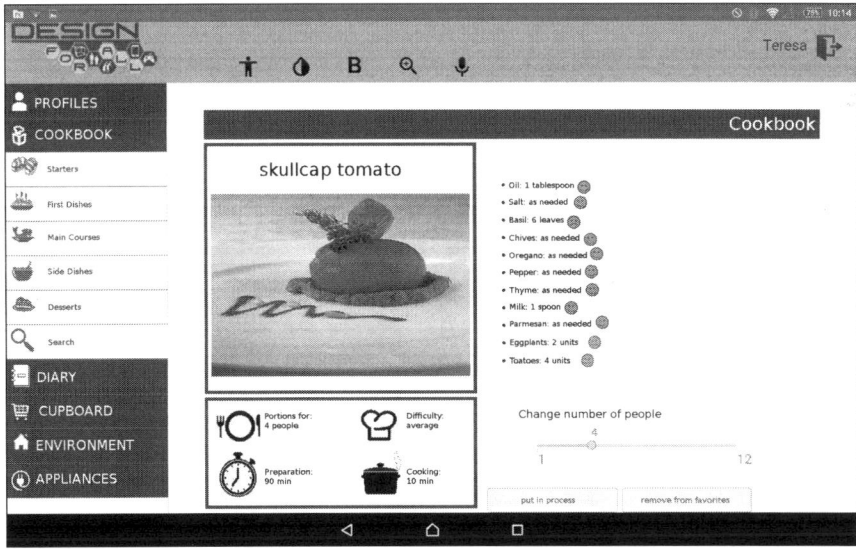

Fig. 2 Cookbook

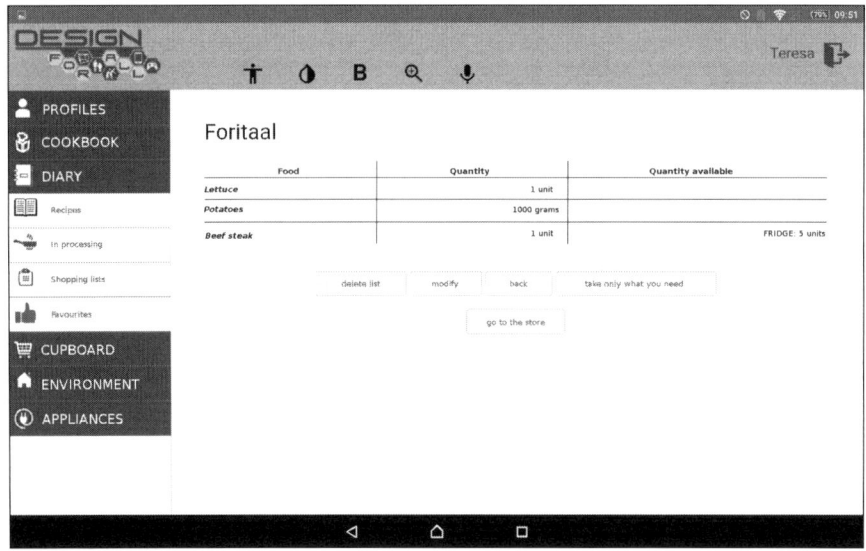

Fig. 3 Diary and shopping list

function can be used to create a new list or to add the ingredients of the selected recipe(s) to an already available list. Information about the quantities in the recipe and what is available in the pantry is made available to help people in deciding what she needs or wants to buy (it may be that she wants to leave a quantity of a necessary ingredient in the pantry), If the measurement units provided by the recipe and the ones used by the user are different, a conversion system is available, at least for a list of basic ingredients. Therefore, it is possible to modify the list of items, to change the quantity to buy or to decide to buy only what is not already in the pantry.

For the Pantry macro-function (Fig. 4), the screen shot shows the three types of storage space: a space at ambient temperature, a refrigerated space and a deep-frozen space. For any item the quantity and the expiry date is shown. Buttons are used to control the lists: (i) to cancel an item, (ii) to add a new one, (iii) to confirm the addition or (iv) to cancel it.

Even if it is assumed that in the future this operation will be automatic, presently the operations after the shopping are simulated, with the explicit addition of new items, even if they are not present in the previously produced shopping list.

For the macro-function control of home appliances in Fig. 5 the oven is used as an example. Some working parameters are shown and can be set. It is possible to choose a cooking program, the cooking temperature, and the switch-on time. Buttons to confirm commands or to correct them, if necessary, are available.

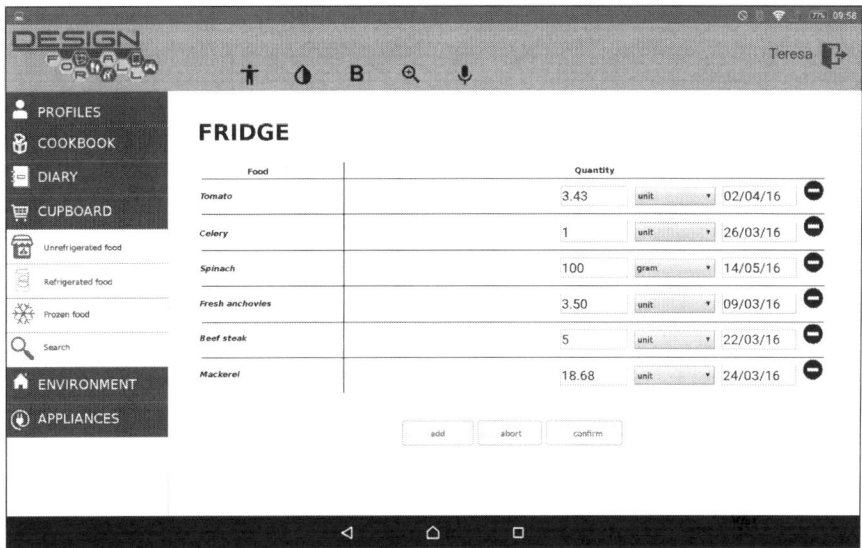

Fig. 4 Pantry

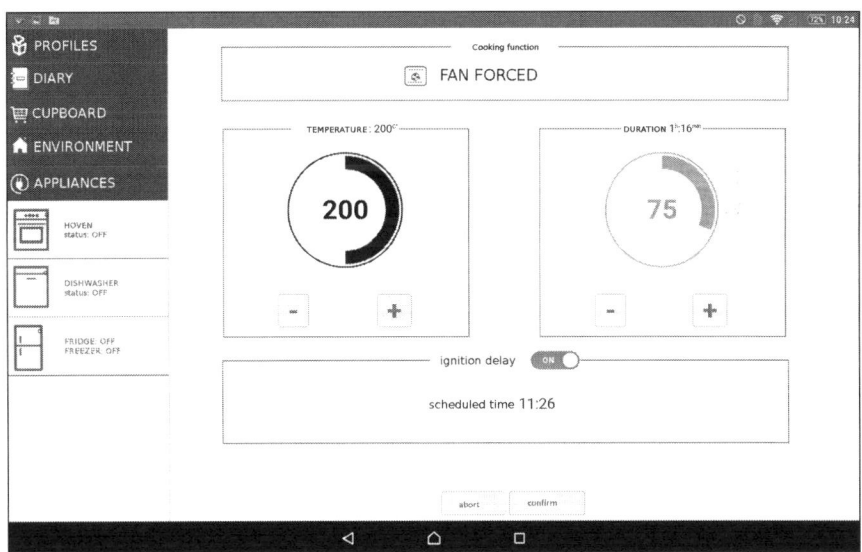

Fig. 5 Appliances

6 Future Work

In this preliminary stage all functions have been arranged on the basis of the evaluation of experienced users. For the future a method to describe these activities in a systematic way, for example through state charts, id under study. With this system it is possible to represent both functionalities and interactions, in a way similar to the one carried out by people when they carrying out their activities. These representations could be simulated and compiled to perform an output in a programming language.

7 Conclusions

The implemented service can be the starting point for the introduction of different sets of functionalities aimed to help people in their daily activities, for example for the automatic production of shopping lists for periodic shopping, based on user habits. It can also include adaptations to individual users, such as the production of warnings related to the specific user health profile (for example diabetes) with automatic suggestions of alternative ingredients. Anyway, the basic concept is that, before studying and applying the adaptation process, it is very important to introduce into the system a sufficient level of knowledge and "intelligent" processing, which is able to emulate carefully the user activity. Otherwise, the adaptation process may result quite limited.

Acknowledgments This material is based upon work supported by the Italian Ministry of Education, Universities and Research for the project "Design4All, Software integration and advanced Human Machine Interfaces in design for Ambient Assisted Living".

References

1. http://www.food-aal.eu/
2. http://www.d4all.eu/en/
3. Antona M, Burzagli L, Emiliani P-L, Stephanidis C (2009) The ISTAG scenarios: a case study. In: Roe PRW (ed) Towards an inclusive future: impact and wider potential of information and communication technologies, ambient intelligence and implications for people with disabilities, ch. 4, sec. 4.1, pp 158–187. COST219ter, Brussels
4. Stephanidis C (2001) Adaptive techniques for universal access. User Model User-Adap Inter 11:159–179
5. Emiliani PL, Stephanidis C (2005) Universal access to ambient intelligence environments: opportunities and challenges for people with disabilities. IBM Syst J 44(3):605–619
6. W3C. http://www.w3c.org
7. WHO (2001) ICF International Classification of Functioning, Disability and Health. World Health Organization, Geneva
8. https://en.wikipedia.org/wiki/Apache_Cordova

Design of a Community-Supported CapAble Microwave System for People with Intellectual and Physical Disabilities

Matteo Zallio, Paula Kelly, Modestas Jakuska, Hicham Rifai and Damon Berry

Abstract Product personalisation has become a central topic and expected part of every day life. Different people have different characteristics and abilities and each user has different needs which means that products have to be tailored accordingly. Microwave ovens are one of the most commonly used home appliances. People use them to quickly heat or cook certain foods. Today, according to the US Bureau of Labor Statistics, more than 90% of U.S. households own a microwave oven. This project seeks to enable people with intellectual disabilities and physical impairments to perform simple cooking tasks. The target group includes ageing people who experience difficulties in using microwave systems, with a particularly low grade of autonomy in preparing foods and meals. In order to address the specific needs of the defined group of users, the research follows the principles of the *Quality Function Deployment* analysis and takes inspiration from the DfA (*Design for All*) theories and the UCD (*User Centred Design*) method. The aim of the research is to find new solutions in order to simplify certain activities of daily living for users who would otherwise be excluded from these actions. In the second stage, the project, seeks to provide a set of tools that enable the interaction with smart appliances to grow the sense of community, by sharing information within a social network and a Cloud-based service system. The main challenge is to create a *"Community Supported Appliance"* that provides technology and settings for enabling users in performing one daily activity. The CSA is intended to be a simple

M. Zallio (✉) · P. Kelly · M. Jakuska · H. Rifai · D. Berry
TPOT Research Group, Dublin Institute of Technology,
Kevin Street Lower, Dublin 8, Ireland
e-mail: matteo.zallio@dit.ie

P. Kelly
e-mail: paula.kelly@dit.ie

M. Jakuska
e-mail: modestas.jakuskas@mydit.ie

H. Rifai
e-mail: hicham.rifai@dit.ie

D. Berry
e-mail: damon.berry@dit.ie

© Springer International Publishing AG 2017
F. Cavallo et al. (eds.), *Ambient Assisted Living*, Lecture Notes
in Electrical Engineering 426, DOI 10.1007/978-3-319-54283-6_5

61

to use, affordable learning system, continuously fed from the community of carers and service users, that has the potential to be used, in the near future, by a wider group of people. A device of this type benefits from added value given from expert users to others in the community, in the form of sequenced multimedia instructions to the person and direct operating instructions to the appliance.

Keywords Design for all · Ageing people · Intellectual disabilities · Physical impairments · Smart home · CapAble microwave · Community supported appliance · User centred design · Ambient assisted living

1 Introduction

Just as every single citizen has a unique set of characteristics and abilities, each user has different needs and in an era of mass-produced goods, people with physical impairments or intellectual disabilities whether those disabilities are life-long or age-related, have to live within a world that is often not tailored for them [1].

Sometimes people with disabilities, are for various reasons, unable to complete what others might consider to be simple everyday tasks, such as eating, bathing, dressing, toileting, and moving—the *Activities of Daily Living* (ADL) [2]. When people are unable to perform these activities, they need help in order to cope, either from other human beings or mechanical devices or both [3].

Innovative technologies are emerging as a support for reacting to problems related to people with disabilities and ageing people, bringing care from hospitals into the community and increasing health services into homes [4]. In particular, smart homes and smart responsive appliances address the promotion of independent living by using assistive technologies for higher quality of daily life, supporting a high degree of autonomy and dignity [5]. In these cases, the help provided by technologies for Smart Living can enhance the level of autonomy for all, they may serve as an enabling mechanism to assist the population, especially in the cognitive and security domains, and also as a mechanism that enhances their daily life [6].

Referring to the ADL activities, one of the main tasks that could enable people with disabilities and ageing people to be more independent, is related to preparing and cooking foods autonomously, by using traditional home appliances like ovens, microwaves or cookers. In order to develop a "*Participatory Design Approach*" a consistent group of users, in particular, people affected by different physical and cognitive impairments, were involved. This was indispensable to provide feedback concerning different types of actions that users perform for eating or preparing meals.

The method used for transforming user needs into specific design inputs for designers and engineers, is the *Quality Function Deployment* (QFD). This method helps to create operational definitions of the specific requirements and prioritizes each product or service characteristic while simultaneously setting development targets for the product or service. There is also a possibility to transform qualitative user demands into quantitative parameters, to deploy the functions forming quality and to deploy methods for achieving the design quality into subsystems and ultimately to specify elements for the design process [7]. By following the results, based on the continuous reverse design approach that has been conducted with the users, the research investigates how to design a user-friendly microwave system that enables people with intellectual disabilities to be more in control of their environment and to live more independent lives by participating in meal preparation.

The aim of the project is to find new solutions in order to simplify certain activities of daily living, in particular those associated with meal preparation, for users who would otherwise be excluded from these actions. This is possible by creating a working example of a *"Community Supported Appliance"* which incorporates a set of smart components with customised interfaces and sequenced instructions for users, in order to enable them to prepare meals independently.

The main challenge is to provide technology and a group of standard settings that give the user a chance to interact with a learning system that could be fed continuously from the user's community.

The research refers to different design approaches, combined with engineering and social sciences and a user requirements analysis borrowed from Ergonomics and Human Factors theories, in order to focus on the main issue and then to develop a prototype of the CapAble Microwave. The role of this device is to facilitate the user's task and to make sure that the user is able to use it with minimum effort [8].

2 Cooking Appliances State of Art: Development and Use of a Microwave

King [9] defined the smart home as "A dwelling incorporating a communications network that connects the key electrical appliances and services, and allows them to be remotely controlled, monitored or accessed". A smart home is equipped with a network and smart technology such as smart lighting system, smart appliances, energy usage monitoring, security system, that enhance people's life in many aspects. Smart technologies have the potential to reduce the burden on caregivers as well as healthcare costs, while maintaining a good quality of life for its users.

Emerging smart technology can facilitate self-care, extend the self-reliance of the ageing population and disabled people, enabling them to perform different actions [10]. Focusing on a kitchen appliance that is expected to change radically in the next few years, the microwave is one of the most common cooking and meal heating systems in use. People use microwave ovens to quickly heat prepared meals, to defrost or cook foods. Today, according to the US Bureau of Labor Statistics, more than 90% of U.S. households own a microwave oven [11].

Contemporary microwave ovens are safer, more convenient and offer a wealth of advanced features. Current models produce about 10% more power than previous versions and many include electronic sensors along with automatic controls for easy programming of cooking commands. They also come in a greater variety of sizes power ratings and styles. From small no-frills models to sophisticated ovens large enough to handle full-size meals, microwave ovens are ready to meet a broad range of consumer needs.

The good news is that some of these advanced features are now available at lower prices [12]. Some vendors have produced what could be considered as the first smart microwaves that are able to interact in a smart, productive way with the users. For example, IBM [13] introduced a concept of central coordination for different appliances for the future kitchen, while Siemens [14] produced a kitchen appliance that gathers important information from the Internet (e.g. cooking recipes or cooking settings). Samsung, is one of the latest producers to release a new microwave which has a series of smart sensors, that work by reading the surface temperature of the food throughout the cooking process to decide when the food is ready, eliminating the possibility of over or under cooked food [15].

However, the evolution of microwaves from the first models produced in the early 1970s, to the latest, integrated units with an assortment of buttons, LCD/LED screens and handles wheels, was not so linear. We can now assume that the level of easy interaction between users and microwave appliances in certain cases decreases exponentially with UI complexity. Bruner [16] assumed that categorisation processes serve to simplify the world, leading people to reserve their refined discriminatory skills only for that with which they are especially concerned. According to this theory, people usually try to simplify processes, in particular those that are repetitive, when they feel confident about using a certain device. This aspect is particularly important because it helps to understand the usability processes that are applied by different people in using the functions of various microwave ovens.

2.1 Microwave Usability Analysis

By analysing the microwave market of the last 2 years, it is possible to find a variety of different models produced by different brands. By taking a small sample of 30 of the most common microwaves starting from €110 up to €340, it is possible to consider what type of user interface system they have.

The analysis shows that microwave appliances have an interface ranging from a minimum of 7 buttons plus hand wheel up, to a maximum of 31 buttons. So, if we think about extrapolating the results of this investigation, to the totality of the microwaves that are available on the world's market, we can estimate that the average quantity of buttons present on a microwave is 16 (Fig. 1).

By using the *Quality Function Deployment* method, with the users from the community and listening to the user group experience, it was possible to notice that most of the time, members of the target group use no more than two buttons, like "add 30s." (which also starts the heat, in our case study) and "Stop/Cancel". If we compare the specific user needs linked to this research project and try to define an

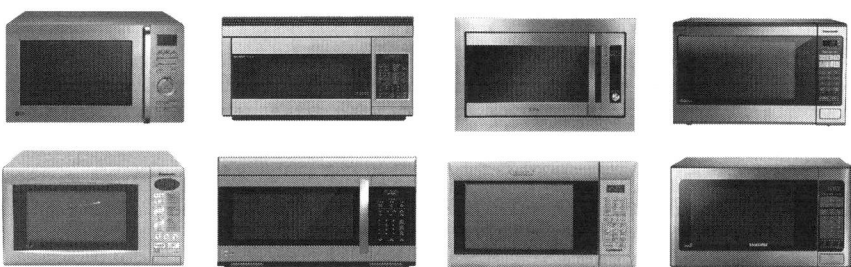

Fig. 1 Example of the most common microwaves interface, which is composed by buttons and hand wheels

average of different users, such as ageing citizens, or people with minor physical disabilities we could say that a significant proportion of the buttons are rarely used (approximately 85% of buttons are not used).

Different aspects like: usability, complexity in interacting with the system and finally affordance, caused a low level of usage of certain buttons. According to D. Norman an "Affordance" is the design aspect of an object which suggests how the object should be used; in particular: "…the term affordance refers to the perceived and actual properties of the thing, primarily those fundamental properties that determine just how the thing could possibly be used…" Affordances provide strong clues to the operations of things. Buttons are for pushing. Knobs are for turning. Slots are for inserting things into. Balls are for throwing or bouncing. When affordances are taken advantage of, the user knows what to do just by looking: no picture, label, or instruction is needed [8, p. 9].

Referring to this theory and according to the microwave analysis, based on the user's request, it has been possible to redesign the physical interface of a general microwave and set up a new interaction method that a community of primary and secondary users could use and implement continuously.

3 Research Methodology for a Community-Designed Device

Understanding user requirements is an integral part of information systems design and is critical to the success of interactive systems. It is now widely understood that successful systems and products begin with an understanding of the needs and requirements of the users [17]. The research, developed in consultation with care staff and service users from a community of people affected by different impairments, aims to identify and develop a new interface and interaction method in order to enable people with cognitive and physical disabilities to learn the cooking process and prepare meals by using a "Smart" microwave.

In the second stage, the project seeks to provide a set of tools that enable the interaction with smart appliances to grow the sense of community, by sharing information with an Internet-based instruction system. This will involve an innovative interface pattern and a set of community-based instructions. Focusing on the type of users, it is important to underline the definition of ID—Intellectual Disability, that includes a broad range of (developing) abilities in the group of people.

Some users may demonstrate language delay, fine motor/adaptive delay, cognitive and social delay and they may, just like any other person, have differing personality traits and temperaments, hyperactivity, disordered sleep and associated behaviours may include aggression, self-injury, defiance, inattention, hyperactivity, sleep disturbances [18].

3.1 Quality Function Deployment Method for a User Centred Design Approach

The *Quality Function Deployment* is a team user-based analysis that provides a way for identifying and transferring user requirements into technical specifications for designing devices, processes and products. The term *Quality Function Deployment* derives from a Japanese translation of this methodology, *hin shitsu* (quality), *ki nou* (function), *ten kai* (deployment). The methodology consists of a structured procedure that starts with the qualities desired by the users, leads through the functions required to provide these products and services and identifies the means for deploying the available resources to best provide, in this particular case, the new microwave interface [19].

In order to address the specific needs of the group of users, while following a path, which provides a usable, and affordable product for ID users, the research takes inspiration from merging the principle dictated from the *Design for All* theories and the *User Centred Design* method. The *Design for All* is the intervention into environments, products and services, which aims to ensure that anyone, including future generations, regardless of age, gender, capacities or cultural background, can participate in social, economic, cultural and leisure activities with equal opportunities [20].

The *User Centred Design* approach originated in Donald Norman's research laboratory at the University of California San Diego (UCSD) in the 1980s and became widely used after the publication of a co-authored book [21]. D. Norman, offers four basic suggestions on how a design should be:

- Make it easy to determine what actions are possible at any moment.
- Make things visible, including the conceptual model of the system, the alternative actions, and the results of actions.
- Make it easy to evaluate the current state of the system.

- Follow natural mappings between intentions and the required actions, between actions and the resulting effect and between the information that is visible and the interpretation of the system state [8, p. 188].

By following the QFD method, the project team employed frequent meetings (one every two weeks for four months) with service users and front line care staff. The meetings were indispensable to gather feedback on the developing system from primary users, a significant number of the 40 people from the community site, in addition to feedback and indications from secondary users (in particular the care-givers and allied health professionals who provide services).

Different instruments were devised in order to collect the feedback and the most useful and productive were: a customized online survey, which was administered by the caregivers, direct interviews with the service users, which occurred during the team meetings with the support of the caregivers and finally a focus group with different persons. The study group was comprised of interviewees and focus group members from one location; overall 10 suitable individuals took part in the inter-views and focus groups out of a community of 40 service users.

A wider group of survey participants was approached across four locations reaching a group of approximately 120 people. One of the groups of interviewees and focus group was made up of 4 individuals ranging in age from 25 to 52 years old. They were identified as they all had differing individual support needs in order to use the microwave however, limited literacy skills affect the 4 participants to varying degrees.

The specifics abilities of those four people are related to:

- Limited literacy to be defined in this instance but not limited to the ability to understand and recognize some words in different contexts, for example on a door push/pull and road signs such as Stop.
- The ability to read/write their own name, but unable to write freely from instruction or memory.
- Recognizing brand names/commonly understood items with support of logos and other environmental clues.

The interviews were conducted on a one-to-one basis in an office environment and were carried out by an experienced and familiar care staff to the interviewees and they were asked about their experiences in using microwaves. The objective of the interview was to:

- Identify positive and negative interactions while using microwaves.
- The possible reasons and barriers that shaped the interactions.
- User patterns/trends, what and when people cook.

All of this information would help in providing data for shaping the "*Persona*" model in the following stage of research. The second, more detailed interviews took place with the same interviewers in a kitchen, which was familiar to the intervie-wees using two different microwaves. The first microwave has two wheels, one for time and one for setting. The second microwave has a digital screen with a number keypad and pre-set functions. In order to capture useful information on the inter-action between person and microwave, users were asked to perform four basic tasks:

- Open door/close door.
- Set up the timer for 2 or 5 min.
- Identify full/half/defrost functions.
- Highlight any dangers while using microwave.

Information was gathered while observing the interactions between each single user and the device. By referring to a reverse process, information was also used to shape the questions and statements in the following focus group. After the initial interviews it was possible to move towards focus groups, which was composed of 6 additional individuals who joined the first 4 users. The objective of the focus group was to ask a wider cross section of user's opinions on the interaction and usage of the microwave. The focus group was held in an office environment, with the presence of the microwaves and 6 additional members; 4 of them were males and 2 females ranged in age from 25 to 57 years old, with similar abilities to the people belonging to the first group of interviewees.

The interview process was the same as the previous one, asking questions related to the usage of the microwave and observing interactions to identify any common problems which were not verbally communicated, in order to collect as much feedback as possible to build the *Persona* model. Finally, support staff joined in at the end of the focus group to help provide insight from their perspective, as they usually provide daily support to the focus group while using the microwave. It emerged from the focus group that users, especially an individual user with cog-nitive disabilities, like to watch cartoons on the TV and so they prefer to look at images, or sketches, rather than reading text or numbers (this is also due to a lack of literacy).

Some of the users also like to interact with apps and games on smartphones or tablets, because those devices provide direct feedback and enroll the user in par-ticipating in an interactive learning process for increasing abilities. From initial interviews and focus group an accessible survey was developed in order to increase the case study size. This was made available across 4 different locations, reaching a group of approximately 120 persons and it was designed to be accessible for people with limited literacy. It has been possible to receive 30 completed surveys, which defined the main user requirement analysis.

Generally, it has been possible to collect feedback related to the request of support for using the microwave and more than the 66% of people responses were positive (Fig. 2).

For ID users, as for older people, the safe use and correct operation of a microwave can be a big challenge, mainly caused by interface usability issues. Settings (product to cook or heat, time and temperature), the often-heavy mechanical catch/interlock on microwave doors, the multi-stage process that they

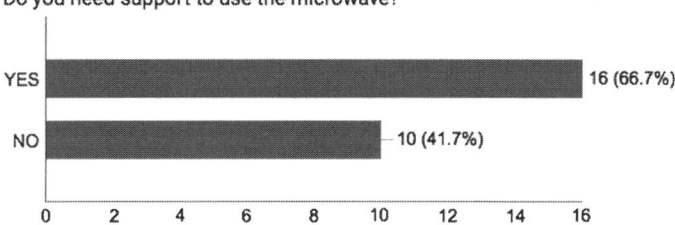

Fig. 2 Online survey for primary users. Do you need support to use the microwave?

have to complete in order to prepare a good quality meal, are some of the main issues identified during the interview, focus groups and online survey.

In these circumstances and for these users, a modified and improved microwave represents an opportunity to be more autonomous, to feel empowered to use technology which was formerly unusable for them and the increased independence of providing hot food by themselves.

3.2 Designing with the "Persona" Model

The set of needs, collected within the interviews, focus groups and survey, were shaped by using the "*User Persona*" model. A *Persona* is a model of a user that focuses on the individual's goals when using an artifact. The model has a specific purpose as a tool for software and product design. The *Persona* resembles classical user profiles, but with some important distinctions. It is an archetypical representation of real or potential users and it is not a description of a real, single user or an average user.

The *Persona* represents patterns of user's behaviour, goals and motives, compiled in a fictional description of a single individual. It also contains made-up personal details, in order to make the *Persona* more "tangible and alive" for the development team [22].

Thanks to this fundamental instrument, it has been possible to summarize the way that people interact with a microwave and what they usually cook for lunch or for dinner in the common microwave room. This was a key topic, because as every experienced microwave user knows, different foods have different heating temperatures and times. In addition, for some foods, like for example soups, popcorn and noodles, the user has to work through a multistage process. They will not just put the prepared meal into the microwave, and switch it on, but they may also need to fill a vessel up with water, preheat an item and stir, then heat again, or for example shake the popcorn box, before and/or in the middle of the cooking process. In addition to the power setting of the microwave itself, food entering the microwave could come from a fridge, freezer or cupboard, necessitating slightly different cooking times.

Finally, it is important to underline that when a food is overcooked there is a serious danger of burns when handling the pot or the food container for this target group. In order to avoid this issue, a humidity sensor that is based on the generation of moisture vapour from the food, could shut off the microwave when a certain level of humidity is reached inside the cavity and a temperature sensor could be also used to determine when the meal is cooked and safe to handle.

For this work three *Persona* models have been created to represent the goals and behaviour of the group of users and synthesized from data collected from interviews with the users.

Maria, *Persona* 1, is a female aged 26. She is extremely independent, she can travel freely in the neighborhood and she is adept in the use of technology such as tablet or smartphone. There are no physical challenges that would Maria in using a microwave but unfortunately she has limited literacy skills and finds it difficult to use numbers in day-to-day life. This aspect has been previously identified during phone training where alternatives for an unlocking pin were required due to his multiple wrong attempts blocking the use of the phone. Finally Maria cannot differentiate between the numbers and setting of the microwave timer correctly, so it is important to solve this issue in order to enable him to use the microwave correctly.

Richard, *Persona* 2, is a male aged 41. He would require extra supports to complete Activities of Daily Living. He uses a motorized wheelchair and has some fine motor skill limitation with handgrip and arm reach across both sides of his body. He also has limited literacy and basic numeracy skills. The identified support needed for Richard is the physical use of the microwave. As the accuracy of touch is decreased at full stretch, he may press the wrong number by accident not by misunderstanding. He finally needs a system that enables the opening of the microwave door with one hand.

Daniel, *Persona* 3 is a male aged 33. He is highly functioning and possesses the majority of skills for independent participation in Activities of Daily Living. He can freely access local areas and has excellent independent skills. He has good numeracy skills that enable him to easily manage money and successfully use the facilities of a bank/ATM. The main support that is needed for Daniel is to understand the effect of the actions/settings on a particular device. It is likely that Daniel set the numbers correctly each time, with the proper sized font, but he might find issue with the functions of the microwave, for example if he cooked the food for the correct time but on the wrong setting.

The results from the interview with primary users and consultations with caregivers allowed the creation of three different representations of the group of users. It is also important to underline that results from the survey (more than 58% of people need support for preparing food packaging, e.g. peel of lid) (Fig. 3) and the main issues related to poor literacy of *Persona* 1 and 2 are very important to understand that not only the cooking process has to be automated by the microwave, but there should be some aid for the process of preparing the food packaging.

In light of this information, the research group focused on defining a common and easy way to use a low cost technology that enables people with intellectual disabilities to use the microwave, but also one that could (according to *Design for*

Do you need support with the instructions on how to prepare the packaging? For example peel of the lid.

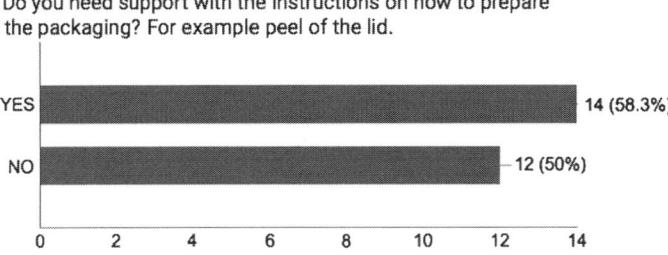

Fig. 3 Online survey for primary users. Do you need support with the instructions on how to prepare the packaging? For example, peel of the lid

What are you using the microwave to do?

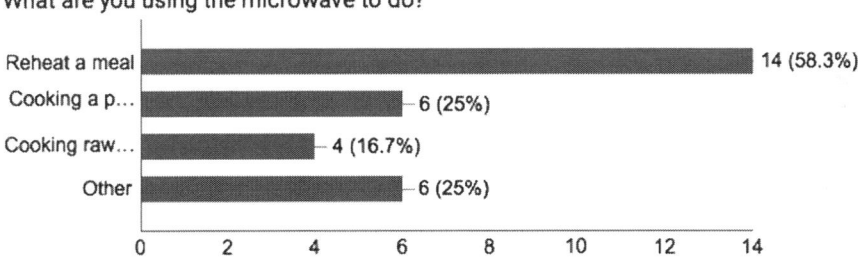

Fig. 4 Online survey for primary users. What are you using the microwave to do?

All and *User Centred Design*) be appreciated by the caregivers and family members as users.

3.3 Preferences from the Users

One of the most important elements that was highlighted by the survey, was that ID people are accustomed to go to supermarkets with the caregivers, where they are given the opportunity to feel independent by choosing prepared meals from the shelves and scanning products at the self-cashier. This is a significant challenge for those people who can, followed by a caregiver, choose and buy foods without any particular help, by using the facilities provided by the supermarkets (automated barcode readers and automatic cashiers).

The results of the survey indicates that more than half of the users use the microwave under supervision, to reheat a meal, that was previously cooked (like prepared meals from supermarkets which have a big portion for just one person) and that 25% use the microwave for cooking a packaged microwave meal (Fig. 4).

These indications brought to light that the majority of the studied users employ a microwave to cook or heat prepared or semi-prepared food, with the help of caregivers. So for the purposes of the work it was possible for the project team to narrow down the field of action of smart systems linked to the microwave.

Packaged and processed food from supermarkets has some drawbacks, but also has the advantage of extensive labelling. Apart from the printed label, the barcode provides important and distinctive information which allows users and (in this case) a capAble microwave, to understand with simply one action, which kind of food is contained in the packaging and provide the possibility to initialise the microwave in the best way. A barcode is a machine-readable arrangement of numbers and parallel lines of different widths printed on a package, which can be electronically scanned at a checkout to register the price of the goods and to activate computer stock-checking and reordering also called Universal Product Code, UPC [23].

Barcodes have a huge potential as an identifier of data related to different products and provide an opportunity to design different pre-sets, for various types of food.

4   The CapAble Microwave

The outcomes of the user analysis, allow us to identify the principles that have driven this smart innovation.

People with disabilities and some ageing people with particular medical conditions have difficulties in recalling very simple sequences of actions. The new microwave device seeks to provide not just cooking assistance, but also a support for independent living, by interacting in a productive way with the user.

As mentioned in the user feedback analysis, some of the users like to interact with apps, games, watching animated movies with the aid of different devices and enjoy scanning products in the supermarkets. One of the key points of the interaction process, which could be researched, is the "gamification" of the cooking process. In recent years, gamification, the use of game design elements in non-game contexts, has seen rapid adoption in the software industry, as well as a growing body of research on its uses and effects [24].

In order to create a smart system by using not only hardware technologies, but also user friendly software, it has been important to design an interface that allows people to easily understand how to use hardware that evokes emotions, feelings and a sort of challenge by performing a particular process. This process is known, as gamification and users and caregivers, were conscious of the potential of this interaction instrument. So, by following these indications, it has been possible to set the hardware structure, which is composed of a barcode scanner, a touchscreen, an audio speaker a *Wi-Fi* module and a *Raspberry PI*, but also understand how to represent the visual feedback on the screen in a communicative way.

One of the simplest and more communicative interfaces, for the users, that they usually like to see and to interact with, are "animations"; simple animations were introduced in the project, to make information accessible in the community. The regular use of Adobe voice (an application for a tablet, which allows for the creation of easy and professional looking animations), gives service users experience with interacting with information in this format.

In other previous experiences, caregivers had positive feedback from using anonymous animated instruction sequences, or simple and clear sketches and drawings in order to communicate some desired interaction to the users. So it was decided, with the help of the caregivers, to move forward on developing a simple and easy "animation based" interface, which could be detailed, but at the same time that would give a clear idea of the sequenced actions that everyone has to perform for cooking a particular meal. The caregivers and users collaborate to create multimedia instructions for the end-users and operating instructions for the associated appliance. These instructions can be managed "in the Cloud" in what we term the instruction management service.

When a user scans a barcode, the barcode information, and information about the device that is requesting instructions are sent to the instruction management service, which responds by sending customised cooking instructions to the requesting device. The device acts in the manner of a browser, by issuing multimedia instructions to the user, prompting them to engage in the cooking process. At certain points in the cooking process, the device also operates the controls of the microwave to cook the product. By enabling users to scan the barcode of foods close to the microwave, the device "understands" what kind of food it is, identifies the appropriate cooking time and temperature and provides visual and audio feedback to the user.

4.1 System Architecture of the CapAble Microwave

The capAble microwave has the potential to give different types of feedback to the user, before starting the automatic cooking process. Two embedded functions are at the core of the interaction system:

1. Suggestion: by pointing out a set of instructions in order to guide the user in the cooking/heating process, the system is able to give instructions not only in directly controlling the appliance presets for temperature, time, but also about what the user could do in order to prepare the food package to be heated. Actions like: peel off the film, add some water, stir the food, shake the bag (for popcorn), etc. can be promoted by the microwave touchscreen interface by enabling user interaction and by making the cooking process more interactive, adaptable and that can be turned into a game, rather than a automatic, boring process.
2. Alerts: it is known that the heating/cooking process has safety concerns, such as e.g. the risk of fire, if someone forgets to turn off the microwave, or the risk of heating the meal too much, or the risk of the food "going off" if the food is left inside the microwave for too long a period. The timer and temperature alerts, settled with the specific information given by the barcode and on-line services,

could be linked to the Cloud network of the community or to the smartphone/tablet of the carer or end user, providing a safer control of the process while avoiding personal security risks.

In order to solve the different user issues, the microwave uses information that is downloaded from the Cloud. Members of the community can upload different user instructions and settings for different types of microwaveable food products to the platform. The platform created on the "easycook.ie." domain (Fig. 5), is a web-service, where people from the community can upload information related to each food (like temperature and cooking time, calories, nutritional information, etc.), bought in supermarkets and simultaneously each microwave of the community can get information thanks to this instruction repository.

This web-based service, alongside this first prototype of the microwave could be seen, not only as a basic information service in the initial stage of the research, but also as a learning tool that enables people to upload additional information and grow the sense of community for different group of users. The capAble microwave effectively becomes an interactive smart object, which provides the required food information and gives help in following the cooking process. So, by interacting with users and redesigning the electronic circuit, the research moves forward on producing a smart add-on module for existing microwaves such as those used by the community. A barcode scanner with a *Raspberry Pi*, a small touchscreen that gives visual feedback a speaker that provides audio feedback and a *Wi-Fi* module are the core elements that comprise the first prototype (Fig. 6).

Another important positive issue that moves on developing the easily accessible, "animation based" interface, is to "keep it simple" and "not personal" (so for example, without showing a particular bowl, taken from just a photo of one user's bowl) it avoids a confusion that occurs when a service user sees a photo of a real bowl. In that case, there was an experience in one of the interviews, that one user could say "it's not my bowl, it's "John's" bowl" and this could be a negative point that could interrupt the process of good interaction between ID user and the smart microwave.

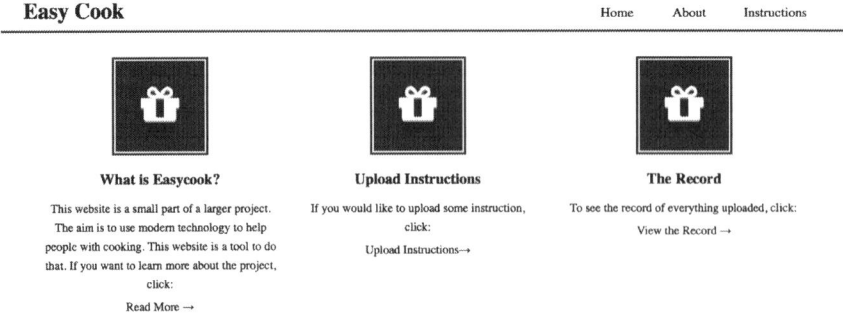

Fig. 5 Prototype of the "easycook.ie." website for the instruction repository

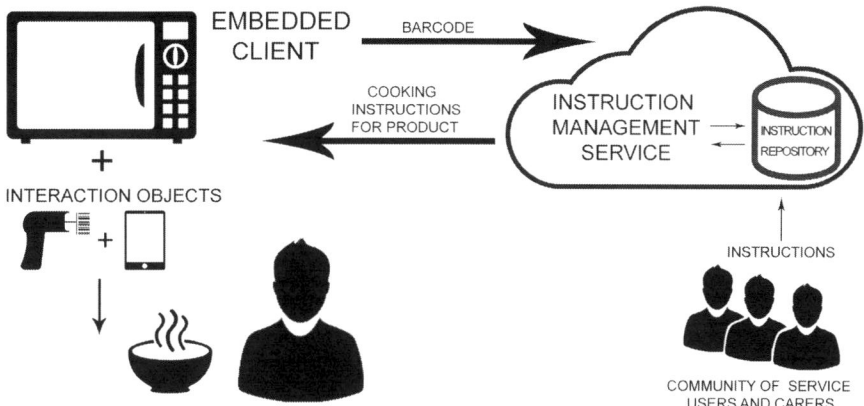

Fig. 6 Architecture diagram of the capAble microwave prototype

The capAble microwave will be enabled to inform the user which food is contained inside the packet just scanned and it will provide assistance for supporting with the instructions on how to prepare the packaging and with the safe opening of the microwave door. By recognising the type of food scanned, which is linked to a set of information (like cooking time, temperature, microwave power) provided on the easycook.ie. website, the microwave will become an interactive device that has the capacity to remind users of the different tasks.

For example: peel off the film, or add some water and then when the user places the product inside the microwave it will automatically start the appropriate cooking/heating process. Basically, by using an integrated barcode scanner, a *Wi-Fi* module, a touchscreen, added to the existing microwave unit and by developing the interaction software, it is possible to transform a classical, difficult-to-use microwave, into an instrument that enables user engagement and that also simplifies the process for varying groups of users to the extent that the required number of buttons is ideally reduced to one.

5 Conclusion

The aim of the project is to find new solutions in order to simplify certain activities of daily living for users who would otherwise be excluded from these actions. This is possible by creating a working prototype of a *"Community Supported Appliance"* which incorporates a set of tools that a community of primary users and secondary users could use and implement, in order to address the main challenge of the cooking process.

By working on the hardware and software technologies and on the interface of the new microwave appliance, it has been possible to share cooking information and to enable people with intellectual and/or physical disabilities to learn from their actions, adding value between members of the community.

The CSA—*Community Supported Appliance* has the potential to become an instrument that enables people to perform actions and to re-design customized interfaces for different home appliances. In perspective, the CSA can be applied within different scenarios, like the home environment or within the public spaces services or private/public transportation context.

The main challenge is to provide the technology and settings that give the possibility to have a learning system that could be fed continuously from the user community of carers and service users. The actual potential of this smart community-based system could be much more significant, if we consider the millions of users that usually operate microwaves just to heat or cook meals. We are conscious that the usage of a barcode scanner could have limits, related to specific foods, but the feedback derived from the first tests with the users group, has shown that the microwave appliance is mostly used not for the "proper cooking" of a meal, but just for heating or preparing "ready-made" foods. So by introducing this small add-on system to a microwave, we could significantly increase the possibility of enabling people with disabilities to independently prepare foods, but at the same time give to everyone a more convenient way to interact with a microwave.

As previously noted, although the focus group in this case was a small group of people with a range of intellectual and physical disabilities, this solution should not be limited only to this cohort. Clearly this type of solution can be applicable to a range of possible user groups. This system could also allow users with other abilities (like ageing people and children) to prepare a safe heated product and finally to save time by reducing the number of actions and the cognitive load that is required to cook/heat a meal in the best way.

Data shows that in 2002 in US, the health related expenditures was more than $61B [25] and the health and caregiver system will be increasingly stressed as those numbers increase. Chronic diseases like Dementia, Alzheimer's and a variety of physical impairments can make ADL very difficult.

For some older citizens, even the simplest of tasks such as cooking a microwaveable meal can become overwhelming due to the complex cooking instructions written in small print on the cooking package and the need for memory and coordination in interacting with the microwave oven [26]. So there is a substantial and growing need to design new interactive systems, based on known actions and known human behaviour, in order to keep people as independent as possible in their environment. This will also affect the process of care provision and the community welfare structure, which will take advantage of these solutions, by reducing the costs and effort associated with private assistance [27]. This research seeks to define a solution related to a particular problem within a community care context and give a suggestion to apply the idea in parallel contexts. Assisted homes and retirement homes users, could help in a further develop of the capable microwave that could become a Universally Designed and functional smart appliance for everyone's house.

This prototype could become an important and useful case study that should be further investigated and integrated in a range of new cooking appliances, by worldwide home appliance producers.

New microwaves, like the Samsung model that was previously mentioned, with additional sensors, will add potential to have smarter community supported cooking appliances with improved safeguards such as warnings to end-users about food temperature. This smart development, apart from the community-support aspect (which is not so developed in the automotive sector) is nevertheless quite similar to the evolution that has already occurred in cars, with new sensors and smart systems.

References

1. Howe MJA (1998) Principles of abilities and human learning. Psychology Press, East Sussex
2. Wiener JM, Raymond JH, Clarck R, Van Nostrand JF (1990) Measuring the activities of daily living: comparisons across national surveys. US Department of Health and Human Services. J Gerontol Social Sci 45(6):S229–S237
3. Fillenbaum GG (1987) Activities of daily living. In: Maddox GL (ed) The Encyclopedia of Aging. Springer, New York
4. Taylor K (2015) Connected health. How digital technology is transforming health and social care. The Creative Studio at Deloitte, London
5. D'Ulizia A, Ferri F, Grifoni P, Guzzo T (2010) Smart homes to support elderly people: innovative technologies and social impacts. In: Pervasive and smart technologies for healthcare: ubiquitous methodologies and tools, 1st edn. Medical Information Science Reference, Hershey
6. Pew RW, Van Hemel SB (2004) Technology for adaptive aging. Steering Committee for the workshop on technology for adaptive aging, National Research Council of The National Academies, p 247
7. Yoji A (1994) Development history of quality function deployment. The customer driven approach to quality planning and deployment. Minato, Tokyo 107 Japan: Asian Productivity Organization
8. Norman D (1988) The design of everyday things. Doubleday, New York
9. King N (2003) Smart home—a definition. Housing LIN Intro Factsheet
10. Chernbumroong S, Atkins SA, Yu H (2010) Perception of smart home technologies to assist elderly people. In: Proceedings of the 4th international conference on software, knowledge, information management and applications (SKIMA 2010), Paro, Bhutan
11. Source, Cox and Alm, Time well spent: the declining real cost of living in America, in Federal Reserve Bank of Dallas—1997. Annual Report; see Exhibit 8 on page 22, 1997. http://www.dallasfed.org/htm/pubs/pdfs/anreport/arpt97.pdf. Cited 10 Mar 2016
12. Liegey Jr PR (2001) Hedonic quality adjustment methods for microwave ovens in the U.S. CPI. Document from: http://www.bls.gov/cpi/cpimwo. Cited 15 Mar 2016
13. Source: IBM Kitchen Demo. http://www.ngi.ibm.com/demos/kitchen.html. Cited 18 Feb 2016
14. Source: SIEMENS Synco living Website: http://www.siemens.com/about/sustainability/en/environmental-portfolio/products-solutions/building-technology/home-automation.htm. Cited 19 Feb 2016
15. Source: Samsung smart oven http://www.which.co.uk/news/2013/10/which-tries-samsungs-smart-microwave-oven-335016/ Cited 19 Feb 2016
16. Bruner JS (1957) On perceptual readiness. In: Psycologycal review, vol 64, pp 123–152

17. Maguire M, Bevan N (2002)User requirements analysis. A review of supporting methods. In: Proceedings of IFIP 17th World Computer Congress, Montreal, Canada. Kluwer Academic Publishers, Dordrecht, pp 133–148. 25–30 Aug 2002
18. Zeldin AS, Bazzano ATF (2014) Intellectual disability. Paper in Medscape, source: http:// emedicine.medscape.com/article/1180709-overview. Cited 24 Feb 2016
19. Guinta LR, Praizler NC (1993) The QFD book. The team approach to solving problems and satisfying customers through quality function deployment. AMACOM Books
20. Citation from: http://designforall.org/design.php. Cited 12 Mar 2016
21. Chadia A, Maloney-Krichmar D, Preece J (2004) User-centered design. In: Bainbridge W (ed) Encyclopedia of human-computer interaction. Sage Publications, Thousand Oaks, pp 445–456
22. Blomkvist SP (2002) Persona—overview, extract from the paper. The user as a personality. Using Personas as a tool for design. Position paper for the course workshop theoretical perspectives in human-computer interaction. IPLab, KTH, 3 Sept
23. Definition from Collins english dictionary—complete & unabridged 2012 digital edition. William Collins Sons & Co. Ltd. Cited 22 Mar 2016
24. Deterding S, Björk SL, Nacke LE, Dixon D, Lawley E (2013) Designing gamification: creating gameful and playful experiences. Paper in CHI'13 extended abstracts on human factors in computing systems. ACM Publisher, pp 3263–3266
25. Koppel R (2002) Alzheimer disease: the cost to U.S Business in 2002. Source: http://www. alz.org/Media/newsreleases/2002/062602ADCosts.pdf. Cited 12 Mar 2016
26. Russo J, Sukojo A, Helal S, Davenport R, Mann W (2004) SmartWave intelligent meal preparation system to help older people live independently. In: Proceedings of the second international conference on smart homes and health telematic (ICOST 2004), Singapore, Sept 2004
27. Zallio M (2013) Home automation and technology: renewal of existing buildings. In: Spadolini MB (2013) Design for better life. Longevità, scenari e strategie, Franco Angeli, Milano, pp 102–110

Work of the Home and Social Relationships as a Guide to Domestic Care for the Elderly

Giulia Frezza, Helen Keefe and Marta Bertolaso

Abstract New technologies might only partially solve the problem of elderly loneliness and social isolation. Ongoing studies analysed by means of a shared perspective promoted by London's Home Renaissance Foundation (HRF) and Rome's Bio-Techno-Practice (BTP) offer a theoretical perspective on this issue that could generate effective guidelines for technology design in this area. The stated goal of the present Italian Forum for Ambient Assisted Living (ForItAAL 2016) refers to "an innovative and integrated approach to address the socio-economic challenges of an aging population, and thus ensure the best fruition of products and services". The vision of HRF is to promote interdisciplinary studies on the home and domestic work, in an effort to create healthy and congenial home environments. Several of these studies address the problem of loneliness and social isolation among aging populations. This research offers a better understanding of the loneliness problem itself as well as more awareness of what thriving homes can offer by way of long-term technological and social solutions for a growing demographic phenomenon. Bio-Techno-Practice (BTP) is a research empowering hub, relying on a renewed philosophy of science recognizing that many constitutive dimensions of the human understanding are simultaneously involved in scientific practice and, conversely, that human practice shapes the direction of scientific investigation (www.biotechnopractice.org/wordpress).

G. Frezza (✉)
Unit of the History of Medicine, Sapienza-University of Rome,
Viale dell'Università 34/a, Rome, Italy
e-mail: giulia.frezza@uniroma1.it

H. Keefe
Home Renaissance Foundation, London, UK
e-mail: hkeefe21@gmail.com

M. Bertolaso
Institute of Philosophy of Scientific and Technological Practice, Faculty of Engineering,
University Campus Bio-Medico of Rome, Via Alvaro del Portillo 21, Rome, Italy
e-mail: m.bertolaso@unicampus.it

© Springer International Publishing AG 2017   79
F. Cavallo et al. (eds.), *Ambient Assisted Living*, Lecture Notes
in Electrical Engineering 426, DOI 10.1007/978-3-319-54283-6_6

Keywords Elderly home care · Ageing health · Social health · Social responsibility · Care · Home environment

1 A Home that Changes Along with a Changing Body

> *Individuals grow and develop at home, so it is in society's best interest to look after it*
> (http://www.homerenaissancefoundation.org/homeorg/about.html).

An essential aspect of the BTP philosophy is the idea of "a home that changes along with a changing body". "The body" in this vision is our first home and it keeps changing throughout life since the very beginning of embryonic development. From that point on, from a biological standpoint the organism can never be described as a perfect equilibrium between cells, tissues, organs, and all the interactions inside and outside the environment, which are also changing.

Our homes (internal and external) are always transforming. Understanding our "changing homes" means to integrate both the idea of the whole mind-body as an interior home as well as the concept of our exterior homes. As a matter of fact, part of the home, or the environment, is definitely made by us and by all other individuals that constantly cooperate to build it up (at the symbiotic, trophic, ecological, cultural and social levels). In other words: we are what we eat but in the meanwhile what we eat is the same environment that we have built, in a continuous feedback loop.

Human beings have been creating home environments since the beginning of time, as part of their culture and history. Houses have been, in this sense, part of human beings' roots, places in which personal biographies are recorded in different ways (pictures, traditions, etc.). Understanding what a home is allows us to identify the right categories, to understand human genuine relations and activities, and their relevance in and for society [1]. In this way, we shift the focus from a thing, i.e. a physical home, to a concrete process, i.e. a natural dynamic relationship. It is *natural* in the sense that it has always characterized human culture and society; *dynamic* because it entails an on-going activity; *relationship* because it implies a constitutive relation among different "players", between a person and his/her environment (i.e. a community). Along these lines *caring* is a typical aspect of a human natural dynamic relationship.

Although it may sound trivial, the human being aspires to autonomy but he/she is naturally dependent and vulnerable. To understand the process of caring, the question, therefore, is clearly about how we can combine these two aspects, i.e. the human tendency to be autonomous with our inherent vulnerability. Avoiding sceptic views about human life and its nature, we can assume that the contradiction is only apparent and that autonomy and vulnerability do not refer to the same feature of human life and behaviour or, at least, not in the same sense. Eventually, this tension for instance has been used by the philosopher Alfredo Marcos to reflect upon the concept of *mutual dependence*, saying that (i) we have to place our autonomy at the service of those who are most dependent; (ii) the form that such service takes is that of caring; and that (iii) as a specification of the latter point, caring means remaining vigilant for someone [1].

2   The Problem of Social Isolation in Elderly Populations

Demographic change—is one of the great challenges of the 21st century, as well as an opportunity. Much depends on how we are going to address it. Europe is the fastest ageing society, the median age is already the highest in the world and the over sixty-five population is supposed to double by 2050 gaining more than 27% of the total population [2]. Consequently cross-cutting concerns emerge, and the need and opportunity to act now.

Moreover, aging in its complexity is revealed as an integral part of an urgency of new accounts of scientific practice in general: new ways of doing science are rapidly emerging, bringing together life sciences and technology, as well as other natural, human and social sciences.

Inherent to our BTP vision lies the idea of identifying a sequence of crucial philosophical issues and questions that are emerging from science, and that inextricably connect Bio, Techno and Practice, emphasizing their reciprocal differences and interdependencies. Interdisciplinary, suitable tools, conceptual as well as technological are needed for developing an overall concept of aging understanding its complexity, and its multifold background (http://www.biotechnopractice.org/wordpress/).

Our paper, integrating the cores of BTP and HRF visions on the topic of home and caring, wishes to highlight that developing better social care technology for the elderly cannot conceal a thorough debate on the more general issue about relational and social problems of aging as a general, multifaceted and interdisciplinary process.

The Home Renaissance Foundation (HRF) promotes research focusing on creating a home which meets the fundamental needs of individual and family and its crucial role in building a more humane society. Moreover, emphasis is given to the recognition of the kinds of work that go into creating healthy and congenial home environments. For HRF, domestic work is not merely a collection of services such as laundry, cleaning, and cooking. It is a values system in which science, art, psychology, culture, skills and an aptitude for management all play a part.

HRF points out the need to understand the *relational* nature of the home and, in such context, the potentialities and risks of home care technologies for the elderly. This reflection, substantiated by best practices that are being gathered by the Foundation, leads towards the emerging direction of *social* care technologies. From this exploratory point of view, HRF organized the international conference series "Excellence in the Home". Several experiences about social care technologies were presented.

Studies collected in the conference's Working Papers have underlined the relevance of social isolation and of a "steady degradation" in companionship care, described as "a fairly neglected element in gerontology, certainly within the area of home care and healthcare technologies for the home" [3]. Works conducted by Intel's Health Research and Innovation Group (HRIG) aimed at exploring the role of technology in helping the elderly remain in their home as long as possible [3]. The approach is based on one fundamental key concept. This developed from overturning the typical engineering approach: first developing technology and then finding uses for the tools produced. Intel's HRIG focus, on the contrary, is based on understanding people's needs and practices before even thinking about developing the technologies. For this reason a team of clinicians and psychologists was enrolled. A group made up of 625 older people were attended to in the designated clinic. At the same time, teams of anthropologists and sociologists interviewed older people and passed time with them (in some cases for days; in other cases, even years).

The result is a direct vision of "what may happen at 3 o'clock in the morning or during the lulls in the day when a person's energy levels are not particularly high" [3]. Between 2006 and 2008 the same team launched an anthropological study on the "Experience of aging" in seven European countries reporting similar results where isolation of older people is shockingly confirmed [3].

Data of "Help the Aged" (now AgeUK: http://www.ageuk.org.uk/) reports that [3]:

- Half of people aged 75 and over in Britain live alone;
- 12% of older people report feeling trapped in their own homes;
- 3% of older people never go out;
- Almost 5 million people consider the TV as their main form of company;
- Over a million UK pensioners ate Christmas dinner alone.

3   Technology and Human Technologies for Elderly Care

The "de Jong Gierveld loneliness scale" [4] for emotional and social loneliness tested on data from 7 countries in the UN generations and gender offers a method for measuring loneliness, which helps better understand the problem.

The scale, developed for older people specifically, divided loneliness into two main constructs:

- *Social loneliness*, which is really about loss of social network or not having a social network;
- *Emotional loneliness* which is that lack of an emotional attachment normally due to loss of a significant other.

If people classify as both socially and emotionally lonely on the de Jong scale they tend to be in the highest risk categories with regards to health.

By means of the de Jong Gierveld loneliness scale, David Prendergast, a social anthropologist leader of the Intel's HRIG project, pointed out a new challenge in home care technologies: how should a well-designed information communication technology help reduce risks of loneliness and social isolation [3]. Indeed technological development should be built from an integrated, wider perspective. As a matter of fact, if one deals with people not even used to computers, the risk of creating a redundant technology increases. Technology dedicated to elderly should be intuitive for them as specific individuals with peculiar idiosyncrasies and limits.

3.1 TRIL Building Bridges (BB) System

A specific communication technology, dedicated to people with little or no experience with computers, could then be developed within the TRIL Building Bridges (BB) system. The project, co-developed with over 150 older people in Ireland following the specific bottom-up approach described above. The BB technological system offers the following [3]:

- Helps people who are isolated have more contact with others;
- Consists of an admin console which is hosted on a server and which deals with all broadcasts and communications between Building Bridges Devices;
- Stores research data from devices and uses Voice over IP technology;
- The in-home device used by the older person is a touch screen computer with speakers and handset.

In this way, the user could contact more people for an on-line chat (up to six people), for messaging (sending greetings and personal messages), for broadcasting (radio and video programs, news, documentaries, music). During the broadcast the user can see who else is listening: an automatic 20 min conference call can be launched when the program is over if they want to join a discussion, or have a phone call with the group. These devices are intended as a "Tea Room" (up to 20 people can enter the tea room any time and chat together), and as a "Window on the World" (they are linked to web cameras in outdoors locations). Moreover, friends and family can be easily added in the BB software connections, sending documents (photos, messages and so on):

- BB is a system that is well suited to the elder who may not be familiar with computers, and who will benefit from increased social engagement;
- BB is a device that helps build bridges between older people, their family and friends, their health and social systems and their communities.

The trials on the system showed an increasing perception of social inclusion revealing a positive metric of success.

3.2 An Option Often Overlooked and Underrated: Inter-generational Living

Other studies, starting from the same concept of the isolation of older people, develop other solutions [5]. As stated by Bryan Sanderson CBE, Chairman of HRF: "Britain has an epidemic of loneliness. Intergenerational living can help ameliorate this for the old and for the young too" [5].

Intergenerational living is indeed a peculiar solution which is not properly technological, but that becomes a technological response when looked from the Bio-Techno-Practice integrated perspective mentioned above.

Cultures look at intergenerational living in different ways. For instance in Japan, up to 65% of older people live in the same home as their children as compared to the rate in the UK of only 16% [5]. Meanwhile in the Netherlands, specific programs allowed students to live rent-free in care homes in exchange for offering companionship to older inhabitants [5, 6].

Studies underline how multigenerational living shows potential in targeting future puzzling care solutions in the UK [5, 7]. In 2013 HRF identified a need for policy research aiming both at describing the challenges of multigenerational households and at outlining how the existing policy infrastructure endorse them [5, 7]. The research showed that intergenerational living is not merely a thing of the past:

- It plays a role in informal care for elderly and for children (47% of interviewed), rather than in supplementing formal care provision (33% of the interviewed);
- Financial incentives can be a strong motivating factor for intergenerational living solutions.

Among other relevant models, intergenerational living represents a non-technical solution, but a solution that takes economics and policy into account. Moreover, one of its potential benefits may be to provide increased dynamism to existing design concepts for the housing stock.

Interviews with intergenerational co-resident families concluded that: "It is imperative that the home environment functionally support the way families interact in response to social changes of an aging parent moving in with an adult child while similarly accommodating the privacy of individual family members" [5]. Along these lines, the courtyard house model common in Scandinavia, China and South America is often considered a model of international best practice design. This intergenerational model can be of help even when rethinking from scratch the issue of technological care for elderly focusing on a human as well as on a technological perspective.

4 Conclusions—Rediscovering the Home

Going back to our initial core metaphor of "a home that changes along with a changing body", we may stress that every home is different also at different times and in the multifarious contexts of life, including the silver time. In light of the physiological process of "changing home" ageing becomes a life span perspective. Moreover, it is a multidimensional process (biological, cognitive and emotional), as well as contextual (individual, gender as well as socio-economical differences may greatly affect the ageing process) (see http://www.cdc.gov/niosh/topics/productiveaging/).

Along these lines, the World Health Organization defines healthy ageing as "the process of developing and maintaining the functional ability that enables well-being in older age" (http://www.who.int/social_determinants/sdh_definition/en). We think that "well-being" is defined according to subjective as well as objective categories which need to be distinctly evaluated and then integrated in one coherent description.

Disruption of an individual's functional abilities occurring with ageing relies mostly on supportive and high-responsive environments. Among the principal factors of a supportive environment there are transportation, social participation and social inclusion, security, education, communication and information, as stressed by priority area 4 of "Health 2020" (the 8th European framework) "Creating supportive environments and resilient communities".

The examples that we described (3.1 and 3.2) are social care technologies as well as peculiar "human-technologies" for dealing with elderly issues. Both solutions are innovative, interesting and built according to the needs of the elderly, and should be implemented according to individuals' and communities idiosyncrasies and standards.

According to our standpoint, intergenerational living is particularly interesting as a kind of solution; considering, for instance, that many might not have access to the Building Bridges technology mentioned earlier. Moreover, it's a long-term solution, because it involves raising awareness about the benefits of (as well as advice about) inter-generational living.

On this basis, a new social care technology for the elderly may be developed, as our ongoing research will try to promote, which especially addresses ageing isolation: allowing "silver people" to remain active, autonomous and fully integrated as well as targeting specific disease prevention strategies (vaccination, injury, mental disruption).

With these insights, we hope to provide some guidelines to assist the development of better social care technologies for the elderly, taking into account the *relational* nature of the home and the lesser known benefits of its promotion.

Acknowledgements The authors wishes to thank Fondazione Alberto Sordi and Home Renaissance Foundation for supporting the project presented in this paper, and making possible its dissemination and discussion at an international level.

References

1. Marcos A, Bertolaso M (2016) What is a home? An ontological and epistemological enquiry. In: Aguirre S, Lastra R, Zamagni S, Argandona A (eds) The home: a complex field. STI & HRF, London
2. WHO-Europe, Regional Committee for Europe 62nd session, Malta 10–13 Sept 2012, Strategy and action plan for healthy ageing in Europe 2012–2020
3. Prendergast D (2011) Home alone: ageing, technology and social isolation. Home Renaissance Foundation Working Papers Number 21, Mar 2011
4. De Jong Gierveld J, van Tilburg T (2010) The De Jong Gierveld short scales for emotional and social loneliness: tested on data from 7 countries in the UN generations and gender surveys. Eur J Ageing 7(2):121–130 (2010)
5. Simpson S (2015) Bricks, mortar and policy perspective for intergenerational living. Report for Housing Learning & Improvement Network, Viewpoint 74, Aug 2015
6. Butts D, Thang LL, Hatton Yeo A (2012) Policies and programmes supporting intergenerational relations. Background paper. UNDESA, New York
7. Simpson S, Callan S (2015) Bricks and mortar across generations: a think piece on intergenerational living in the United Kingdom. Home Renaissance Foundation, London, Mar 2015. http://www.homerenaissancefoundation.org/docs/thinkpiece.pdf

The Design Contribution for Ambient Assisted Living

G. Losco, A. Lupacchini, L. Bradini and D. Paciotti

Abstract The Design role for the assisted living ambient come from the several declinations that design offers into similar branches of knowledge. The centrality of the user is the starting point to the innovation of some design sectors and his physical, psychological, social conditions too. In this context, the research proposed several developments

- The ambient assisted living setting systematization defining its design characters.
- The definition of different levels of intervention according to the components role that make up the main supports of AAL.
- The collection of some case studies proposing solutions in keeping with defined systemic grid.

Keywords Smart glove · Smart object · Interaction design · UCD

1 From Design for All to Design for AAL

The vision of the user as being with an inevitable mental and physical decline that turns him into a social problem, is definitely an obsolete vision and never was true. The properly integrated individual keeps his active social, psychological, and economic contribution at every stage of his live according to the most advanced social realities.

Even in semantic terms the description of separate physical capacity of individuals, not only by age conditions, it is strongly released from the weight of words such as "disabled", "handicapped" "elder" etc.etc.

G. Losco (✉) · A. Lupacchini · L. Bradini · D. Paciotti
Scuola Superiore Sant'Anna, Pontedera, Italy
e-mail: giuseppe.losco@unicam.it

© Springer International Publishing AG 2017   87
F. Cavallo et al. (eds.), *Ambient Assisted Living*, Lecture Notes
in Electrical Engineering 426, DOI 10.1007/978-3-319-54283-6_7

The holistic and inclusive vision of the Design For All has further helped to define the scenarios where space, objects and services are configured as a function of a substantial enlargement of fruition overcoming the issue of skill diversity. The space or the objects are able to be accessible to everybody for their intrinsic and extrinsic characteristics.

This is the purpose that design tries always to reach.

The scenary of Design for AAL overcome the point of view of Design for All because it create a possibility of an Inclusive design including home comfort for unusual conditions of life. The space seems often "heartless" against the user because is just oriented to functional solutions of serious problems.

2   Generating Principles

According to this background, the group of Camerino University, School of Architecture and Design "E.Vittoria" has developed, from long time, several researches in a context where it is proposed a methodology of approach based on some generating principles:

- The definition of the user and his needed not just functional related to its physical, psychological and social conditions but also as a stimulus to a better confort expectation.
- The potentialities of technological innovation, especially digital innovation, to develop innovative solutions for products, components and services to help individuals with disabilities.
- Design as an element of stimulus and final synthesis of a project, able to release the user from a psychological condition of frustration in the use of components, space and objects.

3   The Specific Contributions: Product Design Skills

Three levels of intervention have been identified in this specific context, where the design project can become an original contribution and scientific implementation for industry expertise.

3.1   User Centred Design (UCD) and Interaction Design (ID)

The UCD offers a thorough study of the physical or virtual dialogue systems and use of various products and systems for users with different levels of abilities, through an experimental approach that involves the user in a crucial way, right from the early concept and planning phases of the product.

The inclusion of users in the project (creation of the prototype and use analysis protocol) is strategic and essential especially for users who have a specific medical case, especially when addressed to predict highly customised solutions.

Ill. n° 1, 2, Project by Jessica Pesaresi–audio translator

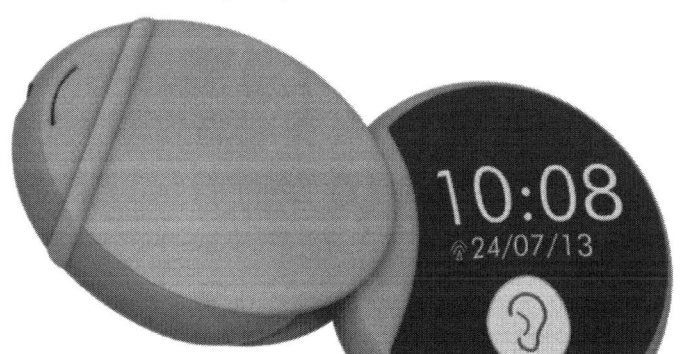

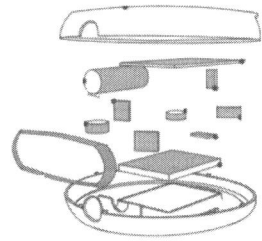

abacus of components

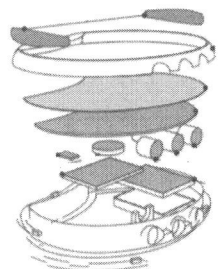

3.1.1 Interaction Design

Addresses the study of interfaces (physical and virtual) in a systematic way with the essential aim of making the product as easy as possible to use in relation to the specific characteristics of users and their pathologies.

The primary objective of ID is to study systems for linking man and product and to optimise the operating procedures, facilitating them (User Friendly) by developing products with features that make them easy to use (Affordance).

Ill. n°3, Project by R. Albertazzi–translator for dumb and blind

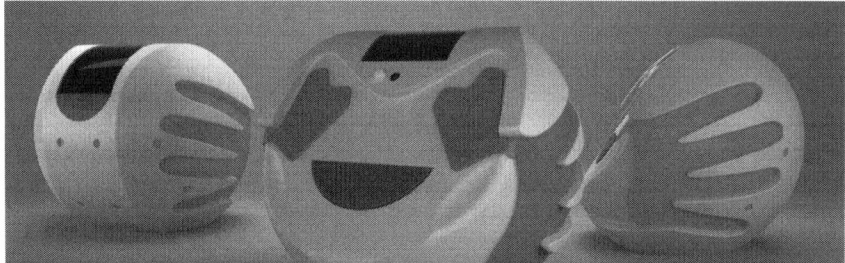

3.2 Technological Implementation Design: Smart Design

Product design acts as a synthesis of technological innovation, particularly informatics and digital, with specific contribution of ICT disciplines, and the potential applied to the concrete project of service and function.

The technology transfer that puts the design in a strategic position is one that defines technological systems that lack the synthetic support of the elements that make it compatible, mainly in anthropic terms, in a context of physical formulas.

An 'intelligent' product (smart object) is the synthesis of this synergistic activity of synthesis, where design is able to create a product that is functional, technological and ergonomic, all thanks to its expertise.

The ongoing dematerialisation of product functions in favour of the massive use of digital technology, requires critical analysis and the proposal of concrete solutions of a formal nature of physical systems capable of materialising the 'smart containers', as well as to propose solutions more closely linked to the needs of a user who has by nature and age, limited inclination to use technological equipment.

3.3 Morphology and Design: The Role of Shape

Seemingly redundant, this term refers to strategically fundamental data that the design can define—the ability to structure a scenario made of new products, in which its expressiveness and inherent communication free the product from the emotional 'medical' and 'rescue' roles and from the frustrating obligation to the use. This would work towards a formal value that best aligns to a normal aspect where form and function do not appear unbalanced but linked to rational necessity.

Several studies show that the emotional approach of the user in difficult physical and movement conditions is extremely critical towards products where the expressive message of the form is medical implant aids, as well as this difficulty being expressed in concrete terms in the refusal of the user to use such aids.

- The design has a very wide intervention margin, in order to define a formal 'normalisation' product that also makes it inclusive as an emotional element.

  The specific areas that make up that margin of intervention are:
  The colour system

- The formal redefinition alluding to the reference products that mitigate the negative impact of the end-user
- The integration of the parties to transform the object in morphological terms from the 'discreet' system to a 'continuous' system
- The interface and the facilitation of the mode of use (see previous section)
- Sensory levers to the reconsideration of materials
- The practical implementation also aimed at encouraging the subject to use and user accept the product, emphasising recreation, leisure and communication.

Ill. n°4 Project by A. Garaguso–sensor for the blind

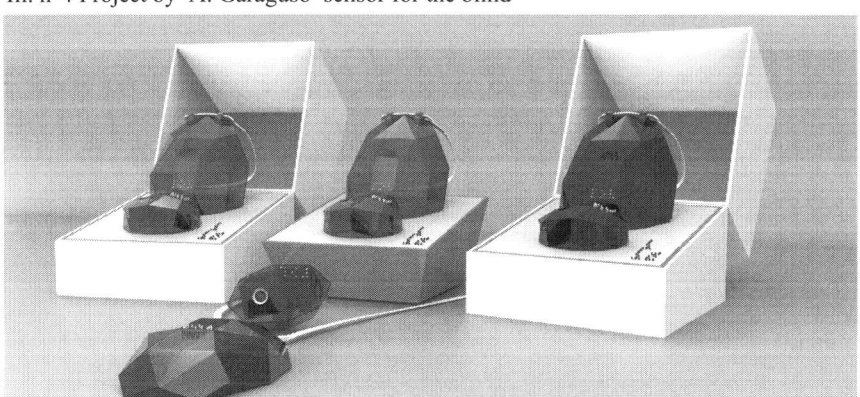

In conclusion, the specific competences of the discipline develop an innovative product that puts the user at the centre of the system, enabling them to determine the choices summarised at a formal level, answering the issues of function, use, ergonomics and formality.

These areas constitute the different declination of the specific design in the field of AAL, considering that in this context more than others, the user is characterised by the specific conditions where the necessity of an accurate study of the product cannot be separated from their areas of design.

4 Specific Contributions: The ALL Intervention Levels

The project is a continuation of previous expertise, defines a system of specific intervention levels for ambient assisted living, always according to the specific abilities of the product design project.

Such levels of intervention correspond to three defined scenarios:

- Objects and intelligent tools (Smart Object)
- Spaces and intelligent contexts (Smart Space)
- Movement and mobility.

In this context they are defined as the specific research projects (case studies).

4.1 Objects and Smart Aids

In systematic terms we can identify a series of useful objects in AAL that can fulfil specific roles for the end-user.

A substantial feature is, as described in the previous chapter, the chance to give articulated functions to the object, both tangible and intangible, or dedicated to digital functionality.

The object of use in this case is able to interact with the user in an articulated manner, supporting an adequate function in relation to the stresses, and from environmental monitoring.

The smart object by its nature has a technological/digital 'heart' capable of reacting, monitoring and giving appropriate functional responses, communicating not only with the end user directly, but also in context, so that if it is equipped with wi-fi connections, it can communicate with remote networks and the Internet (Internet of Things).

The technological potential of these systems is numerous, the need to give a physical form that involves the user is the main characteristic of the design.

The end user with different abilities, more compromised than the average, but more involved and advantageous from the potential of intelligent products, like the users who collaborated with it as a direct or remote assistance (caregiver) represent the research context of this level of approach.

You can take the smart object to different areas of use for AAL:

- Smart objects
- Smart aids
- Smart Prosthesis.

4.1.1 Intelligent Objects

Indicate objects which perform common domestic duties, so nothing special, but that because of their characteristics can adapt to facilitate use by users with different abilities. In this range we can include: appliances, technological equipment, sanitary items etc.

4.1.2 Intelligent Aids

Are part of more complex elements or independent elements that help the use of a particular space or element substantially, or intervene contributing to the active rehabilitation, or supporting a user with a specific pathology. In this context we can find objects or furniture that have thrust interaction technology and we can include: mechanical closets, rehabilitation beds etc.

Ill. n°5 Project by H.Wenwen–bed with lift

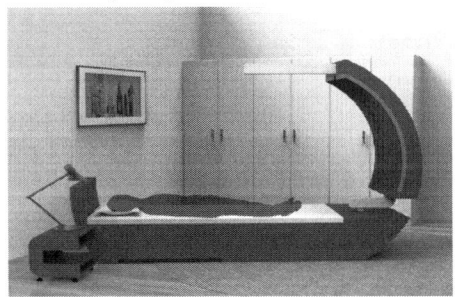

4.1.3 Intelligent Prostheses

Consist of products that directly help the actions of the user with particular pathologies, substituting in a more or less direct way the user's physical function, improving, or reactivating compromised physical functions.

Ill. n°6, 7 Project by G. De Laurentis–tray with robotic arm

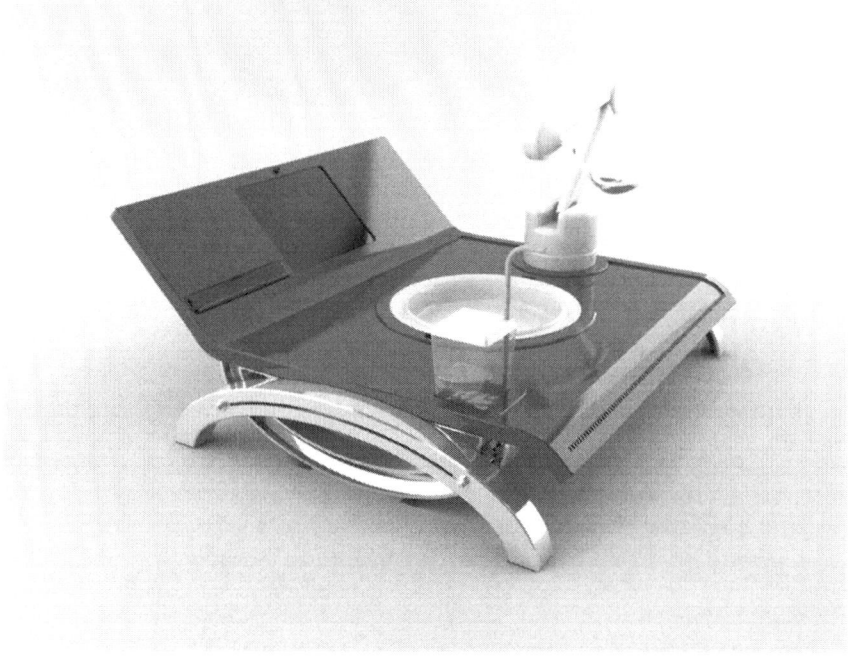

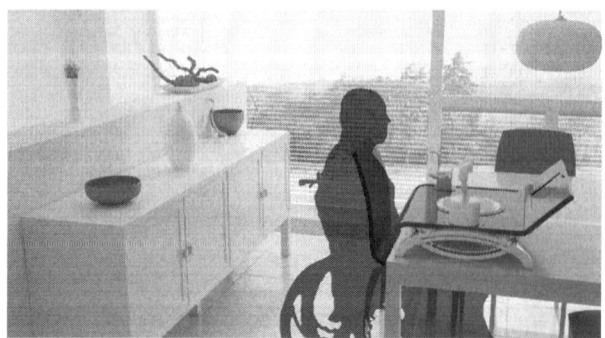

Case Study: Smart Glove

The research project was developed with the development of a prosthesis that helps the rehabilitation of the grip of the upper limbs for those users with specific degenerative pathologies that limit the grip capacity of the limbs.

The specific role of the product proposes, through the exploitation of the fluid-air dynamic characteristics, to replace the mechanical mechanisms with pneumatic mechanisms, decreasing the impact of the mechanisms, as well as the weight and shape.

Ill. n° 8, 9, 10, 11, Project by F. Cotechini–Smart Glove

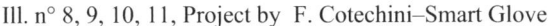

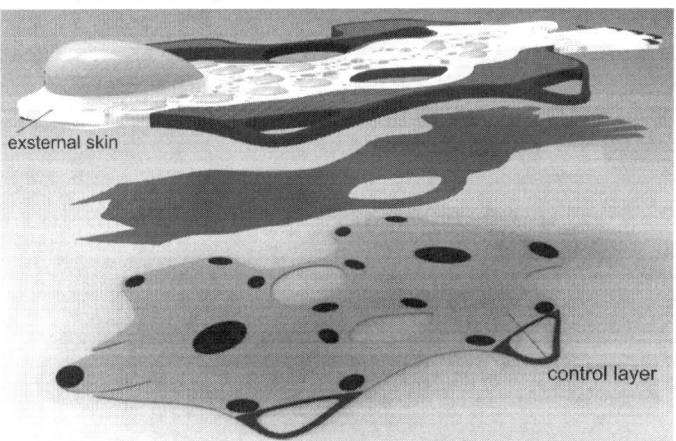

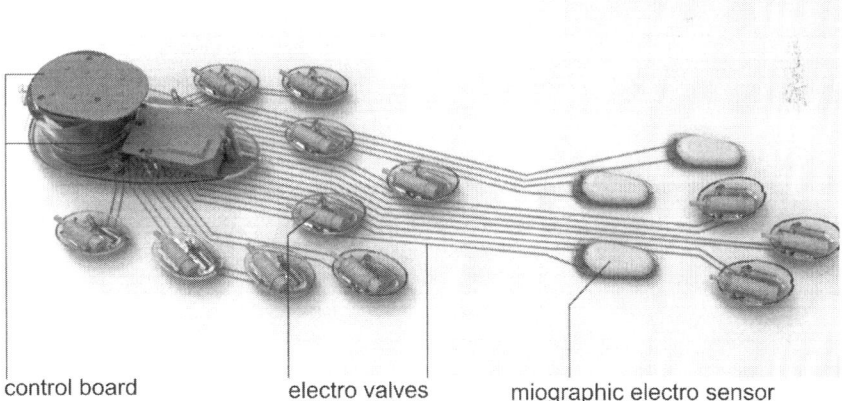

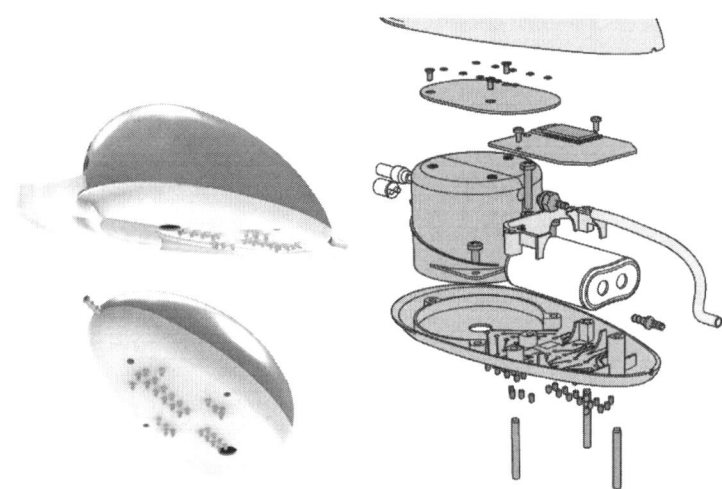

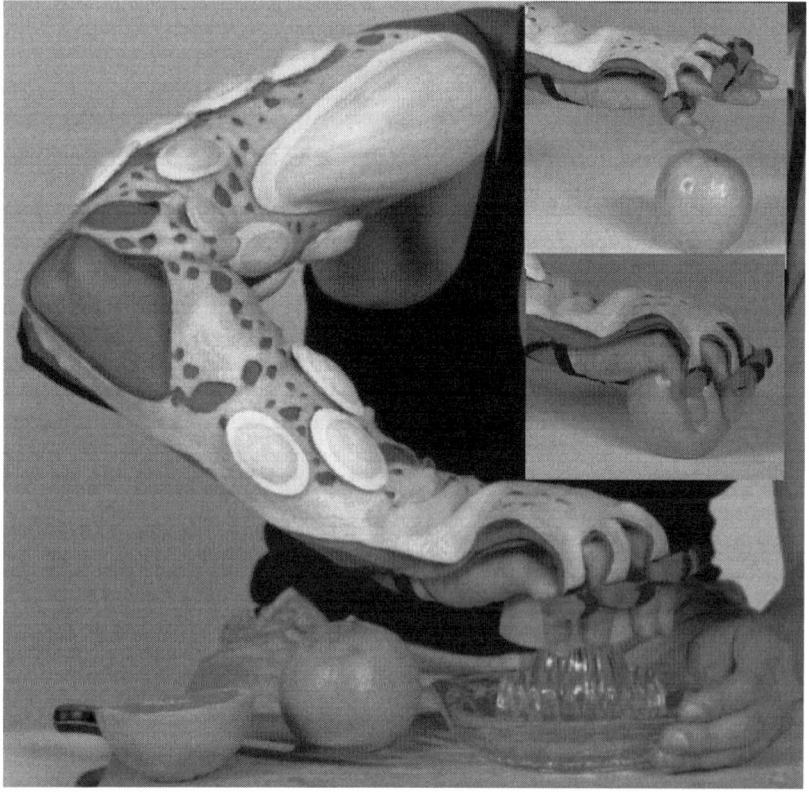

4.2   Residential Spaces and Intelligent Environments

The objects and intelligent assistive devices of which we have just treated, are used within the places of living, whether they are domestic and non-domestic, and with which they must come together in order to provide an integrated environment to measure AAL.

Can be defined in this context two main types of intervention:

- Domestic Context
- Hospital context.

At DOMESTIC level, the research project has suggested the creation of Smart House, through the prefabricated furniture components, modular, multi-functional, technologically implemented, flexible and systematized, acts to rebuild entire domestic areas, or portions of them, up to individual areas functional. These component systems are able to interact with the user and to transform living spaces into dynamic entities, furthering/assist, users, facilitating and optimizing the use of living spaces.

Compared the building envelope, the living space is formed from components capable of performing multiple functions, including that of the delimitation and temporary spatial separation.

Being modular and designed by parametric concepts, the system is able to adapt to any morphological type, to allow an easy integration in domestic environments, whether they are both existing and new buildings. Obviously in the interventions that provide for the possibility of acting building envelope, such as interior work, they can achieve significant results, compared to those of traditional distribution designed layout with fixed scores (partitions).

The "architecture system", must be able to satisfy the needs of a friendly functional spaces, even on very small surfaces, always considering users' issues, well defined in the AAL issues.

These spaces and components can and should adapt to two main requirements:

- Member Fruition independently;
- Member Fruition with direct aid (caregiver) or indirect (remote control systems).

The use can still be considered even with objects and components that have a role REHABILITATION (physical or neurological) or AID AND IMPROVEMENT OF THE USE FOR THE CONDUCT OF ACTIVITIES OF DOMESTIC LIFE.

At HOSPITAL level may be defined the same classifying principles, net of the space characteristics such as environmental units. The hospital setting recognizes several significant moments: the context of care and specific intervention, short-term care, long term care and rehabilitation.

Considering these levels the most functional spaces contiguous with the user (resident) is the admission space (room or ward), services and spaces and rehabilitation components.

Case Study: Housing Unit Minimum 36 Mq

Ill. n° 12, 13, 14, 15 project by S. Angeloni, M. Levitikos

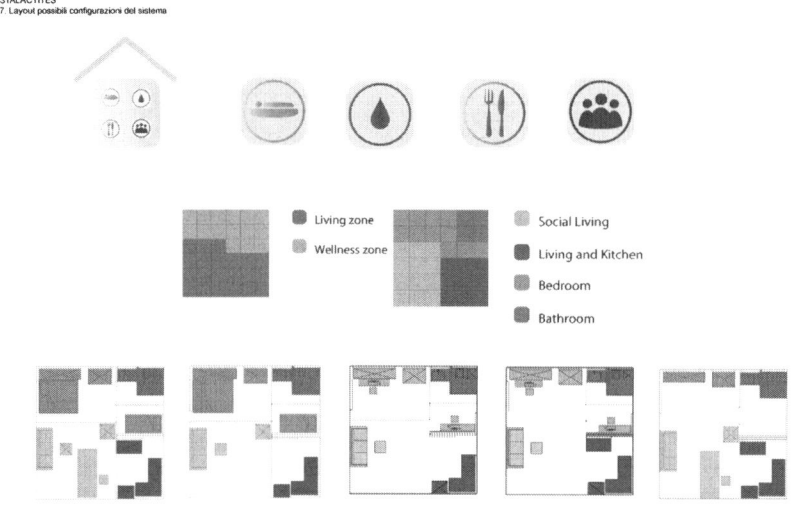

The research project was aimed at the creation of a minimum housing units 6 × 6 × 2.70 m formed by a generic traditional building envelope, inside of which was built a house that can accommodate 2 + 2 persons, to ensure lunch sitting for 8 and living spaces for 8 people seated. Starting from an open-space configuration, the furnishings are distributed to form the functional areas, accompanying over 24 h users. The furniture system is almost all suspended ceiling. This guarantees from a unit area of about 34 m^2 that can take the functional demand connotation (for example we have a living space of 34 m^2, with no architectural barriers, typical of a traditional apartment of 100 m^2, but set in an area total of one third).

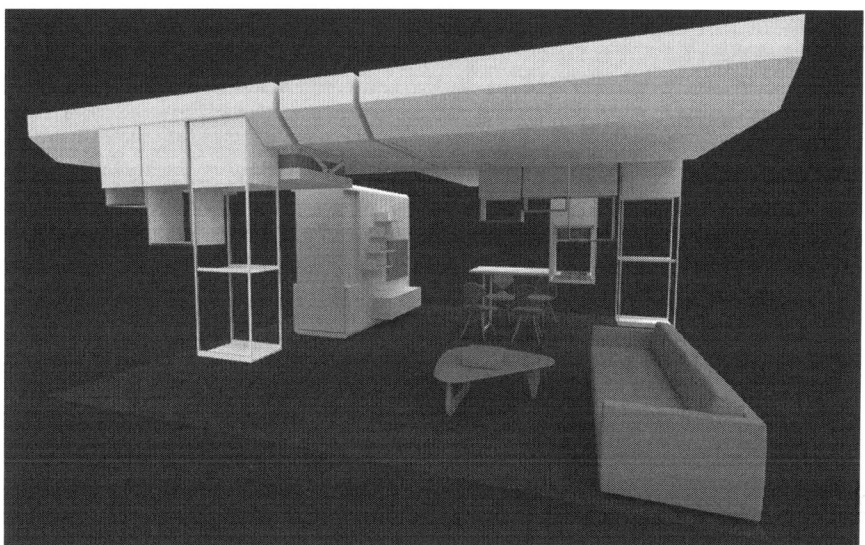

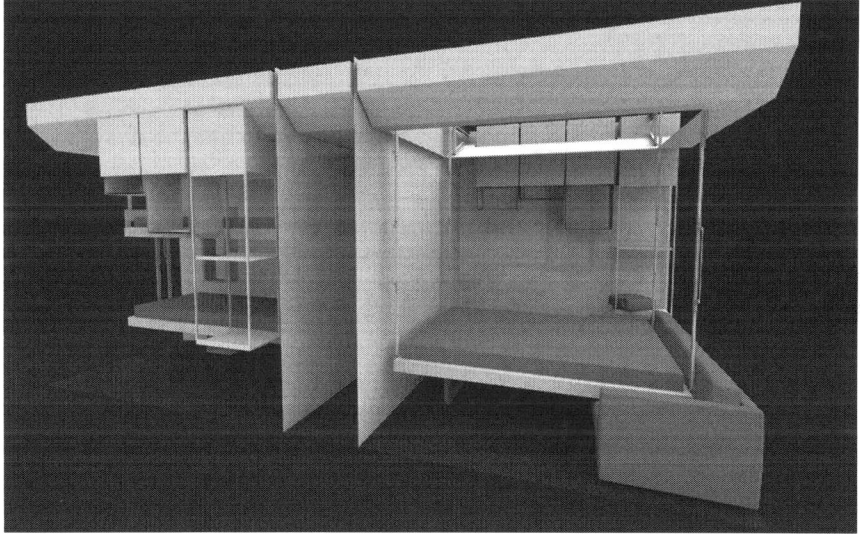

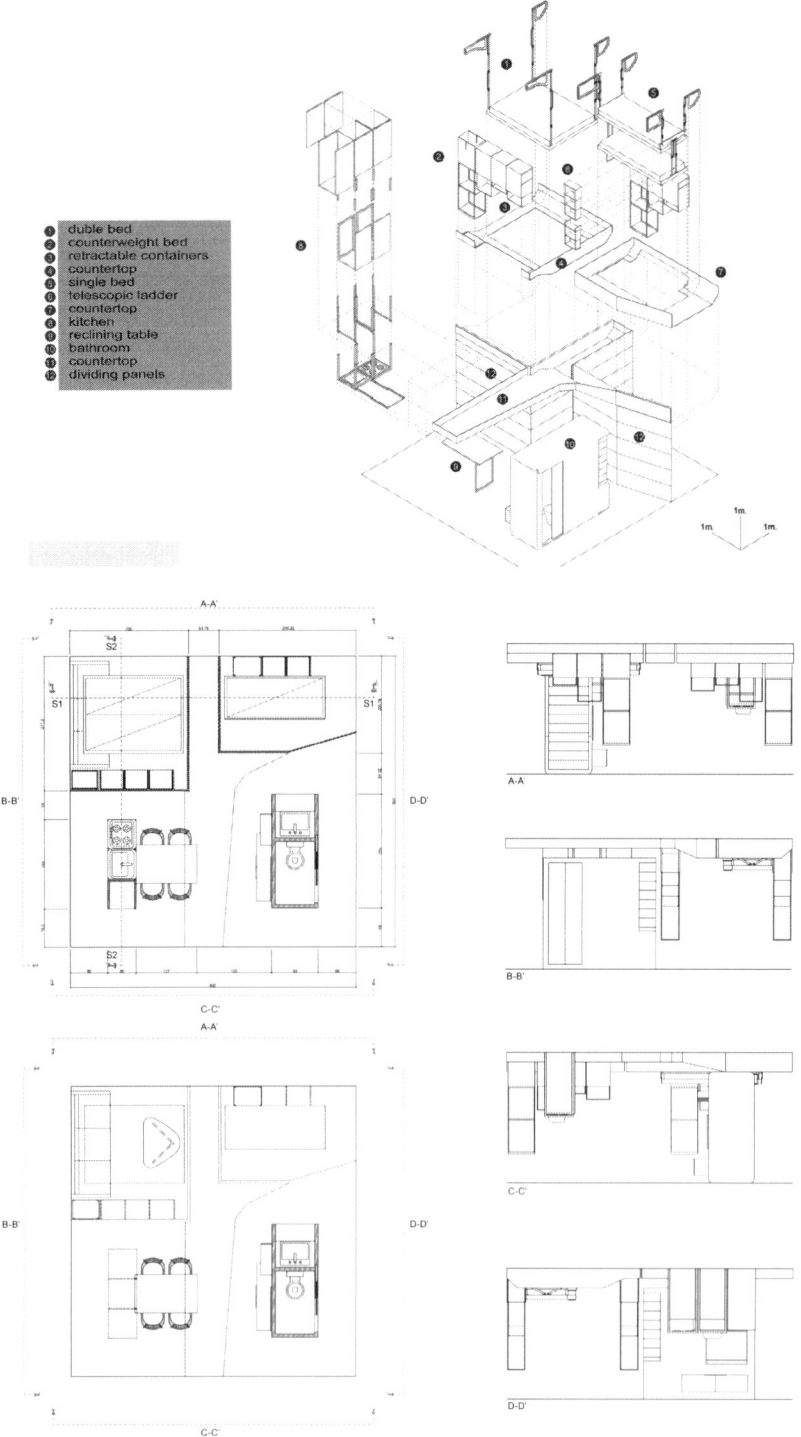

1 duble bed
2 counterweight bed
3 retractable containers
4 countertop
5 single bed
6 telescopic ladder
7 countertop
8 kitchen
9 reclining table
10 bathroom
11 countertop
12 dividing panels

4.3 Movement and Mobility

Mobility is expressed at different levels of complexity, from domestic or personal mobility, to the functional mobility of transport, always taking into account that mobility is one of the first topics of ambient assisted living. This way, different levels of mobility and products can be identified.

4.3.1 Personal Mobility Design (Movement)

This is essentially defined by the domestic space. Mobility can be on-site (if without moving the person) but linked to the mobility of the body in daily activities such as dressing, bathing etc.

In this respect, the design has to deal with the auxiliary product (aid) exploited almost like a real prosthesis able to facilitate some elementary actions.

4.3.2 Domestic and In-Out Mobility Design (Micro-mobility)

This is partially domestic and regards the products and objects needed to move freely within the home, as an aid and as support and security protection, capable of overcoming the users' regular barriers, or supporting the user's safety in an integrated way. Such aids can and must be able to implement the provision of accessibility that does not confine them within the home, and also enables small transfers outside the home. These aids must help the user to overcome even more significant and impactful obstacles and barriers, also allowing movement by using electric engines.

In the mobility aids family two specific categories can be identified:

Integrated Aids

Mobility aids combined with functional expansion technological implementation, for example:

- movement support, lifting with positioning sensors, obstacle detection
- improvement to overcome architectural barriers.

Ill. n° 16, 17 project by D.Paciotti

Integrated Modules Aid

Assistive devices that can be integrated with already existing products that implement functions, for example:

–   wheelchair integration for the use in all weather and digital connections.

Ill. n° 18 project by M.Grelli

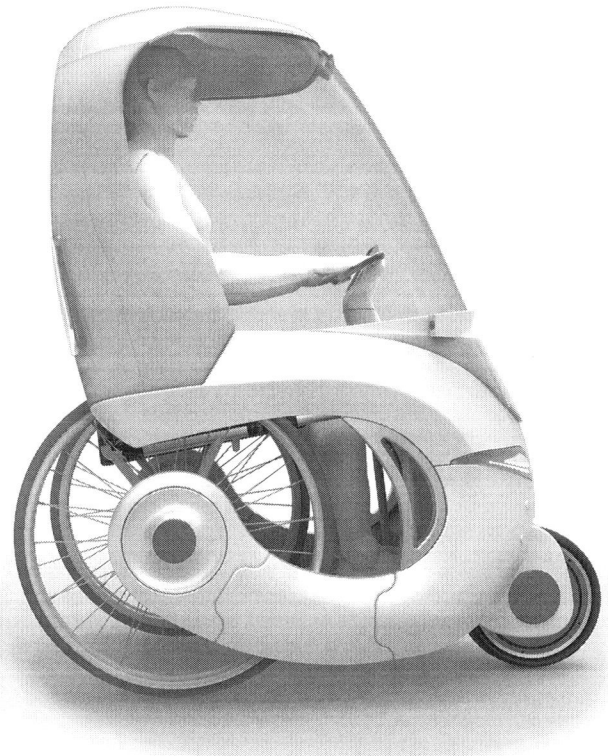

4.3.3 Urban Mobility Design

Short-range urban mobility needs specific requirements for people with pathologies that cause difficulty in movement, the context of current products supports these conditions with the integration of specific systems adaptable to standard cars.

The school's research has developed a mobility product where the primary objective is to propose integrated solutions for the product, from the initial conception of the project, creating an end product that can be used by everyone, including users with greater difficulties.

Specifically, the design project has mainly invested in the ERGONOMICAL and TECHNOLOGICAL fields, developing the following characteristics:

- The concept of a MICROCAR (ELECTRIC QUADRICYCLE) of small dimensions (265 cm in length, same as a Smart For two)
- Increase number of users (3 seats)

- Improving accessibility and internal movement (rotating and shifting seats and opposite double door opening)
- Technological implementation with digital control and monitoring support platform, not only of the vehicle but also the user.

Case Study: Axillary Electric Walker

The product presented was developed by identifying the innovation features in two main functions:

- The underarm support which enables the person to use the upper limbs for other activities.
- The mechanical/electrical change of the user's lifting support from sitting to standing position.

Ill. n° 19, 20 project by A. Garaguso

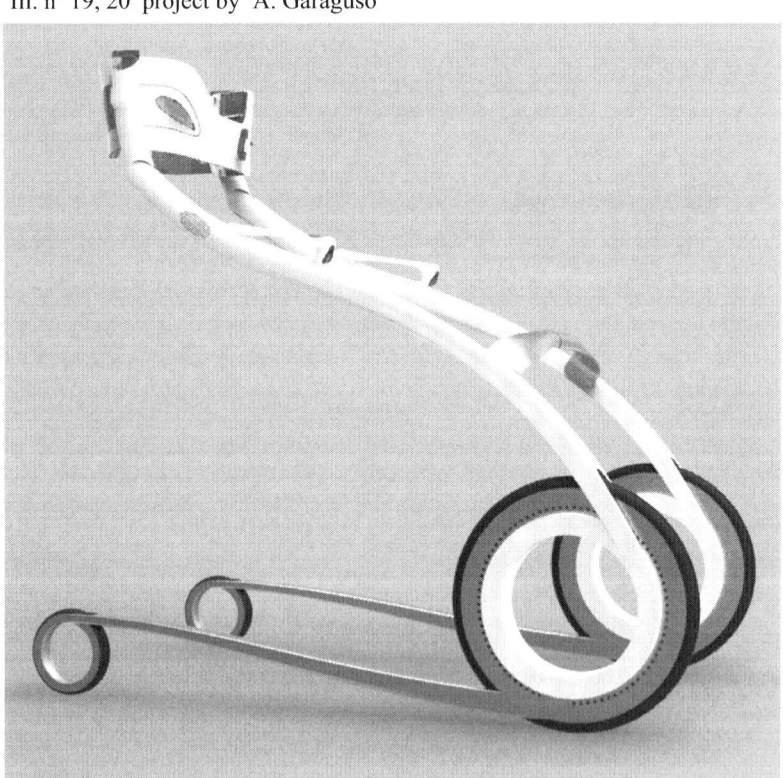

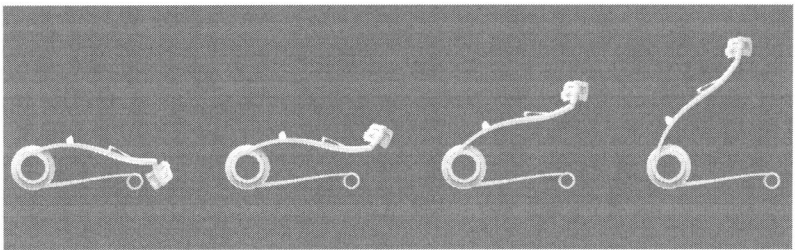

Ill. n° 21, n°22 project by A. Garaguso

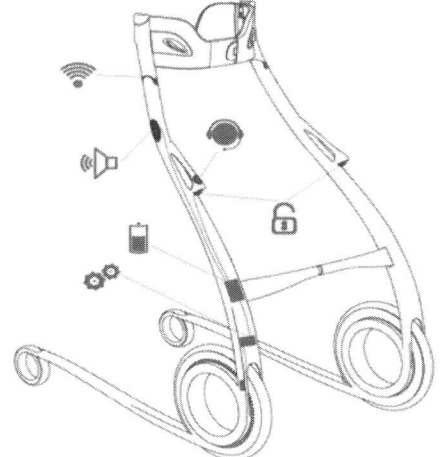

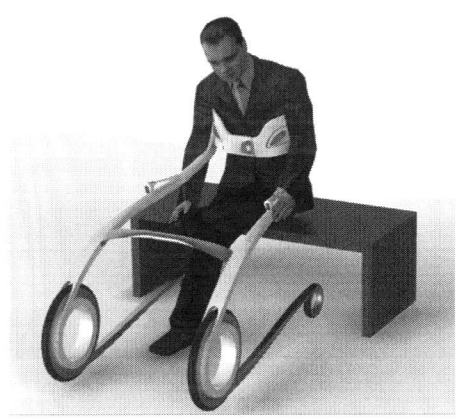

Adaptive Interface for Smart Home: A New Design Approach

Francesca Gullà, Silvia Ceccacci, Roberto Menghi, Lorenzo Cavalieri and Michele Germani

Abstract In an inclusive and accessible smart environments context the implementation of the "design for all" method presents several critical issues. In fact, the universal design represents a difficult challenge for the designer because it depends on the complexity of human intentions in a particular time and place. For this reason, we propose a new approach that aims to support the design of inclusive environments by improving the user-environment interaction.

Keywords Universal design · Adaptable user interfaces

1 Introduction

Research on information technologies has shown in the last twenty years a very fast growth with an increase of attention to the development of solution able to satisfy people with different characteristics and needs. At the present time, one of the main research topics aims at the definition of technologies and tools in accordance to the "design for all" approach. The term Design for All, or Universal Design in Europe [1], is defined as "The design of products and environments to be usable by all people, to the greatest extent possible, without the need for adaptation or specialized design. Hence the extended user concept, which seeks to consider the different characteristics and individual experiences, including the multiplicity of physical, motor, cognitive and contextual, in order to find (as possible) fits-all solutions. Design according to D4ALL means satisfy the seven fundamental principles of

F. Gullà (✉) · S. Ceccacci · R. Menghi · L. Cavalieri · M. Germani
Department of Industrial Engineering and Mathematical Sciences,
Università Politecnica delle Marche, Ancona 6013, Italy
e-mail: f.gulla@pm.univpm.it

S. Ceccacci
e-mail: s.ceccacci@pm.univpm.it

© Springer International Publishing AG 2017
F. Cavallo et al. (eds.), *Ambient Assisted Living*, Lecture Notes
in Electrical Engineering 426, DOI 10.1007/978-3-319-54283-6_8

universal design. These seven principles may be applied to evaluate existing projects, guide the design process and educate both designers and consumers about the characteristics of more user friendly products and environments. These principles are: Equitable Use: The design is useful and marketable to people with diverse abilities; Flexibility in Use: The design accommodates a wide range of individual preferences and abilities; Simple and Intuitive Use: Use of the design is easy to understand, regardless of the user's experience, knowledge, language skills, or current concentration level; Perceptible Information: The design communicates necessary information effectively to the user, regardless of ambient conditions or the user's sensory abilities; Tolerance for Error: The design minimizes hazards and the adverse consequences of accidental or unintended actions; Low Physical Effort: The design can be used efficiently and comfortably with a minimum of fatigue; Size and Space for Approach and Use: Appropriate size and space is provided for approach, reach, manipulation, and use regardless of user's body size, posture, or mobility. In an inclusive and accessible smart environments context the implementation of the "for all" method presents several critical issues. In fact, the universal design represents a difficult challenge for the designer because it depends on the complexity of human intentions in a particular time and place.

A first criticality is represented by the complexity of the users, in terms of physical, cognitive, socio-cultural and attitudinal diversity. The second criticality is represented by the environment complexity; it includes the environment/device typology, context definition and the definition of functional requirements of the environment. Finally, the third criticality, is represented by the complexity of environment interaction.

Therefore, the use of a "design for all" method, today, involves the choice of guidelines that do not effectively support the definition of the design solutions. For this reason, we propose a new approach that aims to support the design of inclusive environments by improving the user-environment interaction. This can be achieved developing an appropriate system that works on three levels: The first level is the technological adaptation that consists of a system custom design into the initial setup which can continuously monitor the user's behavior and mode. The second level are the utilities resulting from the correspondence between the activities performed by the user. This level consists in a study of the proposed service in terms of satisfaction of needs and user's expectations, as well as the technical implementation of specific functions. The last level is the simple and pleasant usability that is based on User-Centered design to create usable products and services.

2 Research Background

Several studies show that exists a certain category of users (i.e. elderly, disabled, user with some limitation) that has a greater number of usability problems than "average" user. However, improving the usability of a program or interface enhances users' efficiency, whether young or old [2]. Requirements and recommendations for human-system interaction have been introduced also by International Organization for Standardization with the ISO 9241-210:2010 [3]. These methods facilitate the design of more effective interfaces better adapted to user's' specifications, but often the outcomes are multiple interfaces for the different types of users. Design for All, as it is called Universal Design in Europe [1], has been introduced in the design of the interfaces as a method by which designers provide their products to be used by the widest possible audience, independently of their age or abilities [4]. It refers to the conscious and systematic work to apply the "Principles of Universal Design" [5] and the related methods and tools [6], in order to develop products and services which are accessible and usable by many people as reasonably possible, avoiding thus the need for later adaptations, or specialized design. Realize successful universal projects is a very big challenge: it means designing products that while having "special functions" result equal or more attractive and usable than common products, so that they are desirable for the average user.

To support the design of products able to accommodate users' variability, the approach known as Ability-based Design has been developed in the context of ICT products [7]. Unlike physical products, computer technology can observe users' performance, model it, and use those models to predict future performance, adapting or making suggestions for adaptations or customization, if automatic adaptation is unwarranted or undesirable [8]. Ability-based design promotes the development of personalized user interfaces that adapt themselves or can be easily adapted by the human user. Langley [9] defines an Adaptable User Interfaces (AdUIs) as "a software artefact that improves its ability to interact with a user by constructing a user model based on partial experience with that user". They are able to alter aspects of their structure or functionality, in order to accommodate different user needs and their changes over time [10]. To achieve this, they have to identify the conditions that necessitate adaptation, and therefore, select and actualize an appropriate course of action. Accordingly, AUIs are able to modify itself at runtime, according to an adaptation state [11].

They can modify all the characteristics, but generally, adaptation is implemented to one of the interface subsystems such as information lay-out (i.e. spatial arrangement, color scheme, image, or text presentation, information content), human-computer dialogue language, and navigation support. According with the nature of adaptation that they provide, adaptive systems are classified into adaptive and adaptable [12]. Adaptable user interfaces are customized directly by the user (i.e. some internet portals in which users can modify the size of characters), while adaptive user interfaces are automatically adapted by the system without direct commands. Adaptive user interfaces are especially interesting for people whose physical or cognitive performance changes over short periods (for instance throughout the day), but however, it should be mentioned that currently there exists only some systems (i.e. health applications) that support this functionality [13].

3 The Design Approach

Designing an adaptive user interface means to define an interactive system able to manage its knowledge about the user (i.e., who is using the system) and the environment (i.e., the context in which the user-system interaction takes place), in order to provide information content, functions, and interaction modalities, in the most adequate way, according to different users and context of use. Therefore, the requirement of a systematic process (flow) which may include alternative decisions making procedures able to accommodate the resulting diversity of individual users, is necessary. To achieve this objective, it is necessary to adopt a design approach which supports the definition of polymorphic design solution, for each system functionalities, so that it allows the definition of how the system should support different users in different contexts of use.

For this purpose, in order to develop our smart adaptive system, a new design approach to adaptive interface has been applied. In particular, the Design of an Adaptive Interface requires to make three fundamental choices:

1. The first level is the choice of the User targets, of the Interface Role and of the Environment Definition. To understand the end-user's capabilities and needs (i.e., user task that need to be supported by the system) and identify the main functionality that the system should have, the Personas method is used [14]. The Personas method is a plain and effective tool useful for designers and developers allowing to gather the strengths and objectives of the user profile. For each profile background, needs and behavior were identified. The interface role and the environment definition are represented by the context of use and by the environment typology and characteristics.

2. The second level consists in the definition of the adaptation goals and rule, the definition of the interaction level and the definition of adaptation variable. The Adaptation goals and rules are intended for those particular objectives we want to pursue due to the process of adaptation (e.g. in order to minimize the number of errors, optimize efficiency and effectiveness, in accordance with the type of application and user for which the final system is intended). Finally, the interfaces adaptation should be activated by several factors, in particular it is necessary to define the "adaptation variables" that consist in the definition of context of use, goal to reach and user expertise.

3. The third level consists in the choice of the adaptation mechanism to use. There are several methods to achieve this level; the most used are the fuzzy logic, the Artificial Neural Network and the Bayesian Networks.

Once defined the three fundamental levels, a new methodology for human-machine interaction and for user interfaces, according to the "design for all" paradigms have been developed. The adaptation system is based on the knowledge provided by three information models: the User Model, the Environment Model (or Domain Model) and the Interaction Model. The system structure allows to:

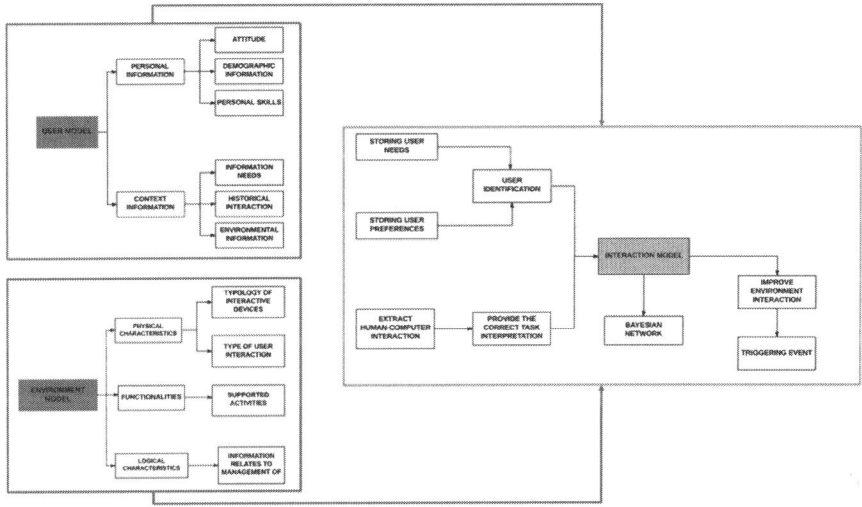

Fig. 1 The adaptation system: user model, the environment model and the interaction model

- Recognize the user;
- Store user needs and preferences;
- Extract information from the human-computer interaction;
- Provide a logic level and task correct interpretation;
- Make more accessible interaction with the environment;
- Define types of events to be triggered (Fig. 1).

4 The Proposed Adaptive System

The global architecture is based on three functional modules, continuously connected each other's: the Database Management System (DBMS), the Application Core and the User Interface (UI). The DBMS provides to store all information about user profile and context data, the Core can easily manage the application routine and apply the adaptive rules implemented by Adaptive Engine. Finally, the user interface allows users to interact with the application functionalities and can be reconfigured according to Core Directives. In Fig. 2 the overall architecture is shown.

4.1 Database

The Database Management System (DBMS) is designed to achieve a large set of structured data inputs and processes the amount of data requested by numerous

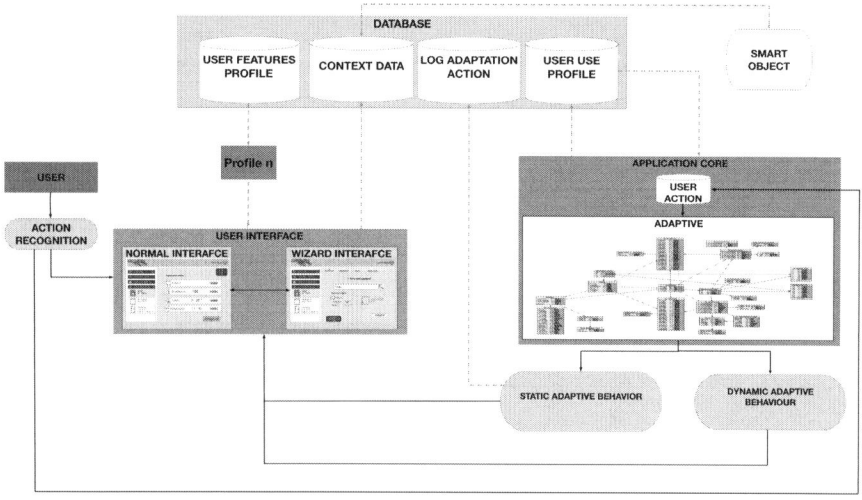

Fig. 2 Proposed adaptive system

users; the information is structured in four semantic areas. (1) User Features Profile (i.e. the User Profile such as personal data and health-related information). This data helps to define an accurate profile decode user's abilities and functionalities according to ICF Model [7]. (2) User Use Profile, where all the user interactions are stored and his/her overall interaction history can be reconstructed. It includes all the context information defined in the User Model. (3) Log Adaptation Actions, that is the collection of all the adaptations provided by the Adaptive Engine during the application usage. Finally, (4) Context Data, where all data related to the context of use are stored (devices status, sensor measurements, time info).

4.2 Application Core

The brain of the application is represented by the core layer that provides to manage the application logic. Besides managing the application routine activities, in the application core the adaptive engine is developed, aimed to make adaptive the proposed system.

The Adaptive Engine represents overall adaptive system pivot: it is composed of an adaptive mechanisms and a monitoring system of changes. Adaptivity consists of change mechanisms which include all dynamic features, such as preferences based on history of user's interaction, information contents, icons, layout, etc. In particular, the adaptive mechanism is based on the Bayesian Belief Network (BBN). Nowadays, Bayesian networks are one of the most comprehensive tools and more consistent for the acquisition, representation and exploitation of knowledge in conditions of uncertainty. A BBN is a probabilistic graphical model that represents a set of stochastic variables with their conditional dependencies through use of a directed graph; each node in the graph represents a random variable, while the edges between the nodes represent probabilistic dependencies among the corresponding random variable.

In order to achieve a proper adaptation action, a Decision Making Algorithm (DMA) is developed [15]. After mapping the net with the UI information and exploiting the power of the Bayesian Network, that allow to obtain inferences about the most probable state from its nodes, the algorithm defines a threshold in order to trigger the adaptation event of the corresponding node. The adaptation routine provides to manage two different information: a real time upgrading of the correlate information to the user interaction, and a storage of complex user interaction flow to track his/her interaction history.

In this way, the system can dynamically adapt the UI configuration and, at the same time, keep track of the user behavior and interface usage. The interaction with the interface items can infer deterministic finding on the mapped node of the net; this event triggers the updating routine of the stochastic distribution of the children nodes. The DMA can be performed and if any probe node returns a dominant state, the corresponding information on interface is automatically updated. Then, when a complete task is completed (i.e. oven setting), the overall findings are stored on database to track the interaction history of the user.

The described mechanism forms the adaptive engine able to define a detailed user use profile and trigger the proper actions in order to minimize the effort and to optimize efficiency in user's interaction.

4.3 User Interface

The User Interface is the module between the system and the end user and, it enables the control of the smart home devices. It has been designed to support the user in the main domestic tasks: the meal preparation, interaction with the appliances and the home environment control. The UI are managed by the Application Core that controls the adaptivity of interface. The adaptation mechanism can operate both (a) on the graphic features and (b) on the contents of the interface. The graphic features (e.g. colour, text and buttons dimension, image size, etc.,) are uniquely related to a disorder (i.e. colour blindness, visual disturbances, motor problem) and they are being designed on the loss of body functionalities with the aid of existing guidelines.

The contents concern the quantity and type of information that the interface gives to the user and they are designed on the abilities of users. In particular, with the aim to support the greater number of end user into management of a smart home, two different modes of information presentation were realized: (I) a Normal Setting for users without cognitive dysfunction and characterized by a good technology attitude and (II) a Wizard Setting for users who have not familiarity with technology and/or have some cognitive dysfunction. Starting from the basis of the standards, guidelines and success criteria contained in the Recommendation of the World Wide Web Consortium [16], the Normal mode is designed to optimize the user interaction. Instead, the Wizard mode is designed in order to simplify the tasks: starting from the Normal mode, the UI has been implemented by the decomposition of the task in more simple and basic actions. In this way, the user must not manage and understand all the information of the appliance or a recipe's procedure. In this case, the system tries to make up for the lack of some user ability and it help him/her to accomplish the activity of daily living independently.

The adaptive system can act during the run time user interaction: if the user chooses, for example, an oven program and the probability of all child nodes of BBN (e.g. temperature, duration, etc.,) exceeds the threshold value, the system automatically sets the most probable values for that oven program, enhancing the interaction efficiency.

5   Conclusion

This paper is the description of an innovative approach to support the design of inclusive environments to improve the user- interaction.

This approach is intended to help the designer to plan environments for smart homes suitable to the requirements of different user groups and contexts of use. It is based on an adaptive system which studies the information provided by three models: the User Model, the Environment Model (or Domain Model) and the Interaction Model. Through this information, the rules and the adaptation mechanisms of the system are established according to the user's skills, expertise and disabilities.

The proposed design approach has been applied to a smart kitchen environment aiming to support users with several impairments (visual, cognitive, motor related) in performing cooking tasks. A decision making algorithm is proposed to manage adaptive behaviour of smart adaptive systems according to the output of the User Model, based on BBN. The validity of the decision making algorithm has been tested through simulation of real users' case scenarios. The results highlight that the proposed decision making algorithm is able to readapt the interface in a reliable and efficient manner [15].

The results of a qualitative experimentation with final users has shown that the proposed interface is suitable for "fragile" users such as elderly with mild to moderate dementia and adult persona with moderate retinopathy and rheumatoid arthritis. In general, it emerged that the proposed adaptive system is able to improve the usability of household appliances, such as oven and dishwasher, as regards the programming and controlling operations. At the same time, it shows how the introduction of smart technologies in the kitchen environment can support users also with unusual attitude to technology [17]. However, the work is not ultimate: the proposed adaptive system has to be evaluated with a greater number of users in order to verify this first qualitative evaluation.

Moreover, it will be necessary to carry out a field study to assess the ability of adaptable features of interface to improve the system usability, as to assess the effectiveness of system to enhance the user's' skills related to cooking activities and to improve users' independent living.

Acknowledgements The work has been developed in the context of the "D4All: Design for all" project, funded by the Italian Minister of University and Research, under the National Technological Cluster initiative.

References

1. Elaine O (2011) Universal design: an evolving paradigm. universal design handbook. W. F. E. Preiser, K. H. Smith, Chap. 1
2. Chadwick-Dias A, McNulty M, Tullis T (2002) Web usability andage: how design changes can improve performance. In: Proceedings of the 2003 conference on Universal Usability (CUU'03). ACM, New York, NY, USA, pp 30–37
3. Kobsa A (2004) Adaptive interfaces. In: Bainbridge WS (ed) Encyclopedia of human-computer interaction. Berkshire Publishing, Great Barrington
4. McAdams DA, Kostovich V (2010) A framework and representation for universal product design. Int J Design 5(1):29–42
5. Connell BR, Jones ML, Mace RL, Mueller JL, Mullick A, Ostroff E, Sanford J et al (1997) The principles of universal design, version 2.0. Center for Universal Design, North Carolina State University, Raleigh
6. Langley P (1999) User modelling in adaptive interfaces. In: Proceedings of the 7th international conference on user modelling. Springer, Banff, pp 357–370
7. World Health Organization (2001) International classification of functioning, disability and health: ICF. World Health Organization
8. Paymans TF, Lindenberg J, Neerinex MA (2004) Usability trade-offs for adaptive user interfaces: ease of use and learnability. In: Proceedings of international conference on intelligent user interfaces, p 301
9. Rothrock L, Koubek R, Fuchs F, Haas M, Salvendyk G (2002) Review and reappraisal of adaptive interfaces: Toward biologically inspired paradigms
10. Benyon DI (1987) System adaptivity and the modelling of stereotypes. National Physical Laboratory, Division of Information Technology and Computer
11. Stephanidis C (2001) Adaptive techniques for universal access. User Model User-Adap Inter 11(1–2):159–179
12. Mace R (1985) Universal design, Barrier free environments for everyone, Designers West, November
13. Wobbrock J, Kane SK, Gajos KZ, Harada S, Froehlich F (2011) Ability-based design: concept, principles and examples. ACM Trans Access Comput (TACCESS) 3(3):1–36
14. Cooper A (1999) The inmates are running the asylum. Morgan Kaufmann, Indianapolis
15. Gullà F, Cavalieri L, Ceccacci S, Germani M (2016) A BBN-based method to manage adaptive behavior of a smart user interface. Procedia CIRP 50:535–540
16. World Wide Web Consortium (W3C) Web content accessibility guidelines (WCAG) 2.0. http://www.w3.org/TR/WCAG20/
17. ISO 9241-210:2010—Ergonomics of human-system interaction—part 210: Human-centred design for interactive systems

Part II
Enabling Technologies and Assistive Solutions

Unobtrusive Technology for In-Home Monitoring: Preliminary Results on Fall Detection

Giovanni Diraco, Alessandro Leone and Pietro Siciliano

Abstract In-home monitoring technologies deployed in personal living spaces are increasingly used for the assessment of health status in older adults, through the measurement of relevant at-tributes ranging from vital parameters to activities and behaviors including mobility, gait velocity, movements in bed, and so on. Several studies agree that unobtrusive monitoring (with the exception of video-recording) is generally well accepted by older adults, especially if non-intrusive technologies are adopted (e.g., not need to wear any device) which do not interfere with daily life (e.g., not need to learn new technical skills, no change in routines, etc.). In order to address the problem of in-home automatic fall detection by continuous unobtrusive monitoring, this study investigates the use of a promising ambient technology, that is the ultra-wideband (UWB) radar sensing, which provides rich information but outside the human sensory capabilities (i.e., not directly usable for obtaining privacy-sensitive information) and thus well acceptable by end-users. Moreover, the problem of performance under real-life conditions has been addressed by suggesting an unsupervised approach not requiring fall-based training but only a subject-specific calibration phase based on observation of daily activities. Preliminary results are very encouraging, showing the effectiveness to achieve good detection performance under real-life conditions through unobtrusive monitoring.

Keywords Fall detection · Unobtrusive monitoring · Ultra-wideband radar sensor · Machine learning

G. Diraco (✉) · A. Leone · P. Siciliano
Institute for Microelectronics and Microsystems, National Research
Council of Italy, c/o Campus Ecotekne, via Monteroni, Lecce, Italy
e-mail: giovanni.diraco@le.imm.cnr.it

A. Leone
e-mail: alessandro.leone@le.imm.cnr.it

P. Siciliano
e-mail: pietro.siciliano@le.imm.cnr.it

© Springer International Publishing AG 2017
F. Cavallo et al. (eds.), *Ambient Assisted Living*, Lecture Notes
in Electrical Engineering 426, DOI 10.1007/978-3-319-54283-6_9

1 Introduction

In-home monitoring technologies deployed in personal living spaces are increasingly used for the assessment of health status in older adults, through the measurement of relevant attributes ranging from vital parameters to activities and behaviors including mobility, gait velocity, movements in bed, and so on. Furthermore, such technologies can also be used to provide more safety (e.g., fall detection) and support with daily activities (e.g., issuing reminders).

Recently, ethical issues concerning technology interventions involving older adults have received increasing attention [1]. Among others, the most common concerns regard privacy (i.e., risks of inappropriate access to personal information) and security (i.e., risks of intrusion through computer systems). However, several studies report that unobtrusive monitoring (with the exception of video-recording) is generally well accepted by older adults, especially if nonintrusive technologies are adopted (e.g., not need to wear any device) which do not interfere with daily life (e.g., not need to learn new technical skills, no change in routines, etc.) [2]. In addition, the good acceptability of unobtrusive monitoring enables the measurement of relevant attributes in continuous modality, producing long-term health data useful for early prediction of heath disorders (e.g., cognitive impairment, dementia, etc.).

In-home monitoring solutions are generally classified into two types: wearable devices and ambient (or context-aware) systems [3]. Wearable-based technologies, typically consisting of embedded MEMS accelerometers/gyroscopes (e.g., fall detection or activity recognition) or skin electrodes (e.g., measurement of vital parameters), suffer from several drawbacks such as limited battery life, the need for on-board processing and/or wireless communication (i.e., both energy-demanding functions), the inconvenience of having to remember to wear a device and the discomfort caused by the device itself. All these drawbacks make the use of wearable devices still far from being suitable for continuous unobtrusive monitoring [4]. On the contrary, the ambient systems are more suitable for this purpose, since they are based on various kinds of sensors deployed in the environment ranging from information-poor but well accepted devices such as simple on/off switches, pressure sensors, infrared sensors and so on, to more information-rich devices, like video cameras, but that raise privacy concerns.

In order to address the problem of in-home automatic fall detection by continuous unobtrusive monitoring, this paper investigates the use of a promising ambient technology, that is the ultra-wideband (UWB) radar sensing, which provides rich information but outside the human sensory capabilities (i.e., not directly usable for obtaining privacy-sensitive information) and thus well acceptable by end-users. Additionally, UWB radar is a multi-purpose technology whose application range spans from detection and measurement of vital parameters to localization, movement detection, and even secure high-throughput wireless communication [5].

2 Materials and Methods

2.1 System Overview

The unobtrusive monitoring system is based on a monostatic sensor module P410 manufactured by Time Domain [6], which is connected via USB to an embedded PC. Both devices are presented in Fig. 1. The P410 is a state-of-the-art UWB radar sensor, working from 3.1 to 5.3 GHz centered at 4.3 GHz, covering a distance range of about 30 m, having good object penetrating capabilities and compact (7.6 × 8.0 × 1.6 cm) board dimensions. The P410 is equipped with an omnidirectional antenna, which in this study has been modified by adding a planar back reflector in order to reduce the azimuth pattern to around 100°. Range data from the P410 are processed by the Embedded PC (EPC), which has low computational profile (i.e., Intel Atom processor based), low power consumption (25 W) and reduced (13.2 × 9.5 × 3.7 cm) dimensions.

The EPC runs the processing algorithms, including (as better explained in the following) preprocessing steps and machine learning, for detection of fall events in real-time.

2.2 Algorithmic Framework for Fall Detection

On the algorithmic side, there are three main stages: preprocessing, feature extraction, event detection. Regarding the preprocessing stage, the scattered radar signal is first filtered by a 16th-order Butterworth (bandpass 3.1–5.3 GHz) and then by a 3-tap FIR motion filter in order to improve the signal-to-clutter ratio. The resulting range profiles are normalized in amplitude and time within a sliding window of time length 1.5 s and distance range up to 5 m. The time duration of

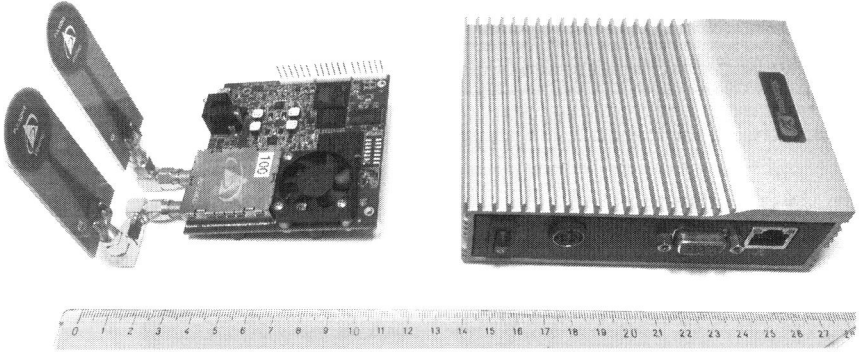

Fig. 1 UWB Radar Sensor P410 (*left*) and embedded PC (*right*)

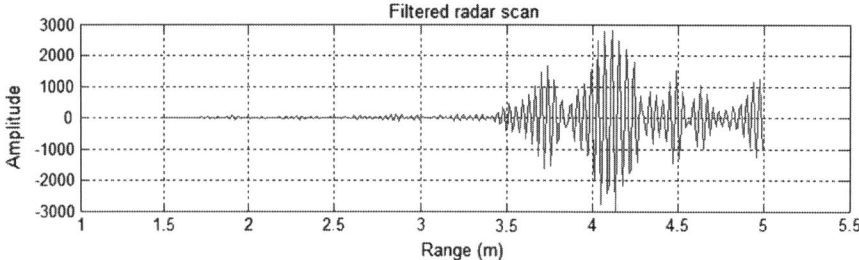

Fig. 2 Preprocessed radar signal referred to a person moving inside a room at a distance of about 4 m from the radar sensor

1.5 s was experimentally determined, as that able to discriminate both fast actions (e.g., falls) and slow ones (e.g., voluntary lying down). Amplitudes and Times-of-Arrival (ToAs) are estimated by peak analysis and tracked with Kalman filter in order to isolate the only target of interest (i.e., the monitored subject). The preprocessed radar signal is shown in Fig. 2.

The extracted features are based on the Micro-Doppler effect which is briefly introduced as follows. As well known, the relative motion between radar and target introduces a Doppler frequency shift which relates directly to the radial velocity: movements towards (away from) the radar introduce a positive (negative) frequency shift. Furthermore, a human target consists of different parts (e.g., head, torso, legs, etc.) which move at different velocities during the same action (e.g., walking, sitting, etc.). The multiple Doppler shifts produced by these smaller motions are referred to as Micro-Doppler features. The feature extraction process starts by computing the Doppler spectrogram which represents the signal power distribution over frequency (x-axis) and distance (y-axis). In Fig. 3, the Doppler spectrograms of radar scans taken during a simulated fall (Fig. 3a) and walking activity (Fig. 3b) are presented. As evident from Fig. 3a, the spectrogram exhibits horizontally aligned peaks (Micro-Doppler) related to movements of body's parts during the fall event. The Doppler spectrogram is computed by applying the short-time Fourier transform to the analytic form of the radar signal. Hence, the Micro-Doppler features are extracted by convolving the spectrogram with a Gaussian filter and summing the power spectrum at all distances for each frequency, in order to obtain one-dimensional Micro-Doppler signatures as those reported in Fig. 3c, d associated with the simulated fall (Fig. 3a) and the walking activity (Fig. 3b), respectively.

The event detection stage deals with the recognition of a fall occurrence from the extracted features. The commonly used methodologies are based on supervised machine learning techniques trained with both positive (falls) and negative (ADL-Activity of Daily Living) samples, both simulated by healthy young subjects. As a result, due to such a training protocol, fall detectors inevitably exhibit lower performance when used in real-world situations, in which monitored subjects are older adults [3]. In order to address this problem and to improve fall detection

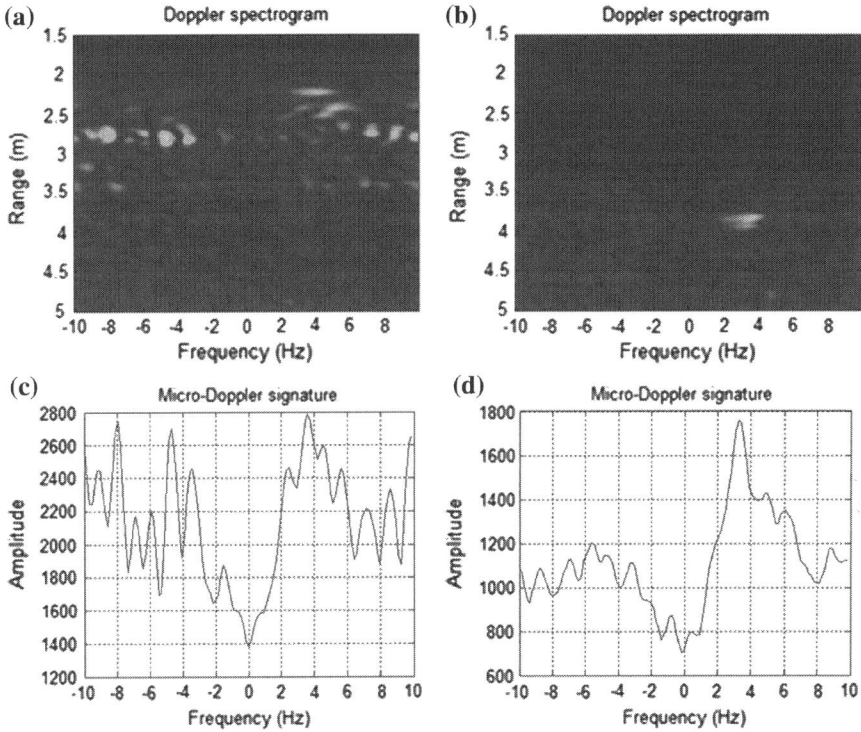

Fig. 3 Doppler spectrum (**a**) and Micro-Doppler signature (**c**) of a radar scan referred to a person falling down at a distance of about 3 m from the sensor. Doppler spectrum (**b**) and Micro-Doppler signature (**d**) of a radar scan referred to a person walking at a distance of about 4 m from the sensor

performance under real-life conditions, an unsupervised approach has been used in which the fall occurrence is detected as a "novelty" with respect the usual daily activities performed by the monitored subject. In the suggested unsupervised approach, novelties are detected using votes casted by multiple one-class K-means classifiers [7]. For evaluation purpose, a classical supervised detector based on Support Vector Machine (SVM) [8] has been also experimented and its performance compared with the unsupervised one.

2.3 Experimental Setup

Both ADLs and falls were performed in a home-like setting, as depicted in Fig. 4, by involving ten healthy subjects divided into two age groups of avg. 24 and 48 years old, respectively. For each participant, a total amount of 436 actions were collected, of which 30 were simulated falls and the remaining were daily activities such as walking, sitting down, standing up, etc. The SVM-based supervised

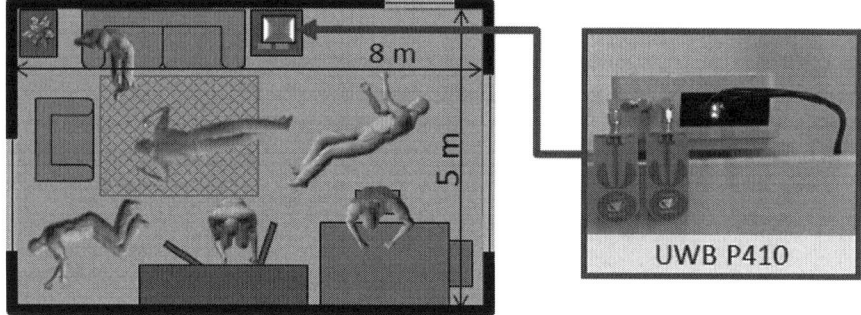

Fig. 4 Experimental setup: home-like setting (*left*) and radar station (*right*)

approach has been evaluated using both intra-group and inter-group strategies. More specifically, the first strategy consisted in training and testing the classifier with actions simulated by individuals belonging to the same group. On the contrary, with the second strategy the classifier has been trained with actions simulated by individuals of the young group and tested by involving individuals of the older group. In both strategies, the SVM classifier was trained with 90 falls and 738 daily actions, and was tested with the remaining 60 falls and 492 daily actions.

Regarding the K-means-based unsupervised approach, since it is oriented to detect falls as novelties among daily "normal" activities (walking, sitting down, standing up, etc.), it has been validated involving the same subject in both observation and testing phases. The observation phase lasted for about 95 min for each subject (i.e., 190 actions), after which the testing phase started and 30 falls/person were performed.

3   Results and Discussion

As summarized in Table 1 the best performance was achieved using the SVM-based supervised approach validated with the intra-group strategy. Although this performance is comparable with previous studies [9], nevertheless there is no guarantee that it could be achieved under real-life conditions since the classifier needs to be trained with simulated falls. In fact, the performance declined with the inter-group validation strategy, in which falls were simulated by young and tested by older subjects (as happens in real-life). More interestingly, the K-means-based unsupervised approach outperformed the supervised (inter group) one without requiring any fall-based training, and thus more reproducible in real-life scenarios. However, it is worth noting that the unsupervised approach requires a preliminary calibration phase during which almost all daily "normal" activities should be observed and labelled as not-fall. In this study, such a calibration phase lasted

Table 1 Experimental results

Approach	Sensitivity (%)	Specificity (%)
Unsupervised[a]	91	89
Supervised intra-group[b]	96	90
Supervised inter-group[c]	86	75

[a]Not trained with simulated falls
[b]Trained and tested with falls simulated involving the same group
[c]Trained with falls simulated by the young group and tested with falls simulated by the older group

95 min per subject, but in real-world it may take much longer depending on habits of monitored subject.

The presented system may find application for continuous indoor monitoring of older adults living alone. In fact, after a period of observation (i.e., unsupervised training), the system can reliably detect fall events against daily activities. The presence of moving objects (e.g., chairs, sofas, etc.) in the room does not interfere with the event detection, since the Kalman filter allows tracking of peaks associated with a human target in the radar signal. Furthermore, it is worth to note that because of the high penetrating ability of the UWB radar, the presence of medium-sized objects (e.g., tables, chairs, etc.) between radar sensor and human target does not raise any occlusion problem. Instead, the most serious noise source in indoor environments is the clutter signal containing reflections from stationary structures (e.g., walls, furniture, etc.). In this study the clutter signal has been strongly attenuated by motion filtering the radar signal. However, this technique is not quite effective for through-wall sensing, in which case more sophisticated clutter removal techniques should be adopted.

As already mentioned, the system reliably detects falls when only one person is present in the room (i.e., a living-alone elderly). When two or more people are present, on the other hand, the system takes into account only the movement patterns of the person nearest to the radar sensor, and thus it is able to detect only falls of the nearest subject. Additionally, when two or more people stay at the same radial distance with respect to the radar sensor, their motion patterns may interfere, affecting the detection performance.

4 Conclusion

The main contribution of this work concerns the investigation and validation in a home-like setting of an unobtrusive monitoring system for fall detection based on UWB radar sensor. Moreover, the problem of performance under real-life conditions has been addressed by suggesting an unsupervised approach not requiring fall-based training but only a subject-specific calibration phase based on observation of daily activities. Preliminary results are very encouraging, showing the effectiveness to achieve good detection performance under real-life conditions through unobtrusive monitoring.

The ongoing work is focused, on one hand, on extending the proposed system to detect falls in multi-user scenarios (e.g., in community dwellings) by facing the multi-target/multi-detection association problem. On the other hand, the future work is to investigate the use the UWB radar sensor also for continuous and unobtrusive in-home monitoring of vital parameters.

Acknowledgements This work was carried out within the project "ACTIVE AGEING AT HOME" (CTN01_00128_297061) funded by the Italian Ministry of Education, Universities and Research, within the National Operational Programme for "Research and Competitiveness" 2007–2013 (NOP for R&C).

References

1. Boise L, Wild K, Mattek N, Ruhl M, Dodge HH, Kaye J (2013) Willingness of older adults to share data and privacy concerns after exposure to unobtrusive in-home monitoring. Gerontechnology Int J Fundam Aspects Technol Serve Ageing Soc 11(3):428
2. Wild K, Boise L, Lundell J, Foucek A (2008) Unobtrusive in-home monitoring of cognitive and physical health: reactions and perceptions of older adults. J Appl Gerontol 27(2):181–200
3. Igual R, Medrano C, Plaza I (2013) Challenges, issues and trends in fall detection systems. Biomed Eng Online 12(66):1–66
4. Hagler S, Austin D, Hayes TL, Kaye J, Pavel M (2010) Unobtrusive and ubiquitous in-home monitoring: a methodology for continuous assessment of gait velocity in elders. Biomed Eng IEEE Trans on 57(4):813–820
5. Nguyen C, Han J (2014) Time-domain ultra-wideband radar, theory, analysis and design, sensor and components. Springer Science & Business Media, New York
6. Time Domain (2015, May 27), PulsON® P410 radar kit. Available: http://www.timedomain.com/
7. Kanungo T, Mount DM, Netanyahu NS, Piatko CD, Silverman R, Wu AY (2002) An efficient k-means clustering algorithm: analysis and implementation. Pattern Anal Mach Intell IEEE Trans on 24(7):881–892
8. Cortes C, Vapnik V (1995) Support-vector networks. Mach Learn 20(3):273–297
9. Liu L, Popescu M, Skubic M, Rantz M, Yardibi T, Cuddihy P (2011, May) Automatic fall detection based on doppler radar motion signature. In: IEEE 5th international conference on pervasive computing technologies for healthcare (PervasiveHealth), pp 222–225

A Neural Network Approach to Human Posture Classification and Fall Detection Using RGB-D Camera

Alessandro Manzi, Filippo Cavallo and Paolo Dario

Abstract In this paper, we describe a human posture classification and a falling detector module suitable for smart homes and assisted living solutions. The system uses a neural network that processes the human joints produced by a skeleton tracker using the depth streams of an RGB-D sensor. The neural network is able to recognize standing, sitting and lying postures. Using only the depth maps from the sensor, the system can work in poor light conditions and guarantees the privacy of the person. The neural network is trained with a dataset produced with the Kinect tracker, but it is also tested with a different human tracker (NiTE). In particular, the aim of this work is to analyse the behaviour of the neural network even when the position of the extracted joints is not reliable and the provided skeleton is confused. Real-time tests have been carried out covering the whole operative range of the sensor (up to 3.5 m). Experimental results have shown an overall accuracy of 98.3% using the NiTE tracker for the falling tests, with the worst accuracy of 97.5%.

Keywords Human posture · Neural networks · Depth camera

1 Introduction

In the recent years, the development of technologies strictly connected to humans increased exponentially. Nowadays, the advent of powerful mobile devices such as smartphones and tablets are a reality, but in the near future smart home technologies will represent a huge market [1–3]. Distributed environmental sensors [4], robots [5], computers and wearable devices [6] will share the home environment with us.

A. Manzi (✉) · F. Cavallo · P. Dario
The BioRobotics Institute, Scuola Superiore Sant'Anna,
Piazza Martiri della Libertà, 33, 56127 Pisa, Italy
e-mail: a.manzi@sssup.it

© Springer International Publishing AG 2017
F. Cavallo et al. (eds.), *Ambient Assisted Living*, Lecture Notes
in Electrical Engineering 426, DOI 10.1007/978-3-319-54283-6_10

These kinds of smart systems need to be aware of humans in order to effectively interacts with them to address several tasks such as energy management or behavioral and health monitoring. In the context of home care application, especially if we consider elderly people, one of the most desirable feature is the ability to detect a falling event. Each year, one in every three older adults falls in their home [7], but less than half talk to their health-care providers about it [8]. Older adult falls lead to reduced functions and premature loss of independence, and oftentimes a fall may indicate a more serious underlying health problem. For these reasons, the importance of the fall detection to have a fast and quick reaction is crucial. In the past, video surveillance systems have been proposed to address this issue, but some of their limitations include the light conditions and the lack of privacy. The recent emergence of depth sensors, so-called RGB-D sensors (e.g. Microsoft Kinect, Asus Xtion, PrimeSense Carmine), has made it feasible and economically sound to capture in real-time not only color images, but also depth maps with appropriate resolution and accuracy. A depth sensor can provide three-dimensional data structure as well as the 3D motion information of the subjects/objects in the scene, which has shown to be advantageous for human detection [9]. Several works about human postures detection with the RGB-D sensors exploit the use of skeleton tracking algorithms for rapidly transforming persons depth information to spatial joints that represent the human figure [10, 11]. Unfortunately, when these methods are used for real world applications the output is not always stable and reliable (see Fig. 1). The reasons that reduce their performance depend on several factors. Among these, we have the distance between the person and the sensor, the occlusions that occur when people interacts with environmental objects and also sideways poses that hides some parts of the user that are not visible to the sensor.

The aim of this work is to develop a system, based on depth cameras, which is able to classify three human postures, including standing, sitting, and lying positions that reliable works in real conditions. In order to do that, we need to deal with the aforementioned problems that afflict the skeleton tracker methods. Therefore, an artificial Neural Network (NN) model is adopted to rely on its generalization ability and its robustness against noisy and missed data. As opposed to other similar works [12, 13], real-time tests, conceived to reproduce realistic and challenging situations

(a)   **(b)**   **(c)**

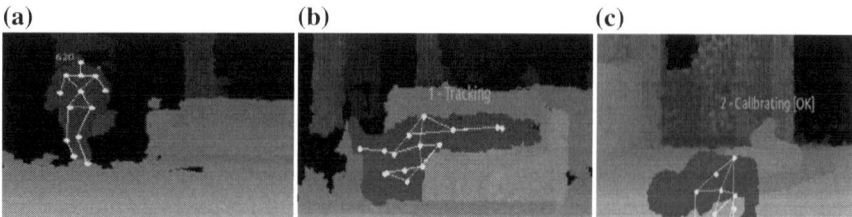

Fig. 1 Examples of worst skeleton detection. **a** The person is far from the sensor and at least two joints are missed. **b** The user is lying on a sofa and the skeleton is fused with the sofa. **c** The person falls down in front of the sensor and the output seems unusable

for the tracker, covering the whole operative range of the sensor, have been carried out. During these experiments, the NN has been continuously fed with all the available joints generated by the skeleton tracker in order to analyse its robustness to unreliable and uncertain joints. At the end of the paper, an application for smart homes and a scenario that includes a domestic robot that integrates the trained NN for falling detection is presented. The paper is structured as follows. Section 2 presents the related work on human postures, while Sect. 3 gives an overview of the proposed system, describing the NN architecture, the dataset, the training and test phases. The real-time experiments are presented in Sect. 4, while the results are summarized in the Sect. 5. A falling event application example for smart environment is presented is Sects. 6 and 7 concludes the paper.

2 Related Work

The importance of detecting human postures, especially for recognize or prevent human falls, is addressed in various previous work. According to Yu [14], a system for the falling recognition must have three main properties, it has to be reliable, unobtrusive and has to preserve the privacy. Several proposed systems make use of wearable devices [15], such as accelerometers [16], gyroscopes [17] and RFID sensors [18]. However, these approaches are often cost prohibitive and they rely on the willingness of the subjects to wear devices, reducing the overall acceptability of the system. Non-invasive methods such as computer vision techniques have been extensively investigated. In [19], a 2-D human posture classification by means of a neural fuzzy network is presented. However, 2-D video based methods generally give not robust and inaccurate results, and they are influenced by the light conditions without providing an adequate privacy.

Recently, the advent of low-cost depth camera received a great deal of attention from researchers. This technology offers several advantages compared to standard video cameras. In addition to color and texture information, depth images provide three-dimensional data useful for segmentation and detection. Moreover, a system that uses only depth information is able to work in poor light conditions (high risk of falling accidents), providing privacy at the same time. In literature, several works address the problem of the posture detection using depth data. Some of these take into account the relation between the human and the ground [20], but, in order to perform floor segmentation, they often assume the floor as a large part of the scene and this assumption seems unrealistic in real home application. Silhouette extraction methods use the centroid as detector feature [19, 21], but the centroid is strong dependent on the posture and on the size of the user. Other works exploit proper skeleton tracking algorithms to use human joints as feature descriptor [22]. However, the depth data are usually affected by noise and the joints are not always available. As it has been pointed out by [11], depending on the quality of the segmented target and the level of occlusion, the skeleton trackers might not detect all the joints and their location cannot be totally reliable. A poor estimation of the skeleton joints occurs when the person is partially occluded or somewhat out of the image, or not facing the sensor (sideways poses provide some challenges regarding the part of the user that is not directly visible), or it is at the far end of the sensor range. For these reasons, it is common to find works based on skeleton tracker, limiting the test phases to samples that are free of excessive noise [12] or performing tests that allow to retrieve easily distinguishable human body features [13]. In order to deal with the aforementioned problems, a feed-forward NN, trained with all the available skeleton joints, is adopted to detect the target postures. During the real-time tests, the NN is fed with the output of a tracking algorithm also when its output is confused and not reliable. Tests have been carried out in order to analyse the behaviour of the NN at different distances, covering the whole range of the sensor.

3   System Overview

The proposed human posture detection relies on a skeleton tracker algorithm that is able to extract the joints of a person from the depth map. Among the most used skeleton tracker we can find the Microsoft Kinect SDK, which works with its namesake device, and the NiTE SDK [23], used in conjunction with the OpenNI framework [24] that is generic and runs both for Kinect and Asus Xtion or PrimeSense device. These software tools are similar and provide the 3D position of the skeleton joints combined with an additional confidence value for each of them. This datum can assume three values: "tracked" when the algorithm is confident, "inferred" when it applies some heuristics to adjust the position, and "untracked" when there is uncertainty. Both SDKs are affected by the same drawbacks when used in real world application. The undesirable conditions happen when the user is too close (<1 m) or too farther from the sensor (>3 m), or when the person assumes sideways poses and occlusions are present. In all these cases, the position of the calculated joints are not reliable and stable, so the associated confidence values are set as "untracked". The Fig. 1 shows three examples of the aforementioned cases. A distant person produces fewer joints than usual, a human lying on a sofa confuses the tracker, while a person that falls down abruptly generates a messy output that seems unusable. Nevertheless, the "untracked" joints are anyway part of the whole skeleton and they have been used to analyse the robustness of the NN against noisy and uncertain values.

3.1   Dataset

The choice of the dataset samples for the training and the validation of the NN is a crucial step. Although there are some online RGB-D datasets about human performing daily activities, unfortunately very few of them contains people in lying

(a)   **(b)**   **(c)**

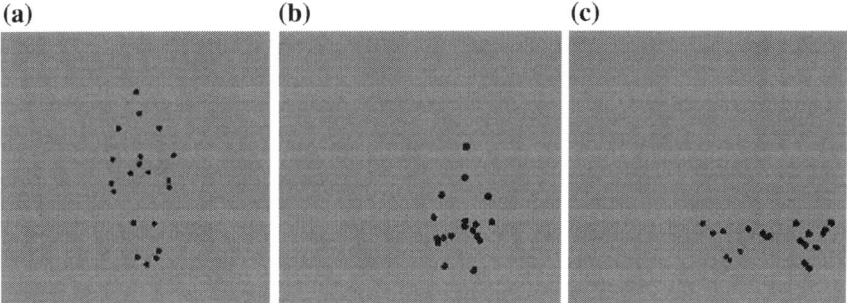

Fig. 2 Three examples of the samples extracted from the dataset: **a** standing, **b** sitting and **c** lying posture

position. For this work, the MSRDailyActivity3D dataset [25] has been chosen. It is recorded with the Kinect SDK and contains 10 subjects performing various activities at the distance of about 2 m. For each frame of the video sequence, the position of 20 skeleton joints is stored in a text file. A total of 120 samples has been taken from these text files to build a set containing subjects in sitting, standing and lying position, equally subdivided (see Fig. 2).

3.2 NN Architecture

The aim of the NN is to detect the three different postures using as input the skeleton joints extracted by the tracker algorithm. The structure of the NN has three layers, with 60 input neurons (3 coordinates for each 20 joints, as provided by the text files of the MSRDailyActivity3D dataset) and 3 output neurons, whose values range from 0 to 1 according to the posture. The neuron number of the hidden layer needs to be minimized in order to keep the amount of free variables, namely the associated weights, as small as possible [26], decreasing also the need of a large training set. The cross-validation technique is adopted to find the lowest validation error as a function of the number of hidden neurons. As a result, an amount of 42 hidden units has been found as sufficient value. The activation function for the hidden and the output layer is the sigmoid, defined as:

$$y = \frac{1}{1 + e^{-2sx}}$$

where x is the input to the activation function, y is the output and s is the steepness (=0.5). The selected learning algorithm is the iRPROP-described in [27], which is an heuristic for supervised learning strategy and that represents a variety of the standard resilient back-propagation (RPROP) training algorithm [28]. It is one of the fastest weight update mechanisms and it is adaptive, therefore does not use the learning rate. The NN is developed in C++ using the Fast Artificial Neural Network Library [29].

3.3 Training, Validation and Testing Sets

In order to estimate the generalization performance of the NN and to avoid the over-fitting of the parameters, the dataset is randomly divided into a training set, to adjust the weights of the NN, a validation set, to minimize the over-fitting, and a testing set to confirm the predictive power of the network. There is no common splitting rule for the dataset. In the present work, we follow the procedure described in [30] in which is stated that the fraction of patterns reserved for the validation set should be inversely proportional to the square root of the number of free adjustable parameters. In our case, these sets are divided in 63, 21 and 36 samples respectively.

All the data are recorded at a distance of about 2 m from the sensor. If the NN is trained with them, the network will produce better result only around 2 m. To overcome this issue, a preprocessing step has been introduced. The NN is trained with normalized joints to ensure a depth invariant feature. Each joint vectors is normalized with the Euclidean norm:

$$\widehat{j} = \frac{j}{\|j\|}$$

where j is the joint and $\widehat{j}$ is the normalized joint.

During the learning phase, the Mean Squared Error (MSE) is separately computed for the training and for the validation set. To guarantee optimal generalization performance, this process is stopped when the validation error starts to increase, since it means that the NN is over-fitting the data [31]. The final errors of the process is 2×10^{-4} for the training and 0.028 for the validation. This process took 339 ms on a Intel Core 2.2 GHz 32bit producing a 100% recognition rate on all the 36 samples of the testing set.

4 Real-Time Tests

As expected, testing the NN with the samples of the dataset gives a True Positive Rate (TPR) of 100%, since the data are well acquired and free of excessive noise. To understand the real performance of the network, real-time experiments have been set up. Since the original dataset is built only with the Kinect SDK tracker, in order to prove the generalization power of the NN tests have been carried out with both Kinect SDK and NiTE tracker of the OpenNI framework. Although these two software behave in a similar way, they have a significant difference. The first one

Fig. 3 Difference between skeleton representation. The Kinect SDK (*left*) uses 20 joints, while the NiTE SDK (*right*) only 15. The missing joints are replaced with the closest

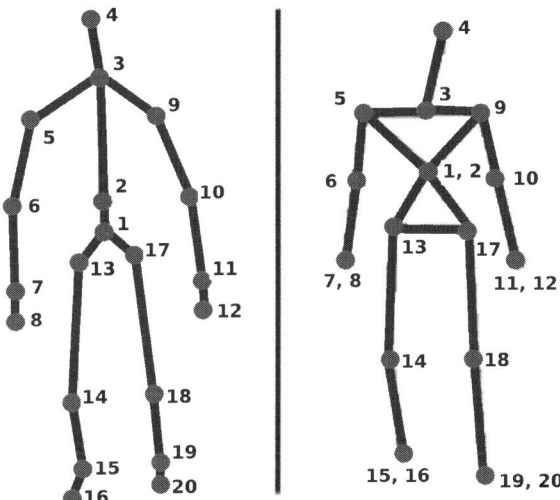

represents the human skeleton with 20 joints, while the latter uses only 15 joints. Therefore, to work with our trained NN, the input is preprocessed to fill the missed joints with the closest available, as depicted in the Fig. 3.

4.1 Experimental Setup

Two different kinds of experiments have been conducted. The first one is about the detection of the three human postures in daily life environment with a sofa, while the second tests how the network behaves when a person falls down. The output of the NN is "standing", "sitting", and "lying" according to the value of the output neuron that is closest to 1. To analyze the results, the outputs are compared with the actual posture of the person, but the intermediate poses between a posture and another are discarded, i.e. when the user is sitting down or standing up. All the tests run at 25 fps. Since the input of the NN is the skeleton data, which are extracted purely from depth maps, the light conditions do not influence the performed experiments.

4.1.1 Sit and Lie on a Sofa

This experiment has been conducted in a real living room with a sofa. The sensors (Kinect and Xtion) have been placed at 1 ms from the ground facing the sofa. A person, starting from the left, goes to the sofa, sits for a while, lies down on it, and then gets up again and goes away. The experiments have been carried out with

6 people (3 male and 3 female) at 3 different distances (3.5, 2.5 and 1.5 m). This setup is intended to address the human trackers problems about the distance (Fig. 1a) and the melting issue between human and objects (Fig. 1b) as already mentioned in Sect. 2.

4.1.2 Falling Tests

Given the lack of available dataset containing falling people, we want to understand the ability of the NN to recognize a falling as a lying posture. Therefore, we set up a series of tests in which a man falls down to the side and to the front of the sensor (Fig. 1c). The device is placed at 1 m from the ground and the NN is fed with all the available joints, even if their confidence value is labelled as "inferred" or "untracked". In this way, the robustness of the NN against data uncertainty has been evaluated. Falling tests are divided in frontal and lateral to take into account also the self-occlusion of some parts of the body. They have been conducted in a kitchen environment with a person that falls down abruptly while its moving toward and sideways and repeated 5 times each. The frontal fall distance from the sensor is about 2 m, while the distance of the lateral fall is about 3 m.

5 Results

The experiment with the sofa has been conducted with 6 persons at different distances and two types of sensors, Kinect and Xtion, and trackers, Kinect SDK and NiTE respectively. The total number of analysed frame are 5214. The NN output with the Kinect SDK proves to be extremely robust and reliable, achieving a 100% for all the three postures. The output with the NiTE skeleton tracker is less reliable and it is summarized with the confusion matrix of the Table 1. As expected, lying is the most challenging posture to classify, since the skeleton tracker provides clearer output with the other two postures. It is worth to know that, in all the cases, the actual lying posture can be misclassified only as sitting, and that neither standing nor sitting is classified as lying. Considering the falling tests, the Kinect tracker yields a TPR of 100% for all the postures, while the NiTE is less reliable, but still satisfactory. Table 2 contains the confusion matrices for these experiments and the results are consistent with the previous tests. To be thorough, since the person falls down quickly, there are not actual sitting posture. Table 3 contains the accuracy calculated for the sofa and the falling experiments. In general, the real standing

Table 1 Confusion matrix of the sofa experiments (NiTE)		Standing (%)	Sitting (%)	Lying (%)
	Standing	100	0	0
	Sitting	0	100	0
	Lying	0	2.8	97.2

Table 2 Confusion matrix for the falling tests (NiTE)

	Standing (%)	Sitting (%)	Lying (%)
(a) Frontal fall			
Standing	100	0	0
Sitting	0	100	0
Lying	0	6.7	93.3
(b) Lateral fall			
Standing	98.9	1.1	0
Sitting	0	100	0
Lying	0	4.9	95.1

Table 3 Accuracy (NiTE)

	Sofa (%)	Frontal fall (%)	Lateral fall (%)
Standing	100	100	99.4
Sitting	99.5	97.6	97.5
Lying	99.5	97.6	98.1
Overall	99.6	98.4	98.3

posture is always recognized even when the user is sideways, given that the output of the tracker is cleaner and reliable in this case. We have to point that these human trackers have been developed for natural interaction and gaming and the players must stand in front of the sensor. As expected, the lying posture is the most challenging to detect, but the rate of the false positive is always null and the actual lying posture is misclassified only with the sitting class and never with the standing. Since the NN is trained with a dataset built on Kinect tracker, using it produces excellent results. However, the use of the NiTE tracker does not involve bad effects. The most interesting result is about the falling test. The NN produces a TPR of 95.1% for the lateral test and 93.3% for the frontal. In particular, if we consider only the lying posture, the frontal fall test has a False Discovery Rate (FDR) of 0%, and the probability of the False Negative Rate (FNR) is 6.7%, while for the lateral fall test the FDR is 0% and the FNR is 4.9%. The overall accuracy is 98.4 and 98.3% respectively. Another important aspect to underline is that, for most of the cases, misclassification happens during postures transitions. These results make it feasible the use of the adopted NN for a falling event application that is described in the next section.

6 Fall Detector Application

Considering the results about the above experiments, a fall detector application has been developed. It is able to generate warning or emergency signals according to the NN output. The Fig. 4 outlines its flowchart. The event generator reads the outputs of the NN storing them with an associated timestamp. When a lying posture is detected and its internal state is not equal to warning, it finds the last standing

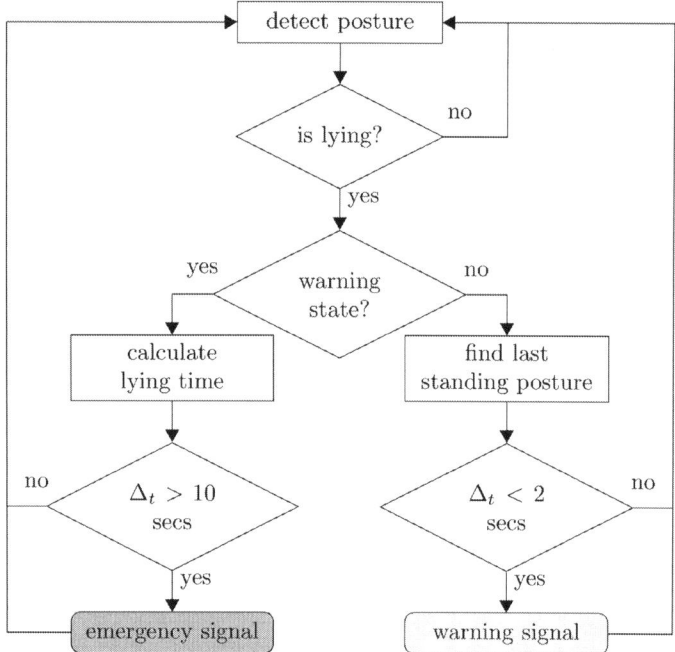

Fig. 4 The fall detector module reads the output of the neural network continuously. According to the posture and to appropriate threshold, it is able to send warning or emergency signals

detected posture and computes the delta time. As already stated by Fu et al. [32], if this value is less than 2 s, the system considers it as a falling event and generates a warning signal. The detector still continues to check the input and if the posture stands in lying position for more than 10 s, it sends also an emergency signal. Currently, we are simulating this system with a domestic robot, which is able to retrieve these kinds of events and react consequently. When the robot receives a warning signal from the falls detector, it moves to the area of interest and starts an interaction procedure with the person to ask him/her if an help is needed. If no answer is received it warns a specific person (i.e. a caregiver or relatives) through a video-call mechanism. If the robot receives an emergency signal, it starts soon an automatic video-call and at the same time it moves to the area of interest to provide as much information as possible to the caregiver.

7   Conclusion and Future Work

In this paper, a feed-forward artificial Neural Network to detect three target postures (i.e. standing, sitting and lying) by means of an RGB-D sensor is presented. The NN is trained with samples extracted from a public dataset recorded with the

Kinect SDK, while the real-time tests are carried out both with the Kinect and the Asus Xtion Pro Live device using the Kinect proprietary skeleton tracker and the NiTE tracker respectively. The input data are preprocessed and normalized in order to be depth invariant, improving the results of the NN all along the field of view of the sensors. The output of these skeleton tracker algorithms in real world application is not always stable and accurate, especially when the user is not standing and parts of the human body are occluded by the person itself or by external objects. A series of real-time experiments, conceived to analyze the behavior of the trained NN in challenging situations, have been conducted. During these tests, the NN processes continuously the output of the skeleton tracker also when the joints are labelled as unreliable. Our results demonstrate its high robustness against the uncertainty of the data, achieving an accuracy of more than 98% for the falling tests. The NN, trained with a Kinect dataset, demonstrates its power of generalization also when it is fed with data produced by a different tracker (NiTE software). Following the results of the experiments, a fall detector application which integrates the NN is also presented. The proposed system runs in real-time and, since it is based only on depth maps that do not use color information it guarantees the privacy of the person and it is able to work also in poor light conditions. Further improvements can be obtained creating an ad hoc database containing fallen people in a real environment. For our best knowledge, an RGB-D dataset of this type is not yet available, and it will concern one of our next works. In this way, it will be possible to train a model using more realistic data. Future developments will also focus on the development of a multiple depth cameras system, which covers areas of the home with high risk of fall, such for example bathroom and bedroom. Moreover, additional depth cameras give the possibility to estimate the user position in the home.

Acknowledgements This work was supported in part by the European Community's 7th Framework Program (FP7/2007–2013) under grant agreement No. 288899 (Robot-Era Project) and grant agreement No. 601116 (Echord++ project).

References

1. Aquilano M, Cavallo F, Bonaccorsi M, Esposito R, Rovini E, Filippi M, Dario P, Car-rozza MC (2012, August) Ambient assisted living and ageing: preliminary results of RITA project. In: 2012 Annual international conference of the IEEE engineering in medicine and biology society, pp 5823–5826
2. Atzori L, Iera A, Morabito G (2010) The internet of things: a survey. Comput Netw 54 (15):2787–2805
3. Suresh S, Sruthi P (2015) A review on smart home technology. In: Online international conference on green engineering and technologies (IC-GET), IEEE, pp 1–3
4. Bonaccorsi M, Fiorini L, Cavallo F, Saffiotti A, Dario P (2016) A cloud robotics solution to improve social assistive robots for active and healthy aging. Int J Soc Robot 1–16
5. Di Nuovo A, Broz F, Belpaeme T, Cangelosi A, Cavallo F, Esposito R, Dario P (2014, October) A web based multi-modal interface for elderly users of the Robot-Era multi-robot

services. In: IEEE international conference on systems, man, and cybernetics (SMC), IEEE, pp 2186–2191

6. Moschetti A, Fiorini L, Esposito D, Dario P, Cavallo F (2016) Recognition of daily gestures with wearable inertial rings and bracelets. Sensors 16(8):1341

7. Tromp A, Pluijm S, Smit J, Deeg D, Bouter L, Lips P (2001) Fall-risk screening test: a prospective study on predictors for falls in community-dwelling elderly. J Clin Epidemiol 54 (8):837–844

8. Stevens JA, Ballesteros MF, Mack KA, Rudd RA, DeCaro E, Adler G (2012) Gender differences in seeking care for falls in the aged medicare population. Am J Prev Med 43 (1):59–62

9. Sung J, Ponce C, Selman B, Saxena A (2011) Human activity detection from rgbd images. Plan Act Intent Recogni 64

10. Chen G, Giuliani M, Clarke D, Gaschler A, Knoll A (2014) Action recognition using ensemble weighted multi-instance learning. In: IEEE international conference on robotics and automation (ICRA), 2014, pp 4520–4525

11. Munaro M, Ghidoni S, Dizmen DT, Menegatti E (2014) A feature-based approach to people re-identification using skeleton keypoints. In: IEEE international conference on robotics and automation (ICRA), 2014, pp 5644–5651

12. Patsadu O, Nukoolkit C, Watanapa B (2012) Human gesture recognition using kinect camera. In: IEEE international joint conference on computer science and software engineering (JCSSE), pp 28–32

13. Le TL, Nguyen MQ, Nguyen TTM (2013) Human posture recognition using human skeleton provided by kinect. In: International conference on computing, management and telecommunications (Com-ManTel), pp 340–345

14. Yu X (2008) Approaches and principles of fall detection for elderly and patient. In: 10th International conference on e-health networking, applications and services. HealthCom 2008, pp 42–47

15. FATE (2016) Fall detector for the elderly. http://fate.upc.edu. Accessed 25 May 2016

16. Bourkeφ A, Scanaillφ CN, Culhaneφ K, OBrien J, Lyonsφ G (2006) An optimum accelerometer configuration and simple algorithm for accurately detecting falls, 2006

17. Bourke AK, Lyons GM (2008) A threshold-based fall-detection algorithm using a bi-axial gyroscope sensor. Med Eng Phys 30(1):84–90

18. Chan M, Est`eve D, Escriba C, Campo E (2008) A review of smart homespresent state and future challenges. Comput Meth Programs Biomed 91(1):55–81

19. Juang CF, Chang CM (2007) Human body posture classification by a neural fuzzy network and home care system application. Syst Man Cybernet Part A Syst Huma IEEE Trans 37 (6):984–994

20. Bian ZP, Chau LP, Magnenat-Thalmann N (2012) A depth video approach for fall detection based on human joints height and falling velocity. In: International conference on computer animation and social agents, 2012

21. Rougier C, Auvinet E, Rousseau J, Mignotte M, Meunier J (2011) Fall detection from depth map video sequences. In: Toward useful services for elderly and people with disabilities. Springer, New York, pp 121–128

22. Schwarz LA, Mkhitaryan A, Mateus D, Navab N (2012) Human skeleton tracking from depth data using geodesic distances and optical flow. Image Vis Comput 30(3):217–226

23. "NiTE GitHub." https://github.com/PrimeSense. Accessed 25 May 2016

24. "OpenNI GitHub." https://github.com/OpenNI. Accessed 25 May 2016

25. Wang J, Liu Z, Wu Y, Yuan J (2012) Mining actionlet ensemble for action recognition with depth cameras. In: IEEE conference on computer vision and pattern recognition (CVPR), 2012, pp 1290–1297

26. Priddy KL, Keller PE (2005) Artificial neural networks: an introduction, vol. 68. SPIE Press, Bellingham

27. Igel C, Hüsken M (2000) Improving the rprop learning algorithm. In: Proceedings of the second international ICSC symposium on neural computation (NC 2000), Citeseer, vol 2000, pp 115–121
28. Riedmiller M, Braun H (1992) Rprop-a fast adaptive learning algorithm. In: Proceedings of ISCIS VII, Universitat, Citeseer
29. Nissen S, Nemerson E (2000) Fast artificial neural network library. Available at leenissen. dk/fann/html/files/fann-h. Html, 2000
30. Guyon I (1997) A scaling law for the validation-set training-set size ratio, AT&T Bell Laboratories, pp 1–11
31. Floreano D, Mattiussi C (2008) Bio-inspired artificial intelligence: theories, methods, and technologies. MIT press, Cambridge
32. Fu Z, Culurciello E, Lichtsteiner P, Delbruck T (2008) Fall detection using an address-event temporal contrast vision sensor, in circuits and systems, 2008. In: IEEE international symposium on ISCAS 2008, pp 424–427

A Tilt Compensated Haptic Cane for Obstacle Detection

Bruno Andò, Salvatore Baglio, Vincenzo Marletta and Angelo Valastro

Abstract Several Electronic Travel Aids (ETA) have been developed to improve the autonomy of impaired people, with specific regard to visually impaired. Such systems often perform a good job in detecting obstacles, identifying services and, generally, obtaining useful information from the surroundings, thus enabling a safe and effective exploitation of the environment. The main drawback of systems developed in the Ambient Assisted Living framework is related to the form and the degree of information provided to the end-user. The arbitrary codifications, often adopted, lead to a diffidence of the user against the proposed solutions. This paper deals with a study on a haptic device aimed to provide the user with information on the presence of obstacles inside the environment. The haptic interface is intended to reproduce the same stimuli provided by a traditional white cane, without any contact with the environment. A real prototype of the system, implemented through a short cane with an embedded smart sensing strategy and an active handle, is presented. The tests performed, with users in good health and blindfolded, confirm the suitability of the proposed solution.

Keywords Assistive systems · Mobility · Visually impaired · Haptic interface · Electronic cane · Navigation aids

B. Andò (✉) · S. Baglio · V. Marletta · A. Valastro
DIEEI—University of Catania, v.le A. Doria 6, 95125 Catania, Italy
e-mail: bruno.ando@dieei.unict.it

S. Baglio
e-mail: salvatore.baglio@dieei.unict.it

V. Marletta
e-mail: vincenzo.marletta@dieei.unict.it

A. Valastro
e-mail: angelo.valastro@gmail.com

© Springer International Publishing AG 2017
F. Cavallo et al. (eds.), *Ambient Assisted Living*, Lecture Notes
in Electrical Engineering 426, DOI 10.1007/978-3-319-54283-6_11

141

1 Introduction

Many systems have been developed with the aim of assisting impaired people in performing daily activities. "Most human activities are carried on in particular places, and no matter how skillful a person may be in other respects, he or she will be excluded from participation in those activities by the inability to get to where they are carried on" [1]. Prestigious reviews of the state of the art in this field can be found in [2–7]. Interesting approaches to assist visually impaired users in mobility tasks include the Russell Pathsounder, the Polaron™, the Kay Sonic Torch, the Sonicguide and the Sonic Pathfinder [8–10], the Mowat Sensor [11], the Nottingham Obstacle Detector, the Laser Cane [12], the Infrared (IR) based Clear Path Indicators described in [13], the Talking Signs, the Sonic Orientation Navigation Aid system and the Kahru Tactile Outdoor Navigator [14, 15]. In [16] an electronic device to be attached to a traditional white cane and aimed to alert users of low-hanging obstacles is presented. The system uses a ultrasonic range sensor and an eccentric mass motor to deliver information about detected obstacles by haptic alerts.

Other approaches exploit vision systems to translate the environmental contents into different forms of perception such as auditory or tactile [17, 18]. Recently, many attempts have been made by researchers to develop effective mobility and navigation aids exploiting new Information and Communication Technology (ICT) based solutions [19–25], also in the field of context-aware systems [26, 27].

In line with the Ambient Assisted Living (AAL) policy, mobility aids should improve the life quality and the well-being of impaired people providing self-confidence and autonomy. To this end, the form in way the information generated by a mobility aid is provided to the end-users strongly affects the approach in developing such kind of helps. In this framework, and as emerges from above examples, the information is often codified in arbitrary forms using tactile or auditory sense. In the last two decades, there has been a growing interest in non-visual forms of presentation. Different solutions based on touch and tactile devices, force feedback joysticks, sound, or smell to represent information, have been proposed [28]. Among these, haptic interfaces play a fundamental role in developing electronic assistive systems for the visually impaired. Gibson (1966) defined haptics as "The sensibility of the individual to the world adjacent to his body by use of his body". Haptic includes both the capability to sense the environment through touch and kinesthesia, meaning the ability to perceive body position, movement and weight (by receptors located in muscles, tendons and joints) [29]. A state-of-the-art survey on haptics is available in [30], while a comprehensive review and classification of haptic methods is given in [31].

Numerous solutions for the realization of haptic interfaces for the visually impaired are available in the literature. In [32] the authors proposed a force-field haptic rendering method for converting videos of 3D maps (used by schools for the visually impaired to teach students how to navigate buildings and streets) to haptic data for off-the-shelf haptic devices. An application of a haptic interface in a tool for orientation and mobility training for visually impaired users is presented in [33]. In this two works authors used a commercial desktop haptic device providing the user with a force feedback. A haptic vision substitution system for visually impaired people, exploiting image processing capabilities of a smartphone platform, was presented in [34]. A vibrotactile stimulator is used in the solution based on a fingertip-mounted camera recently presented in [35]. The proposed solution acts as a sensory substitution system for the user's sense of sight and allows visually impaired users to remotely identify objects of interest and to navigate through natural environments. Anyway no attention was paid to the natural codification of the information provided by the presented solution. The development of haptic interfaces assisting impaired users is discussed in [36–38]. Results from tests of haptic interfaces for visually impaired children are reported in [39].

The above preamble highlights the need for novel "haptic" approaches aimed to provide the end user with information on the perceived environment, by a natural form of codification. This strategy supports avoiding the masking of natural echoes (the user must be always able to "visualize" the environment). The research team of the SensorLab at the DIEEI-University of Catania (Italy) is focusing on advanced multi-sensor systems for AAL and suitable solutions for the user interaction. As an example, in [6] the possibility to make regular contrasted images (fully accessible to normally sighted people while becoming under-threshold stimuli for the visually impaired) accessible to persons with a reduced visual sensitivity, by selectively adding noise to image pixels, is investigated. In [40–42] smart algorithms exploiting inertial data from a multisensor system for the ADL classification, with particular regards to fall events, were presented.

The same group is involved in the development of haptic interfaces to provide visually impaired people with a suitable form of information on the surroundings.

As an example, in [43] the authors proposed a model to convert obstacle positions into a suitable stimulation of the hand palm. Basically, the system exploits a matrix of strain gauges on the handle of a white cane to record the palm deformations due to the interaction between the cane and the obstacles.

In [44] a first implementation of the Haptic Cane is presented. The device exploits a tactile interface to provide information about incoming obstacles and their position within the environment. The haptic tool is installed in the cane handle and provides the user with a codification on the palm similar to the one provided by a traditional white cane bumping against an obstacle. Limitations were related to the adopted smart processing architecture, the cross-interference between actuators installed in the cane handle, and the absence of a cane-floor interaction model allowing for the dynamic setting of the obstacle perception threshold.

In [45] a new obstacle stimulation model is introduced along with the implementation of a cane-floor interaction model to perform an adaptive adjustment of the perception threshold.

In this paper a renewed release of the Haptic Cane is presented, where the cane-floor model has been optimized and implementing auto-calibration features to compensate for the effect of users characteristics.

The terrific advantage of this solution is strictly related to the natural form of user-cane interaction adopted to transfer the information on the obstacle position to the user, compared to traditional forms of codification. This strategy allows for avoiding the masking of natural echoes, improving user confidence in the device and reducing training. Moreover, the proposed methodology avoids unwanted user-environment interactions thus improving the user acceptability of the assistive tool.

2 The Haptic Cane Architecture

The Haptic Cane basically consists of a short cane with an active handle and an embedded smart sensing and processing unit. A real view of the device is shown in Fig. 1.

Although a deep description of the sensing and haptic architecture implementing the assistive tool is given in [44, 45], in the following some notes on the system are provided for the sake of completeness.

In order to detect obstacles and recognize their position in the space in front the user two dual-element high-performance ultrasonic distance ranger modules, Devantech SRF08, have been installed on a short cane (covering the left and right areas in front of the user). Each module employs two ultrasound transducers working at 40 kHz implementing the transmitter (Tx) and the receiver (Rx), respectively. The SRF08 uses an I2C interface for communication with the processing unit. The main task of the sensing tool is the estimation of the obstacle's distance from the user, D_i (where $i = 1, 2$ counts for the ultrasound sensors). The two modules have been installed by assuring the partial overlapping of the conical beam of the two ultrasound transmitters. This strategy assure the detection of obstacle on center.

Conversely to a traditional white cane, the adopted sensing strategy allows for detecting the obstacle position without sweeping the cane from left to right and vice versa. Actually, on the basis of the response of the left-right sensors the obstacle is detected as belonging to the left/central/right position with respect to the user.

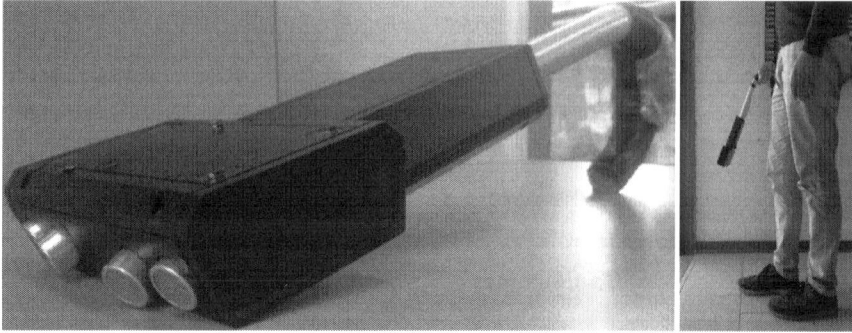

Fig. 1 A real view of the Haptic Cane

A basic assumption is that the user is aware of the cane inclination and hence of the obstacle position along the vertical dimension. Actually, the vertical scanning of the environment is in charge of the user. Visually impaired people sense the position of an obstacle with respect to their body reference frame via proprioception under active exploration, i.e., they move the cane in the space and perceive the position of the cane through the position and orientation of their arm holding the cane.

The Haptic Cane prototype uses a set of 6 flat vibrating actuators, Solarbotics VPM2, which are distributed along the interface between the cane handle and the palm to provide the user with a sensation miming the one produced by a white cane bumping against obstacles. The actuation system has been developed by following a user-centered design approach assuring the user comfort during the system operation. More details on the haptic interface are available in [44, 45]. The total length of the Haptic Cane, L_{HC}, including the sensor head, is 40 cm.

In case an obstacle is detected by the ultrasound sensors, the pattern shown in Fig. 2 is used to provide the haptic stimuli to the user. As it can be observed, three sets of actuators have been used to codify obstacles in the Left, Center and Right positions independently on the vertical position of the obstacle.

A low power three-axis ADXL335 accelerometer has been used for the cane tilt estimation. The system is managed by a Droids Multi Interface Board (MuIn) equipped with a PIC18F2520 Microchip running at 40 MHz, which supports also a wireless link with a dedicated PC station adopted during the development phase and for the sake of system debugging. To such aim a LabVIEW Virtual Instrument (VI) implementing a suitable Graphical User Interface (GUI) has been also developed. The wireless link is implemented through an XBee-PRO module by MaxStream, Inc., which supports the ZigBee transmission protocol (IEEE 802.15.4).

3   The Detection/Stimulation Paradigm

The operation of the Haptic Cane is based on the comparison between distances D_i, measured by the sensors and a threshold D_{TH}. In case one or both the two measured distances are lower than D_{TH} the system reveals the presence of an obstacle along the user path. Since also the floor can be erroneously detected as an obstacle, in

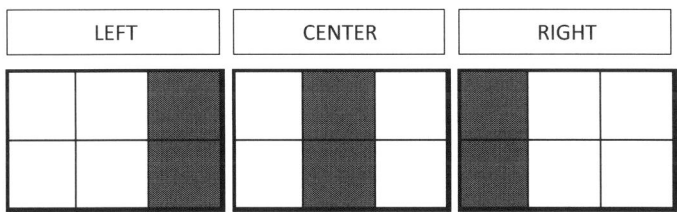

Fig. 2 The matrix of actuators embedded in the cane handle. The actuators activated in case of a Left/Center/Right obstacle is detected are indicated in *dark*

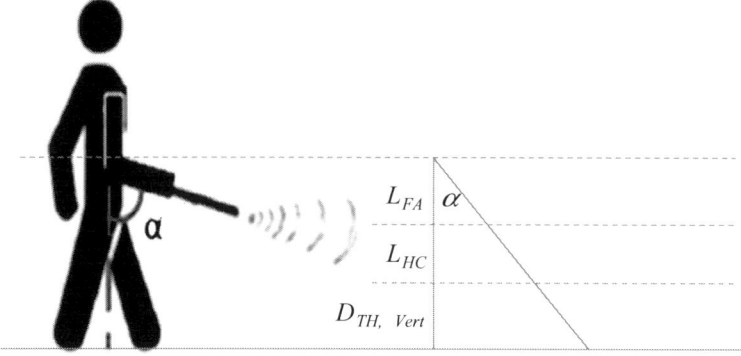

Fig. 3 The effect of the tilt during the Haptic Cane operation

order to avoid false alarms due to the cane-floor interaction, an adaptive estimation threshold D_{TH} has been implemented [44, 45]. The methodology presented in [44, 45] was based on the use of a linear model between the threshold D_{TH} and the cane tilt, α.

In this paper an advanced compensation strategy has been used which requires a calibration phase to fit the compensation model on the user characteristics.

Figure 3 schematizes the effect of the tilt during the Haptic Cane operation. As it can be observed the threshold D_{TH} depends on the cane tilt.

As first, it must be considered that in order to mimic the operation of a traditional cane the working range of the device has been fixed around to 110 cm. When the Haptic Cane is in the vertical position the threshold, D_{TH}, is set to $D_{TH,Vert}$.

In case the cane is tilted, the threshold value, D_{TH}, can be estimated by the following model:

$$
D_{TH}(\alpha) = \begin{cases} \frac{D_{TH,Vert} + L_{HC} + L_{FA}}{\cos(\alpha)} - (L_{HC} + L_{FA}) & \text{if } 0 < \alpha < ar\cos\left(\frac{D_{TH,Vert} + L_{HC} + L_{FA}}{110 + D_{TH,Vert} + L_{HC} + L_{FA}}\right) \\ 110 \text{ cm} & \text{if } \alpha \geq ar\cos\left(\frac{D_{TH,Vert} + L_{HC} + L_{FA}}{110 + D_{TH,Vert} + L_{HC} + L_{FA}}\right) \end{cases}
$$

$$(1)$$

where L_{FA} is the user forearm length.

In order to estimate L_{FA} for each user a calibration procedure has been implemented which requires the user to perform a first measurement with the cane in the vertical position and a next one with an arm-forearm position of 90°. The results of these two measurements, $D_{TH,Vert}$ and D_{Hor}, are acquired by the microcontroller platform in order to estimate the forearm length as:

$$
L_{FA} = D_{Hor} - D_{TH,Vert}
$$

$$(2)$$

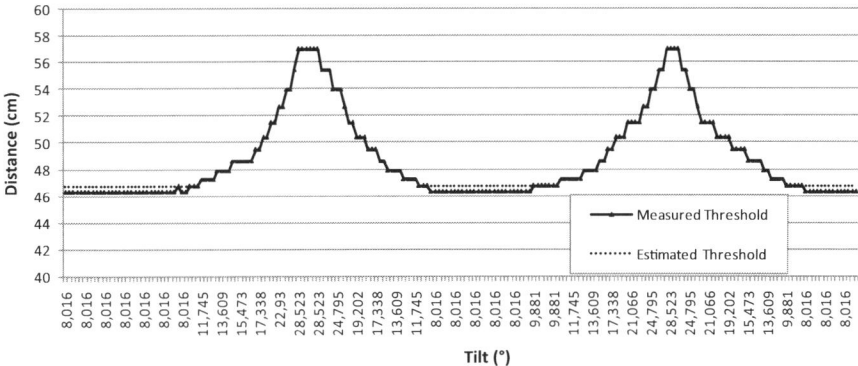

Fig. 4 The comparison between the measured threshold and the one estimated by the system in case of two consecutive repetitions of the cane sweep up to about 20°

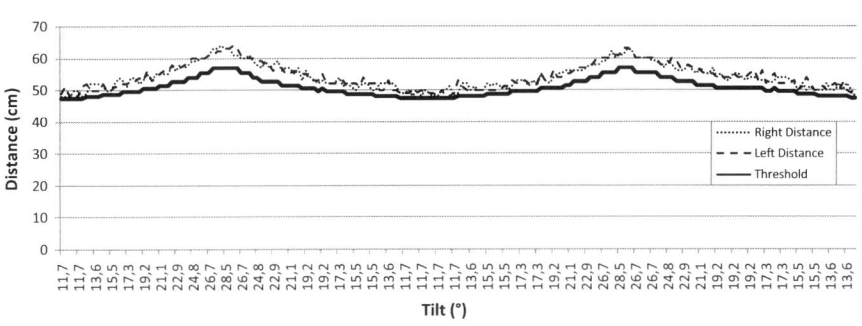

Fig. 5 Tests performed in the absence of obstacles to assess the tilt compensation strategy. The floor distance detected by the two sensors during two consecutive repetitions of the cane sweep of about 20° and the threshold estimated by the system

In order to test the above compensation strategy a number of tests have been performed with real users. Examples of results obtained during the experimental survey are commented in the following notes.

The comparison between the measured threshold and the one estimated by the system in case of two consecutive repetitions of the cane sweep up to about 20° is shown in Fig. 4.

Figure 5 shows the floor distance detected by the two sensors during two consecutive repetitions of the cane sweep of about 20° and the threshold estimated by the system. As it can be observed the threshold is always below the target distances thus avoiding false positive results.

4   Results and Conclusions

The Haptic Cane functionality in the presence of obstacles has been tested by dedicated experiments. Figure 6 shows the distance measured by the ultrasound sensors during a cane sweep in case of (a) a left positioned obstacle, (b) a right positioned obstacle and (c) a center positioned obstacle.

As it can be observed and as expected, in the case of the right/left obstacle one on the two distances measured by the ultrasound sensors are below the threshold, while in case of the central obstacle both distances are under threshold. Experimental results like examples shown in Fig. 6 demonstrated the system reliability.

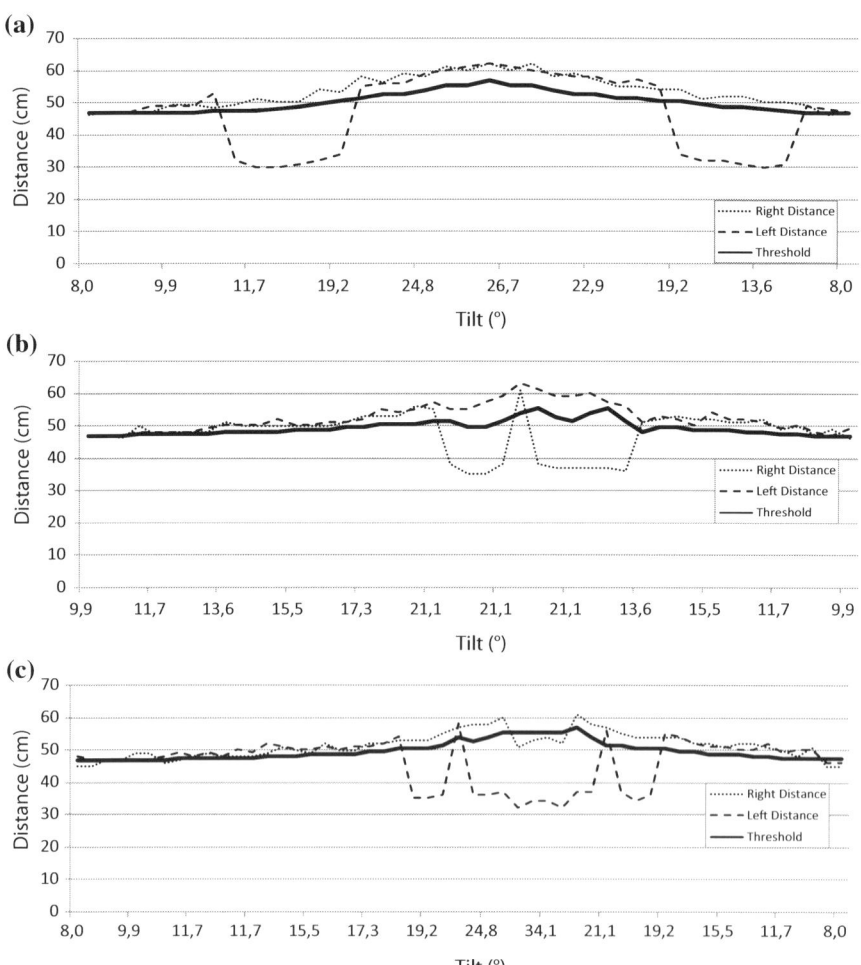

Fig. 6 Tests performed in the presence of obstacles to assess the cane functionality. **a** Left positioned obstacle; **b** Right positioned obstacle; **c** Center positioned obstacle

In conclusion, in this paper an improved version of the Haptic Cane [43–45] has been presented. In particular, a novel compensation strategy has been implemented and tested. The main advantage of the proposed solution consists in the robustness of the device behavior against different characteristics of the user, such as the height.

Moreover, the use of a Haptic interface aims to provide the user with a tactile feedback on the obstacle position which resembles the feeling provided by the traditional white cane. Finally, it must be observed that the sensing architecture do not require sweeping the cane from left to right and vice versa, while the vertical scanning of the environment is left in charge of the user.

Above features, coupled with the possibility to use a short multi-sensor cane which avoids unwanted cane-environment interactions, aims to improve the life quality and the autonomy of visually impaired people.

Considering that the prototype developed aims to the proof of concept of the methodology proposed, future efforts will be dedicated to improve the haptic interface and to extend the system functionality in terms of environment perception and tilt estimation as well as to implement solutions for energy harvesting from human related activities to provide a supplementary power source to the sensing and sensing electronic thus reducing the need for periodic batteries replacement [46–49]. Moreover, a wide set of experimental supervised tests with real users will be performed.

References

1. Committee on Vision (1986) Electronic travel aids: new directions for research. National Academy Press, Washington, D.C.
2. Hersh M, Johnson MA (eds) (2008) Assistive technology for visually impaired and blind people. Springer, London, GB
3. Bujacz M, Baranski P, Moranski M, Strumillo P, Materka A (2008) Remote mobility and navigation aid for the visually disabled. In: Sharkey PM, Lopes-dos-Santos P, Weiss PL, Brooks AL (eds) Proceedings of 7th international conference on disability, virtual reality and association technologies with art abilitation, Maia, Portugal, 8–11 Sept 2008, pp 263–270
4. Velázquez R (2010) Wearable assistive devices for the blind. In: Lay-Ekuakille A, Mukhopadhyay SC (eds) Wearable and autonomous biomedical devices and systems for smart environment: issues and characterization. LNEE 75. Springer, Chap. 17, pp 331–349
5. Farcy R, Bellik Y (2002) Comparison of various interface modalities for a locomotion assistance device. In: Miesenberger K, Klaus J, Zagler W (eds) Computers helping people with special needs. Springer, Berlin, pp 421–428
6. Andò B, Ascia A (2007) Navigation aids for the visually impaired: from artificial codification to natural sensing. IEEE Mag Instrument Meas 10(3):44–51
7. Andò B, Baglio S, La Malfa S, Marletta V (2011) Innovative smart sensing solutions for the visually impaired. In: Pereira J (ed) Handbook of research on personal autonomy technologies and disability informatics. Med. Inform. Science, Hershey, PA, pp 60–74
8. Kay L (1964) An ultrasonic sensing probe as a mobility aid for the blind. Ultrasonics 2:53–59
9. Kay L (1966) Ultrasonic spectacles for the blind. In: Dufton R (ed) Sensory devices for the blind. St. Dunstans, London

10. Russell L (1965) Travel path sounder. In: Proceedings: Rotterdam Mobility Research Conference. American Foundation for the Blind, New York
11. Pressey N (1977) Mowat sensor. Focus 3:35–39
12. Nye PW (1973) A preliminary evaluation of the bionic instruments-veterans administration, C-4 Laser Cane. National Research Council, Washington, D.C., National Academy of Sciences
13. Andò B, Graziani S (2009) Multisensor strategies to assist blind people: a clear-path indicator. IEEE Trans Instrument Meas 58(8):2488–2494
14. Loughborough W (1979) Talking lights. J Vis Impairment Blindness
15. Gemperle F, Ota N, Siewiorek D (2001) Design of a wearable tactile display. In: Proceedings of 5th international symposium on wearable computers, Zurich, CH, pp 5–12
16. Wang Y, Kuchenbecker KJ (2012) HALO: haptic alerts for low-hanging obstacles in white cane navigation. In: IEEE haptics symposium, Vancouver, BC, 4–7 Mar 2012, pp 527–532
17. Meijer P (1992) An experimental system for auditory image representations. IEEE Trans Biomed Eng 39(2):112–121
18. Velazquez R, Fontaine E, Pissaloux E (2006) Coding the environment in tactile maps for real-time guidance of the visually impaired. In: Proceedings of IEEE international symposium on micro-nanomechatronics and human science, Nagoya, Japan, 5–8 Nov 2006, pp 1–6
19. Prudhvi BR, Bagani R (2013) Silicon eyes: GPS-GSM based navigation assistant for visually impaired using capacitive touch braille keypad and smart SMS facility. In: 2013 world congress on computer and information technology (WCCIT), Sousse, 22–24 June 2013, pp 1–3
20. Ahmetovic D (2013) Smartphone-assisted mobility in urban environments for visually impaired users through computer vision and sensor fusion. In: 2013 IEEE 14th international conference on mobile data management, Milan 3–6 June 2013, pp 15–18
21. Tahat AA (2009) A wireless ranging system for the blind long-cane utilizing a smart-phone. In: 10th inteneration conference on telecommunications, ConTEL 2009, Zagreb, 8–10 June 2009, pp 111–117
22. Bujacz M, Baranski P, Moranski M, Strumillo P, Materka A (2008) Remote guidance for the blind—a proposed teleassistance system and navigation trials. In: 2008 conference on human system interactions, Krakow, 25–27 May 2008, pp 888–892
23. El-Koka A, Hwang DK (2012) Advanced electronics based smart mobility aid for the visually impaired society. In: 14th international conference on advanced communication technology (ICACT), Pyeongchang, 19–22 Feb 2012, pp 257–261
24. Andò B, Baglio S, Marletta V, Pitrone N (2009) A mixed inertial & RF-ID orientation tool for the visually impaired. In: IEEE SSD'09, 6th international multi-conference on systems, signals and devices, Djerba, Tunisia, 23–26 Mar 2009, pp 1–6
25. Andò B, Baglio S, Lombardo CO, Marletta V (2014) An advanced tracking solution fully based on native sensing features of smartphone. In: IEEE sensors applications symposium (SAS) 2014, Queenstown, New Zealand, 18–20 Feb 2014
26. Andò B, Baglio S, La Malfa S, Marletta V (2011) A sensing architecture for mutual user-environment awareness case of study: a mobility aid for the visually impaired. IEEE Sens J 11(3):634–640
27. Andò B, Baglio S, Lombardo CO, Marletta V, Pergolizzi EA, Pistorio A (2013) RESIMA: a new WSN based paradigm to assist weak people in indoor environment. IEEE M&N2013, pp 1–4
28. Loftin RB (2003) Multisensory perception: beyond the visual in visualization. IEEE J Comput Sci Eng 5(4):56–58
29. Klatzky RL, Lederman SJ (1999) The haptic glance: a route to rapid object identification and manipulation. In: Gopher D, Koriats A (eds) Attention and performance XVII. Cognitive regulations of performance: interaction of theory and application, Mahwah, NJ, Erlbaum, pp 165–196
30. Varalakshmi BD, Thriveni J, Venugopal KR, Patnaik LM (2012) Haptics: state of the art survey. IJCSI Int J Comput Sci 9(5, 3):234–244

31. Panëels S, Roberts JC (2010) Review of designs for haptic data visualization. IEEE Trans Haptics 3(2):119–137
32. Moustakas K, Nikolakis G, Kostopoulos K, Tzovaras D, Strintzis MG (2007) Haptic rendering of visual data for the visually impaired. IEEE Multimedia 14(1):62–72
33. Schloerb DW, Lahav O, Desloge JG, Srinivasan MA (2010) BlindAid: virtual environment system for self-reliant trip planning and orientation and mobility training. In: IEEE haptics symposium 2010, Waltham, Massachusetts, USA, 25–26 Mar 2010, pp 363–370
34. Akhter S, Mirsalahuddin J, Marquina FB, Islam S, Sareen S (2011) A smartphone-based haptic vision substitution system for the blind. In: 2011 IEEE 37th annual northeast bioengineering conference (NEBEC), pp 1–2, Troy, NY, 1–3 Apr 2011
35. Horvath S, Galeotti J, Bing W, Klatzky R, Siegel M, Stetten G (2014) FingerSight: fingertip haptic sensing of the visual environment. IEEE J Trans Eng Health Med 2
36. Hayward V, Astley OR, Cruz-Hernandez M, Grant D Robles-De-La-Torre G (2004) Haptic interfaces and devices. Sens Rev 24(1):16–29
37. Cassidy B, Cockton G, Coventry L (2013) A haptic ATM interface to assist visually impaired users. In: Proceeding of the 15th international ACM SIGACCESS conference on computers and accessibility, pp 1–8
38. Yoshino K, Shinoda H (2014) Contactless touch interface supporting blind touch interaction by aerial tactile stimulation. IEEE haptics symposium (HAPTICS), Houston, TX, 23–26 Feb 2014, pp 347–350
39. Patomäki S, Raisamo R, Salo J, Pasto V, Hippula A (2004) Experiences on haptic interfaces for visually impaired young children. In: Proceedings of the 6th international conference on multimodal interfaces (ICMI'04), 13–15 Oct 2004, pp 281–288
40. Andò B, Baglio S, Lombardo CO, Marletta V (2015) An event polarized paradigm for ADL detection in AAL context. IEEE Trans Instrum Meas 64(7):1814–1825
41. Andò B, Baglio S, Lombardo CO, Marletta V (2016) A multi-sensor data fusion approach for ADL and fall classification. IEEE Trans Instrum Meas 65(9):1960–1967
42. Andò B, Baglio S, Lombardo CO, Marletta V, Pergolizzi EA (2015) Fall & ADL detection methodologies for AAL. In: Proceedings of the second national conference on sensors, Roma 19–21 Feb 2014. Lecture notes in electrical engineering, vol 319. Springer, pp 427–432
43. Andò B, Baglio S, Pitrone N (2008) A contactless haptic cane for blind people. In: Proceedings of 12th IMEKO TC1 & TC7 joint symposium on man science and measurement, 3–5 Sept 2008, Annecy, France, pp 147–152
44. Andò B, Baglio S, Lombardo CO, Marletta V, Pergolizzi E, Pistorio A, Valastro A (2015) An electronic cane with a haptic interface for mobility tasks. In: Andò B, Siciliano P, Marletta V, Monteriù A (eds) Ambient assisted living, Italian forum 2014, biosystems and biorobotics. Springer, pp 189–200
45. Andò B, Baglio S, Marletta V, Valastro A (2015) A haptic solution to assist visually impaired in mobility tasks. IEEE Trans Hum-Mach Syst 45(5):641–646
46. Andò B, Baglio S, Bulsara AR, Marletta V, Medico I, Medico S (2013) A double piezo—snap through buckling device for energy harvesting. In: IEEE 17th international conference on solid-state sensors, actuators and microsystems (TRANSDUCERS & EUROSENSORS XXVII), Barcelona, 16–20 June 2013, pp 43–45
47. Andò B, Baglio S, Bulsara AR, Marletta V (2013) A bistable buckled beam based approach for vibrational energy harvesting. Sens Actuators, A 211:153–161
48. Andò B, Baglio S, Bulsara AR, Marletta V, Ferrari V, Ferrari M (2015) A low-cost snap-through buckling inkjet printed device for vibrational energy harvesting. IEEE Sens J 15 (6):3209–3220
49. Andò B, Baglio S, Bulsara AR, Marletta V (2014) A wireless sensor node powered by nonlinear energy harvester. IEEE Sensors 2014, Valencia, Spain, 2–5 Nov 2014

Improved Solution to Monitor People with Dementia and Support Care Providers

Laura Raffaeli, Carlos Chiatti, Ennio Gambi, Laura Montanini,
Paolo Olivetti, Luca Paciello, Giorgio Rascioni and Susanna Spinsante

Abstract Assistive Technologies offer the possibility to develop services aimed at improving the Quality of Life of patients and caregivers. Specifically, this work refers to the case of persons with dementia who can live in their homes but need to be assisted. This paper describes a monitoring kit that provides alarms to the caregiver in case of dangerous situations or unusual events detected by the sensors. It is composed by a set of non-intrusive sensors installed within the house, and can be configured in order to best fit with the needs of each patient. The proposed system could have the potentiality to reduce the stress that usually affects the caregivers, due to the continuous effort required and the worry about the patients' safety. The improved system results from an existing solution that has been re-visited according to the feedbacks obtained from a pilot trial.

L. Raffaeli (✉) · E. Gambi · L. Montanini · S. Spinsante
DII, Università Politecnica Delle Marche, Ancona, Italy
e-mail: l.raffaeli@univpm.it

E. Gambi
e-mail: e.gambi@univpm.it

L. Montanini
e-mail: laura.montanini@univpm.it

S. Spinsante
e-mail: s.spinsante@univpm.it

C. Chiatti · P. Olivetti
INRCA, Ancona, Italy
e-mail: c.chiatti@inrca.it

P. Olivetti
e-mail: p.olivetti@inrca.it

L. Paciello · G. Rascioni
ArieLAB Srl, Ancona, Italy
e-mail: l.paciello@arielab.com

G. Rascioni
e-mail: g.rascioni@arielab.com

© Springer International Publishing AG 2017
F. Cavallo et al. (eds.), *Ambient Assisted Living*, Lecture Notes
in Electrical Engineering 426, DOI 10.1007/978-3-319-54283-6_12

Keywords Dementia monitoring · Caregiver support · Mobile app · Data analysis

1 Introduction

The design of so-called Assistive Technologies (ATs) is driven by the aim of improving the Quality of Life (QoL) [1] of end users, including patients, caregivers, and healthcare operators, through the possibility of supporting each of them with specific functionalities and services [2]. This is particularly true for persons with dementia (PwDs), as the lack of an effective and definitive cure makes maintaining or increasing their QoL the primary care goal.

Dementia is a *syndrome*, meaning that it is possible to identify groups of characteristic symptoms, rather than a disease process, with the exception of some types of dementia, such as Alzheimer's Disease (AD). Among the most common symptoms it is possible to mention progressive loss of cognitive functioning, including decision making, mathematics, communication, memory and spatial reasoning. Each PwD experiences dementia symptoms uniquely, and this fact reflects on highly individualized care needs. A nurse or caregiver taking care of a PwD adjusts to his/her symptoms, noticing changes in the person throughout the day, and over longer periods. A certain quality of care is attained when the caregiver is able to interpret behavioral symptoms and, in turn, communicate with the PwD appropriately [3].

Given the above premise, context-aware Ambient Assisted Living (AAL) technologies emerge as the most viable approach for the seamless adaptation of the living environment to the fluctuations of the user's conditions. The design of ATs for dementia looks for technologies that can achieve the same goals of residential caregiving, taking into account the person's level of need, the way ATs are perceived and used, and the resulting outcomes. Four classes of technologies are typically identified [4]: (i) prevention and engagement technologies; (ii) compensation and assistance technologies; (iii) care support, (iv) enhancement and satisfaction.

Home caregiving provided by relatives, or residential caregiving delivered by nurses, may benefit from a smart environment equipped to predict and minimize safety risks, and to contact help when needed. This can be made possible by gathering information on user patterns and environmental risks, by assessing the individual's needs, and activating proper actions to alert when a safety threshold is breached. All these functions pose specific requirements: sensors are needed to collect data [5, 6]; proper communication capabilities are necessary to send alerts and notifications [7]; reasoning algorithms shall be applied to generate knowledge from raw data, by identifying patterns and anomalies [8].

A smart home system may collect biosignals and physiological data which help detect behavioral changes, as well as variations in the user's interaction with the home devices or appliances. A requirement of utmost importance is the possibility to collect such a huge amount of data unobtrusively, and without the need of user's cooperation. Minimizing the interaction required by the user is especially important with dementia, as declines in procedural memory hinder the capabilities of the user itself. Zero Effort Technologies (ZETs) use algorithms to collect, analyze and apply data autonomously and unobtrusively.

This paper presents the technological evolutions in the design of a ZET kit [9] to unobtrusively monitor PwDs, who are still able to stay at home, but need to be assisted, usually by a relative (spouse, husband, son), or a caregiver. The aim of the kit is to support caregivers in monitoring the PwD, trying to reduce the burden of caring, and ensuring a continuous supervision that can automatically generate alarms and prevent risks by analyzing and detecting anomalous behaviors. The original kit was equipped with sensors and sound/visual alarms; the evolved version of the kit, discussed in this paper, supports remote communication and a set of functionalities running locally on a high-performance embedded board. Some of the improvements related to the sensor network have already been applied and tested for the realization of another project [10]. In that case, however, the kit was employed for the monitoring of patients in a nursing home, so the scenario was different.

The paper is organized as follows: Sect. 2 discusses state-of-art projects and technologies for PwD and their caregivers, whereas Sect. 3 provides a detailed description of the proposed system architecture and functionalities. Preliminary results on the proposed system are discussed in Sect. 4; finally, Sect. 5 concludes the paper.

2 Related Works

In this Section, a closer look at ATs for elderly people living at home or in care institutions, typically suffering from different stages of cognitive decline or frailty, is provided. There is a need to distinguish between:

- integrated solutions *versus* solutions looking at single specific aspects;
- systems that act preventively and try to predict potentially harmful incidents *versus* systems that detect either short-term emergencies (e.g. falls), or long-term trends (e.g. changing of eating behaviors).

The majority of the applications developed up to now has been focusing on handling immediate needs, like detecting an emergency situation. In fact, several emergency calling systems are available in the market. Some of them are designed for indoor use [11, 12], others also operate outdoor [13, 14]. Most of the commercially available solutions rely on a worn sensor, typically an armband or necklace, equipped with an emergency button that needs to be pressed to call for help. This raises some concerns: if the person cannot act on the button, because unconscious, or does not wear the device, the emergency situation is not automatically detected and no alarm is activated.

Especially for people with cognitive and memory problems, solutions have been developed to automatically turn off potentially hazardous electrical devices, such as a running oven or iron.

Other solutions initially developed for professional institutions working with PwDs deal with area monitoring, access control, and location tracking. They use Radio Frequency IDentification (RFID) technologies, to detect people entering or exiting areas and rooms in a building [15]. Some of these systems observe and track the paths people walk to raise warnings or alarms in case anomalies are detected. Low power, low cost, and high precision indoor localization systems are still under research.

Algorithms for activity recognition and behavior prediction analyze the data collected by a set of sensors installed in the home of the monitored elderly, to find out what the person is, or has been doing, and detect abnormal situations, emergencies, and anomalous trends. This information is delivered to informal or formal caregivers, to timely react with proper counter-measures. Typically, off-the-shelf sensing technologies are used, such as magnetic sensors for doors and windows, and presence detectors, to acquire the data needed [16, 17]. Sometimes, additional sensors such as pressure based bed sensors, floor mats, or depth cameras [18] are utilized. The aim is to detect so-called Activities of Daily Living (ADLs), and Instrumental ADLs (IADLs) (e.g. cooking, cleaning, managing medication and financial issues), but also basic tasks (walking, dressing, eating, personal hygiene etc.) that directly relate to the level of dependency of the older person [19].

Some projects address their monitoring to detect the symptoms of dementia, such as wandering [20], depression, memory loss [21, 22], counting toilet visits (incontinence) or especially focusing on the sleep patterns and the behavior during the night, as people tend to lose their day-night rhythms with the progress of the syndrome [23].

In general, AAL systems for PwDs should be designed in a way that they work unobtrusively in background, implicitly interacting with the user. However, sometimes explicit user interaction is inevitable or even wished. In this case, the design of User Interfaces (UIs) for people at different stages of dementia shall be carefully addressed.

Compared to other existing solutions, the proposed system does not recognize activities and does not analyze the trend of the patients' conditions. Even if in the system configuration, as will be explained in Sect. 3.4, the caregiver can set some parameters to best adapt his/her needs, however the cognitive stage of the patients does not affect how the system works. Summing up, the system has the following characteristics:

- it is essentially an alarm system for the detection and notification of dangerous events;
- it is a support tool addressed to the caregivers;
- behavior analysis is not provided: only evident abnormal events are recognized;
- it is a passive system, the patients do not interact with it.

3   System Architecture and Functionalities

As already hinted in the Introduction section, this work describes the evolution of a kit for PwDs' monitoring at home. In this section, the system architecture is described (see Fig. 1), and the main applied changes and improvements are discussed.

The core of the system is the so-called "box", composed by a processing unit and two wireless communication interfaces (SubGHz and GSM/GPRS modules). Environmental sensors detect events and contextual information (such as temperature and humidity), and send them to the central unit, through the SubGHz technology. Once the data have been acquired and processed, the box notifies if an alarming event has occurred, by sending an SMS to the subscribed caregivers. The subscription, i.e. the registration of the caregiver's phone number, and the setting of other parameters can be managed through a smartphone application designed to enable both a caregiver and a technician interact with the box, for configuration and installation purposes. Finally, at the end of the day, a report summarizing the most relevant events happened during the day is sent by the box to the remote server through the GPRS module.

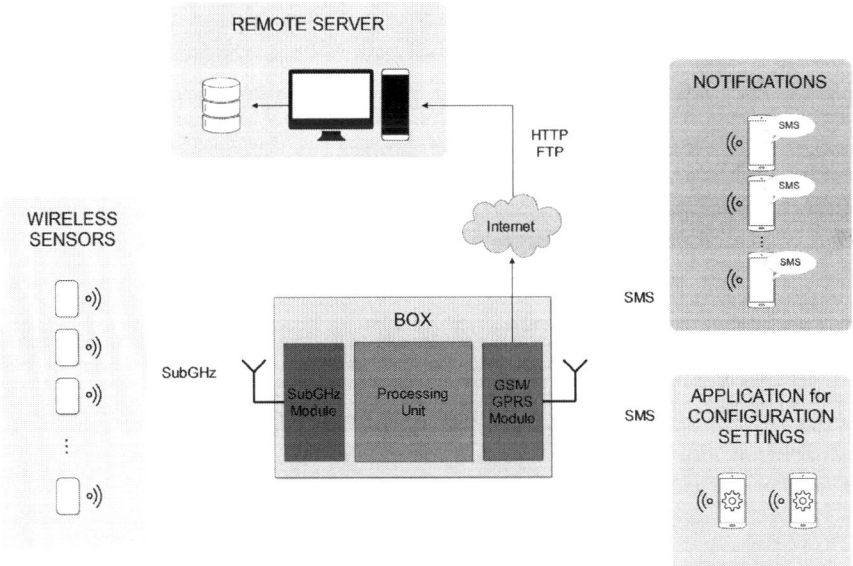

Fig. 1 System architecture representation

3.1 Data Acquisition

The system provides a set of sensors installed within the home, to monitor different aspects of the patient's daily life unobtrusively. In order to keep the installation as simple as possible, a wireless transmission technology has been chosen, specifically a SubGHz technology operating at 868 MHz. Each sensor is connected to a small board in charge of simple processing and data transmission toward a central node. This node is able to identify the data sender thanks to the unique identifier (id) assigned to each sensor. The available sensors are:

- bed presence: a force sensor to detect the patient's presence in bed;
- water: to detect a flooding condition;
- smoke: standard smoke detector;
- magnetic sensors: to be placed on doors and window fixtures, and on the refrigerator door;
- presence sensor: passive infra-red (PIR) sensor to detect the patient's presence in the bathroom;
- temperature and humidity sensors.

Furthermore, a smart control unit, the box, is placed at home to manage the entire monitoring system. The core element of the box is a single-board computer, and is equipped with a module operating in the SubGHz band, to acquire sensors data, and with a GSM/GPRS module for sending voice and text messages, and also for data uploading to a remote server. Finally, a switch enables and disables the alarms for the detection of the events. The detailed mode of operation of the box is described in the following sub-section.

3.2 Data Processing

As highlighted in Fig. 2, the software architecture of the platform is composed by different blocks, that communicate with each other. In particular there are:

- modules that listen for events (such as events generated by wireless environmental sensors, or incoming SMS);
- modules that elaborate events/data;
- modules that execute real time or scheduled actions, through the GSM/GPRS module.

The box represents the central unit that receives information from the sensor network built around the monitoring area, and also manages the user interaction. At the system startup, the configuration phase runs, in which the software activates all the modules appointed to monitor different situations or events, and discovers the enabled sensors. At the end of this phase, the "Events Elaborator Module" (the real core of the application) is started.

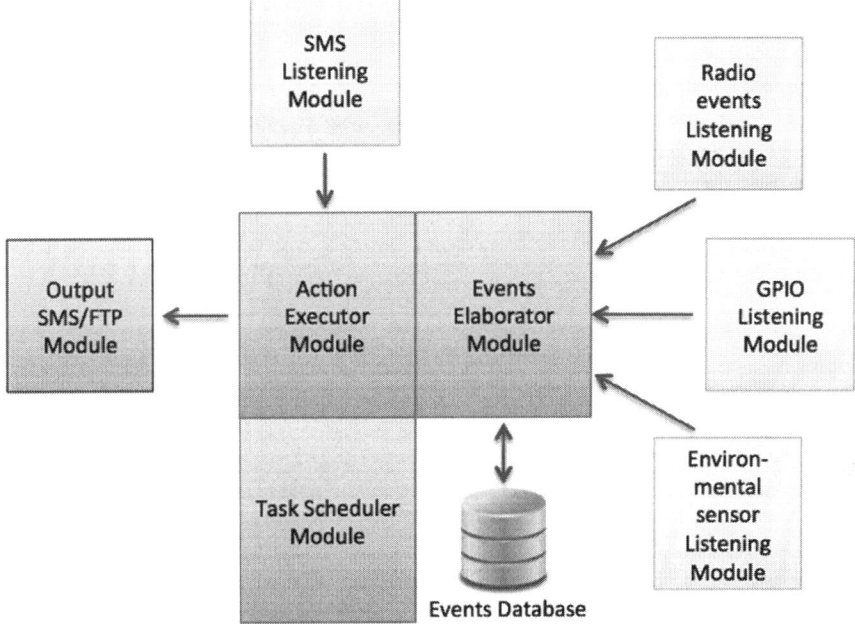

Fig. 2 Main blocks of the platform software architecture

This module runs cyclically, checking for new events every 5 s: if an event is arrived, it is managed by undertaking specific actions in accordance with its type, as described later. The Events Elaborator Module applies a check, called "One Minute Check", to monitor the state of the system (peripherals, database) and the state of all the enabled sensors, analyzing, for example, if there are communication errors. Each sensor has to be treated in a different way, by following a logical workflow describing the behavior modeled for that type of sensor. In general, for every sensor different types of events can occur:

- *birth* event, related to the startup of the radio board;
- *scenario* event, related to the activation/deactivation for digital sensors, or to the acquired value for analog sensors;
- *alive* event, created with a certain frequency (in this case fixed to 6 h) in order to ensure the system that the radio board connected to the sensor is powered and active.

In order to explain how the system works, the workflows of operations associated to two different sensors are described. The former refers to the "access" sensor typology, for example a magnetic sensor located adjacent to door and windows in order to monitor if a person has opened or closed them. The evaluation is different depending on the arrival of an event or a One Minute Check. The One Minute Check evaluates only if there are communication errors, while in case of an event, it is possible to distinguish if the board has restarted or if the magnetic contact has been opened or closed. Obviously, only the opening event is considered as an alarm. The latter case refers to the "bed" typology, where the alarm condition is related to the fact that the user is not returning to bed over a certain time interval, during the night period defined by the caregiver. This means that a scenario event is treated in a completely different way with respect to the case previously described.

This way the system is really flexible and it is possible to manage every type of sensor or condition in a seamless way. From the functional point of view, another important part of the software concerns the actions performed by the system, as a reply to events. These actions are controlled by the "Action Executor Module" that exploits the GSM/GPRS module for the communication. Besides, the software is completed by the "Scheduler Module" which is able to manage scheduled actions, in this case regarding the creation of a daily report to send to the caregiver, in order to inform him/her about the state of the monitoring.

3.3   Notification Management

The control unit handles the generation of notifications caused by several types of events. It is able both to send a text message (SMS) to the caregiver, and to perform a call, sending him/her a pre-recorded voice message that varies depending on the specific event to notify. One of the main differences between the solution described in this paper and the system developed previously concerns the confirmation of the notification delivery to the caregivers or patient's relatives. In fact, it is important to ensure that the caregiver has received the message and distinguish a true answer from an answering machine. For this reason, the improved version of the kit requires the person called to confirm the receiving of the message by pressing a key on the phone.

The system foresees the configuration of two lists of people: the former can include up to six caregivers, the latter includes two installers. Notifications can be related to the events generated by the sensors, or to the configuration requests issued by a caregiver or installer. In the first case, the processing unit evaluates each event in order to classify it as an alarm or not. The following situations are considered as "alarms":

- the door or window is open;
- the patient wakes up and does not get back to bed within a certain time interval (during nighttime);
- the refrigerator door has not been opened for a long time (over a fixed time interval);
- the patient has not accessed a certain area of the house for a defined time interval;

- activation of smoke and water detectors.

Moreover, other two alarm conditions can be detected by the environmental sensors:

- the temperature is above or below a threshold;
- the humidity rate exceeds a certain threshold.

If an alarm event is recognized, the first person in the caregivers' list is called; in case of no answer, the control unit tries with the following one, till the end of the list. If none of the persons answers, an SMS is sent. Another function offered by the system is the daily dispatch of a message containing the most important events occurred during the day: in this case, it is sent to all the caregivers.

The second notification type is referred to the configuration requests made by means of a mobile application, which is described widely in Sect. 3.4. In fact, as visible, several parameters have to be set, such as time intervals and thresholds, that are properly formatted and sent to the box as SMSs. Likewise, an SMS is sent back from the box to the user with a response.

Finally, in order to increase the system reliability, if the detected event concerns the system operation, such as a malfunctioning, a text message is provided, addressed to the phone numbers of the installers included in the list.

3.4 System Configuration

In order to allow the ongoing dynamic configuration of the kit, an Android application for tablet and smartphone devices has been implemented. A mechanism which allows to configure the processing unit was already provided in the previous version of the project. It gives the possibility to modify some parameters through a web interface, accessible by connecting the box to a computer, with an Ethernet cable. Such a solution was designed to be used as a one-off operation, only by installers. In fact, caregivers could not customize the kit in its first version according to their needs and to those of the elderly to be monitored.

The application presented below is intended to overcome this lack, permitting to dynamically configure the system wherever the user is, in a simple and convenient way. It foresees two access modality: installer and caregiver, selectable via an initial login form. The user interface[1] is the same both for caregivers and installers, but some more technical features are available exclusively to the latter.

As shown in Fig. 3, the functionalities are divided into three main topics: *general*, *notification*, and *account*. The three topics can be selected by a tab bar located on the top of the view.

---

[1]Most of icons provided by Icons8.

Fig. 3 Android application
interface for the settings
management: on the *top view*
there is a tab bar to select the
type of settings; on the central
part of the interface all
functionalities related to the
chosen topic are shown;
finally on the *bottom*, a button
allows to save the changes
and send them to the
processing unit

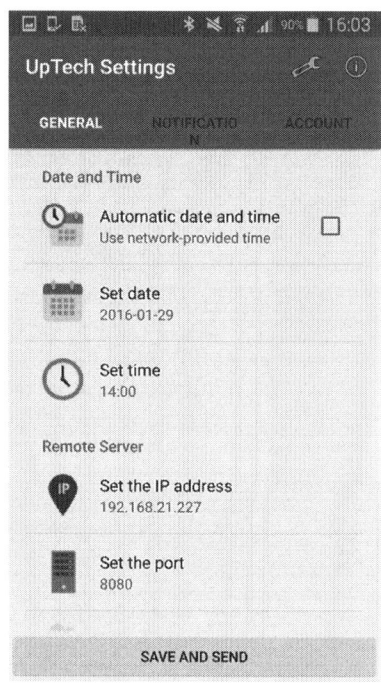

In the *general* tab there are all features referring to the system general functioning. More specifically, they allow the user to:

- set date and time;
- set parameters to access the remote server;
- check the residual credit on the box SIM card;
- set values for the box functioning and request information about its current state;
- request to forward data reports to the remote server;
- request the sensor configuration.

Naturally, all the features related to the setting of specific operating parameters, and the report or configuration requests, can be acted upon only by the installer, who has the appropriate skills to manage and use them.

The *notification* section allows, instead, to modify values concerning the detection of alarms, or to disable notifications from one or more sensors. Specifically, the user can:

- set thresholds (e.g. temperature and humidity limit values);
- enable/disable the receipt of notifications from some or all sensors;
- set timeout values, i.e. the time interval required in some particular situations, as listed in Sect. 3.3.

Finally, the *account* tab enables to modify the information about the users who interact with the system. Particularly, it is possible to:

- modify the personal password;
- add/remove the caregivers' phone numbers;
- add/remove the installers' phone numbers.

The last feature is available only for installers.

Once the user has applied the desired changes, he/she can save and send them to the box by clicking the "save and send" button on the bottom of the screen. In such a case, it is possible to check the modified settings from a summary window (Fig. 4) and decide whether to transmit them or apply further changes.

The Android application communicates with the box through SMSs. The communication protocol is conceived with the aim to reduce the number of characters sent, and consequently the costs. When the caregiver or the installer wants to change a setting or submit a request to the box, the message will be forwarded in the following format:

TECHHOME#FeatureCode#[Parameters]

The SMS starts with the "TECHHOME" keyword, followed by an hash symbol, a numerical code, and then another hash symbol. Optionally it is possible to add some parameters separated by commas. The numerical code allows to establish the desired feature. In fact, for each functionality an identification code and, in some cases, specific parameters are provided. To submit multiple commands on the same message, the "feature code—parameters" pairs must be appended until the number of characters available for a message has finished.

For example, to issue a command to the box for editing the maximum and minimum temperature thresholds and the disabling of notifications coming from a certain sensor, a message as follows is sent:

TECHHOME#0007#MAX-30,MIN-15#0009#DIS-10

where 0007 is the numerical code identifying the temperature threshold feature, the number 30 is the maximum value in degrees, and 15 the minimum. The 0009 code represents, instead, the enabling/disabling of a sensor; the "DIS" keyword indicates the disabling and the number 10 is the id of the sensor to disable. The same message format is adopted also when the box needs to forward information to the smartphone, for example the sensors configuration.

3.5 Remote Storage

The project foresees the adoption of a remote server that collects data of several users. The introduction of this element, which was not present in the previous architecture, is mainly due to the following reasons:

- the availability of information about a patient enables to perform a long-term analysis of his/her condition;

Fig. 4 Summary window to
check the modified settings
before sending them to the
box

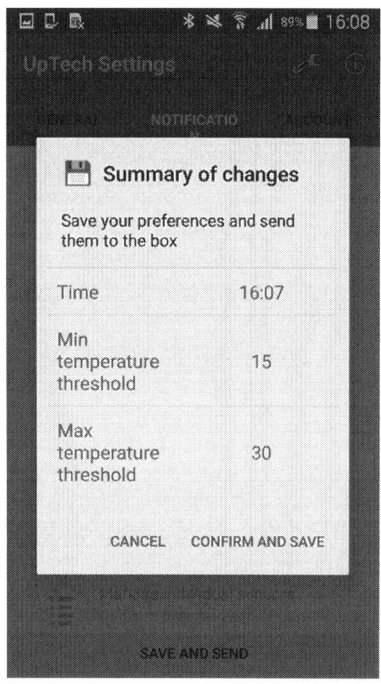

- to allow care providers and medical personnel to access the patient's data for monitoring purpose;
- to access information remotely;
- to overcome memory space problems of the home box.

Each evening, the processing unit creates a report containing all the information related to the daily activities. It includes the events collected by the sensors, the requests made through the configuration app, and the notifications, in addition to status information of the box. This report is sent to the remote server over a GSM/GPRS connection, through the File Transfer Protocol (FTP). The report structure follows a JSON formatting (JavaScript Object Notation), whose main fields are:

- box_number,
- report_date,
- last_boot_date,
- last_boot_state,
- sensors,
- notifications,
- requests.

The box that have sent the file is recognized by means of a unique identifier, the "box_number". The "last_boot_date" indicates day and time of the last boot of the box, which is currently in the "last_boot_state" (e.g. "Configured"). Each element of the array "sensors" corresponds to one of the sensors installed in the house. Some specific information are included: id, name, type and minimum RSSI value (Received Signal Strength Indicator) registered during the day. Furthermore, the sensor events are listed, grouped by type: Activations, Deactivations, Errors, Births, Timeouts. As an example, the structure of one element of "sensors" could be the following:

```
{
"sensor_id": 11,
"name": "sensorName",
"sensor_type": 1,
" rssi_min": "low_value",
"activations": [
{"id_event":112233,   "date_event":"18-01-2016 08:57:07"},
{"id_event":112234,   "date_event":"18-01-2016 09:45:07"},
]
"deactivations": [...],
"births": [...],
"errors": [...],
"timeouts": [...]
}
```

All the events have their own id, which is unique within the box. The RSSI value is helpful to recognize whether the sensor battery is low. Some arrays can be empty in the report: in fact, it is possible for example that no errors have occurred during the day. Moreover, different sensors provide different types of events: for example, the temperature and humidity sensors just provide activations and errors, or the timeout event is not present for water and smoke sensors.

The array "requests" contains the operations performed by the system installer or caregiver through the configuration application described in paragraph 3.4. A unique identifier is associated to each request, which is also composed of the timestamp of the operation, the user identification and type (installer/caregiver), the requested parameters and the result (success or not).

All the events and requests that have generated a notification are listed in the "notifications" array. Thus, each item includes the id of the corresponding event or request. Notifications can consist of a call or an SMS toward the mobile phone numbers provided during the system configuration. The first choice is generally the call, and in case of no answer an SMS is sent, as explained in Sect. 3.3. The outcomes of this procedure are reported as follows:

```
"called_caregivers": [
{"number": "3331234567", "answer": 0},
{"number": "3474142433", "answer": 0},
{"number": "3382122233", "answer": 0}
],
"sms_notification": 1
```

Both the numbers and results of the calls are present, and also the indication of the SMS notification (1 if sent, 0 if not sent). In this example, none of the caregivers answered, thus an SMS has been sent.

The creation and forwarding of the JSON file is only the first step in the remote storage and data management. The authors are also working on the set up of a server with a twofold purpose: not only to store the file with the patient's data, but also to provide a web interface to display information. On one hand, the FTP connection for the daily report exchange is replaced by the HyperText Transfer Protocol (HTTP). The server processes the requests by extracting information and inserting it in a database. On the other hand, a web interface is provided, in which a user (e.g. caregiver) can log in with his credentials and access the various sections: events, requests, notifications and RSSI values. The contents are organized in different web pages and in a tabular fashion, in order to display the information more clearly.

4   Preliminary Tests and Discussion

At the end of the previous pilot, participants filled in a satisfaction questionnaire which has allowed to understand the strong and weak aspects of the technological kit. Among the weak aspects, it has emerged for example that some sensors showed operating problems and caused false alarms [24]. To overcome these problems, the bed and water sensors have been replaced. In fact, the new bed sensor provides a calibration that adapts the sensing to the patient's weight. As for the flooding detection, a different type of device have been chosen to avoid the false alarms due to high humidity rates. Additionally, these events generate acoustic alarms locally, that in some cases have frightened the users, and therefore have been removed.

With respect to the first realization, other sensors have been included in the kit to enhance the degree of monitoring. A presence sensor is used to monitor the user's presence in a room, for example to verify that he/she enters the bathroom periodically. Moreover, a magnetic sensor placed on the refrigerator door can detect its opening and thus give information about eating.

In the first kit, in case of unexpected energy blackout, the processing unit shut down abruptly. In order to avoid this situation, a battery pack have been added to the box, so that the processing unit can continue its normal operation for a certain time interval. Then, if the interruption prolongs over time, it shuts down in a controlled and correct way.

As already described, one of the main improvements brought by the new kit is the remote communication toward a server, to send data related both to users and system operation. From the reliability point of view, this makes possible a continuous monitoring, the detection of eventual malfunctions and a prompt intervention if necessary. In the feedbacks received by the users, some have pointed out that the box is quite big, so it does not look good and occupies space. Thanks to more accurate design and technical choices, it has been possible to remove some elements and thus significantly reduce the dimension of the box. Finally, at the caregivers' opinion, the system should be more flexible, and adaptable to the patient's needs. Therefore, the configuration of some parameters has been made easier and user-friendly thanks to the mobile application.

After the implementation of the new kit, a prototype composed by a complete set of sensors and a central unit has been tested in a laboratory environment. The test is divided into three parts.

The first, lasting two weeks, consisted in the installation, configuration and normal daily usage of the system. All the dangerous situations requiring alarm notifications (see Sect. 3.3) have been verified in the laboratory. Several tests have been performed in order to check the capability if the control unit to contact the selected phone numbers in the expected order, through a call or SMS, and in different possible conditions, such as phone off, rejected or missed calls, for both home and mobile phone numbers. One of the goals of the proposed solution is to try to reduce care burden and stress among caregivers through the use of technology. In order to do this, the home monitoring kit must have as few problems as possible, avoid false alarms, and promptly notify malfunctions. Also thanks to the data log created in the normal system operation, it has been possible to detect and solve a few minor problems that occurred during the test. After completing these interventions, no technical issues emerged at the end of this first stage, as the system correctly detects and notifies alarms.

For the second part of the test, the transmitter boards have been disconnected from the sensors and connected temporarily to another board to perform a "stress" test. This board has been programmed to simulate signals corresponding to the ones generated by the sensors, but with such a frequency that the number of events of a whole year have been generated in a few hours. Despite the high number of events generated with a frequency absolutely impossible for real-life situations, the system continued to work correctly. The only effect observed was a delay between the event detection and its notification, due to the increasing queue of events to be processed.

A third significant test has been done, by switching on/off the system around 100 times randomly, so to prove the behavior of the new solution to sudden and not expected power-leaks.

The solution described in this paper takes part in a wider project, that will test the impact of the designed technology to support the caregivers of PwDs who are still living in the community. The hypothesis is that technology can substitute in part the time caregivers spend in supervision and monitoring activities for patients. The decreased time is expected to reduce the caregiver burden, and thus result in an overall improvement of quality of life for carers and PwDs.

5 Conclusion

This paper presents a system aimed at supporting the caregivers in monitoring the PwDs. It consists in a ZET kit, able to ensure the continuous monitoring of the subject, the automatic generation of alarms, and the prevention of dangerous situations, simply by analyzing the data collected by environmental sensors and sending notifications to caregivers. The system described so far is an evolution of a previous solution, tested on a large group of users. The feedbacks obtained allowed the authors to make significant improvements oriented toward the caregivers' specific needs.

The new solution presented in this paper has been thoroughly tested by both functional and stress tests in a laboratory environment.

The project foresees a controlled trial lasting 12 months, which will start soon and will take place in Sweden, thanks to an international collaboration. A total of 320 dyads including PwDs and their primary informal caregivers (640 participants in total) will be recruited. They all will receive home visits from a dementia nurse in charge of data collection. Among them, an "intervention" group will also have the technological monitoring kit installed in their homes.

References

1. Logsdon RG, Gibbons LE, McCurry SM et al (2002) Assessing quality of life in older adults with cognitive impairment. Psychosomatic Med 64:510–519
2. Mitseva A, Peterson CB, Karamberi C et al (2012) Gerontechnology: providing a helping hand when caring for cognitively impaired older adults—intermediate results from a controlled study on the satisfaction and acceptance of informal caregivers. Curr Gerontech Ger Res. doi:10.1155/2012/401705
3. Peterson CB, Prasad NR, Prasad R (2012) The future of assistive technologies for dementia. Gerontech 11(2):259
4. Van Bronswijk JEMH, Bouma H, Fozard JL (2002) Technology for quality of life: an enriched taxonomy. Gerontech 2(2):169–172
5. Gasparrini S, Cippitelli E, Spinsante S et al (2014) A depth-based fall detection system using a kinect sensor. Sensors 14(2):2756–2775
6. Gasparrini S, Cippitelli E, Gambi E et al (2015) Performance analysis of self-organising neural networks tracking algorithms for intake monitoring using kinect. In: Proceedings of 1st IET international conference on technologies for active and assisted living (TechAAL), November 5th, 2015, Kingston (UK), IET Conference. doi:10.1049/ic.2015.0133
7. De Santis A, Gambi E, Montanini L et al (2015) Smart homes for independent and active ageing: outcomes from the TRASPARENTE project. In: Proceedings of the 2015 Italian forum on ambient assisted living, Lecco (IT), May 2015
8. Spinsante S, Gambi E, Montanini L et al (2015) Data management in ambient assisted living platforms approaching IoT: a case study. In: Proceedings of the 1st international workshop on internet of things for ambient assisted living (IoTAAL)—IEEE Globecom 2015, December 6th, 2015, San Diego (USA)

9. Chiatti C, Rimland JM, Bonfranceschi F et al (2014) The UP-TECH project. An intervention to support caregivers of Alzheimer's disease patients in Italy: preliminary findings on recruitment and caregiving burden in the baseline population. Ag Men Health 1–9

10. Montanini L, Raffaeli L, De Santis A et al (2016) Overnight supervision of Alzheimer's disease patients in nursing homes—system development and field trial. In: Proceedings of the 2nd international conference on information and communication technologies for ageing well and e-Health (ICT4AWE). April 21–22, 2016, Rome (Italy)

11. TeleAlarm (2016) TeleAlarm security and telecare. http://www.telealarm.com/en. Retrieved 14 Mar 2016

12. Tunstall (2016) Tunstall Healthcare. http://www.tunstall.co.uk/. Retrieved 14 Mar 2016

13. NEAT (2016) NEMO portable alarm trigger with GPS and GSM. http://www.neatgroup.com/se/en/carephones/nemo/. Retrieved 14 Mar 2016

14. Limmex (2016) Limmex emergency watch assistance at the push of a button. https://www.limmex.com/intl/en. Retrieved 14 Mar 2016

15. Kaba (2016) Kaba TouchGo—open doors with just a touch. http://www.kaba.com/care. Retrieved 14 Mar 2016

16. RelaxedCare Consortium (2016) RelaxedCare: connecting people in care situations. http://www.relaxedcare.eu/de/. Retrieved 14 Mar 2016

17. ALLADIN Consortium (2016) ALLADIN Project. http://www.aladdin-projecteu/. Retrieved 14 Mar 2016

18. Gasparrini S, Cippitelli E, Spinsante S et al (2015) Depth cameras in AAL environments: technology and real-world applications. In: Theng LB (ed) Assistive technologies for physical and cognitive disabilities. IGI Global, Hershey, Pennsylvania

19. Tapia EM, Intille SS, Larson K (2004) Activity recognition in the home using simple and ubiquitous sensors. In: Ferscha A, Mattern F (eds) Pervasive computing: second international conference, PERVASIVE 2004, Linz/Vienna, Austria, April 21-23, 2004. Proceedings, Springer, Berlin, Heidelberg

20. Future-Shape (2016) SensFloor in care, large area sensor system provides support in the event of fall detection or wandering behaviour. http://www.future-shape.de/. Retrieved 14 Mar 2016

21. MyLife Products AS (2016) Memas, your memory assistants, coordination, pleasure and safety. https://www.mylifeproducts.no/en/. Retrieved 14 Mar 2016

22. MyLife Consortium (2016) MyLife, technology for participation, wellbeing and quality of life. http://www.karde.no/mylife-project.org/. Retrieved 14 Mar 2016

23. Wang H, Zheng H, Augusto JC et al (2010) Monitoring and analysis of sleep pattern for people with early dementia. In: 2010 IEEE International conference on bioinformatics and biomedicine workshops proceedings, pp 405–410

24. UpTech Project final report (2014)

Open Source Technologies as a Support for Community Care

Giada Cilloni, Monica Mordonini and Michele Tomaiuolo

Abstract According to current definitions, health can not be merely intended as the absence of disease or infirmity. In this sense, for maintaining health, the coordination and collaboration among social and health systems is becoming essential, and it can happen only though the harmonization of existing and new integrated information systems. In this study, we will discuss the main requirements which are usually expected from applications for health and social care. For this purpose, the features of a number of commercial applications will be presented. Finally, we will confront these requirements and features with those obtainable trough available open source projects, when opportunely integrated.

Keywords Community care · Well-being and active ageing · Disability and rehabilitation · Health

1 Introduction

The environment in which health care and social services are being provided is changing by the day. In fact, significant societal changes are the mark of these years including ageing of population, growing value attributed to personal care, preference for living at home also when needing assistance, interconnection and integration of diverse services.

The concept of self-care is founded on the representation of an ill person not as a simple passive receiver of health services but, on the contrary, as the first and main "operator" of the care work towards his own health. M. Stacey was among the first

G. Cilloni (✉) · M. Mordonini · M. Tomaiuolo
University of Parma, Parma, Italy
e-mail: giada.cilloni@studenti.unipr.it

M. Mordonini
e-mail: monica.mordonini@unipr.it

M. Tomaiuolo
e-mail: michele.tomaiuolo@unipr.it

© Springer International Publishing AG 2017
F. Cavallo et al. (eds.), *Ambient Assisted Living*, Lecture Notes
in Electrical Engineering 426, DOI 10.1007/978-3-319-54283-6_13

persons to acknowledge the importance of including the patient into the health work: "*A patient can be said to be a producer as much as a consumer of that elusive and abstract good: health*" [1]. Self-care regards the maintenance of personal health: it includes all the choices that people adopt for themselves and their families to stay in good shape, physically and mentally.

Care provision is usually based on either the effort of relatives, or hospitals and care centers. Since recent years, both those approaches are being questioned and the situation is changing. In fact, the support of relatives is becoming less viable, as family members are frequently occupied with work. On the other side, the relocation of patients, elders and people who need social care, outside of their communities, is not desirable for their own wellness; in many cases it is not even necessary, as they preserve enough strength and capabilities to stay at home. Moreover, rooms in hospitals and care centres are in a limited number and the trend is toward their reduction, in spite of a growing number of elders. As a consequence, the traditional approach to provide cares and social services in hospitals and institutional centres is being paralleled with a growing tendency to provide cares in the community, directly. In this kind of "community care" or "domiciled care", services to assisted people are provided directly into their home or into their habitual environment, allowing them to continue to live as much independently as they can. Home-care (or family-care) is founded on the role of caregivers and it is characterized by their strong affective involvement towards the ill person. An important fact, which is not always emphasized enough, is the large support provided by family, community members and other informal carers who can be paradoxically excluded from the rest of the community care. In fact, two types of caregivers can be easily identified:

- an "informal" caregiver, also called primary caregiver, can be a son or daughter, a spouse or more rarely another relative or friend; an informal caregiver performs a non paid work and, in most cases (about 73% [2]), is a female person, usually a wife or a daughter;
- a "formal" caregiver is instead a nurse or any other health care professional.

The range of services varies from the delivery of meals and other goods to domestic help, from generic home monitoring and assistance to nursing and medical care. Until the recent past, health care was meant mainly in terms of services provided by public agencies. Today it is possible to distinguish at least six sources from which it can be originated:

- sociological and health assistance provided by public services;
- voluntary associations and social cooperatives;
- informal care provided as family help;
- mutual-assistance groups;
- profit-making private assistance;
- local programmes of neighborhood assistance (voluntary organizations, churches, etc.).

Usually, those services are supplied by a number of organizations and agencies, which act largely in an independent way, with different responsibilities and goals. However, all those agencies and informal carers need to coordinate their actions, in order to avoid serious service inefficiencies, and so they need the availability of systems to share information about the recipient, without breaching the official confidentiality requirements [3, 4, 5]. The coordination of these autonomous bodies and individuals in a comprehensive information system is a challenging problem, that could result in misunderstandings among the involved professionals, ignorance of important notions about the patient, fragmentation of care, overlapping and duplication of assessments. Involving autonomous entities, the communication process aimed at reaching a mutually accepted agreement on the overall care management often takes the form of a negotiation process [6].

In fact, the main aim of this paper is to analyze these various problems, advancing some possible solutions. In particular, it will deal with the organization and coordination of information and services among social and health systems, from both the points of view of their actual opportunity and their technical feasibility.

First, in the following sections, the need for an holistic care management is explained and an overview of existing software for community care is illustrated. Then, the main use cases and their implementation in a case study on an open-source platform are presented. Finally, a functional evaluation of the tested prototype and some conclusions close the article.

2 The Need for Holistic Care Management

The article 25 of the declaration of human rights says: "*Everyone has the right to a standard of living adequate for the health and well-being of himself and of his family, including food, clothing, housing and medical care and necessary social services, and the right to security in the event of unemployment, sickness, disability, widowhood, old age or other lack of livelihood in circumstances beyond his control.*" This way, it puts social assistance and health care on the same level, for guaranteeing the wellness of an individual. World Health Organization defines health as "*a complete state of physical, mental and social well-being, and not merely the absence of disease or infirmity*". Maintaining health thus requires more than what the traditional health-care systems can provide. Social assistance systems, including personal hygiene and nutrition, are essential to maintain in good health a number of individuals, especially elders [7]. Thus, the coordination and collaboration among social and health systems is becoming essential, and it can happen only though the harmonization of existing informative systems and new integrated ones. Nowadays informatics solutions have been mainly oriented towards formal health-care services, and much less towards social assistance.

The current tendency is to manage the provision of cares in complex systems, based on the interaction of a number of different entities, including neighbourhood and institutional care centres, daycares and social security institutions, each of them involving people with various roles e.g. health care professionals, social care assistants, assisted people and their relatives. Social assistance is directed towards anyone in need of help, either because of an illness, physical or psychic disturbs, or social and financial adversities. Therefore, assisted people may have different ages, from children to elders. Overall, the current tendency is not mainly driven by technology, but nevertheless technology will play a fundamental role in the realization of the underlying information systems, for the holistic care management. Computer networks and innovative software tools, in fact, are able to support the realization of integrated systems which greatly ease the collaboration among the various involved agencies and persons, driving the evolution of those systems towards so-called "virtual organizations", in which the various involved humans operate as part of a virtual community [8].

In general, organizational structuring is a coordination technique which allows the definition of the organization that governs the interaction among the system agents, i.e., the organization that defines the information, communication, and control relationships among the system agents [9, 10, 11]. Aside of specific health and social services, relevant important changes are happening also at the production and distribution level, with many supply chains that are changing their structures and dynamics. Some of those changes can help to solve some typical problems of social services, such as delivering meals and products at home, providing assistance at home or in the neighborhood, etc. In fact, other than cost efficiency and on-shelf availability, additional parameters are acquiring importance in the design of supply chains, such as traffic congestion in urban areas, energy consumption, carbon emissions and the permanent rise in transportation costs. As a result, there is a trend toward information sharing in collaborative supply chains, collaborative warehousing, especially in the form of consolidation centres at the boundary of cities, collaborative distribution and neighbourhood delivery, in cities as well as non-urban areas, including home delivery and pick-up [12].

Moreover, technological changes intertwine into this scenario, with widespread adoption of various types of computing devices, ranging from laptop and lighter mobile devices to mobile phones, accompanying users through different locations and different countries. Accordingly, e-health deals naturally with mobile users, e.g., in teleassistance scenarios, and it is common understanding that e-health should transparently accommodate fixed and mobile users. So called m-health services should be accessible to anyone, anywhere, anytime, anyhow. In mobile scenarios, various devices can be used to collect, transmit and process vital patients' data, e.g., heart rate and blood pressure, in real time [13, 14]. Such systems are especially important in applications that remotely monitor patients with chronic ailments or in homecare [15, 16].

Broadly speaking, such systems are designed to access medical information in a mobile and ubiquitous setting. This access may be either (i) the retrieval of relevant medical information for usage by healthcare practitioners, e.g., a hospital doctor on his/her ward round [17]; or (ii) the acquisition of patient-generated medical information, e.g., telemonitoring the patient's health state outside the hospital. In both cases, it is extremely important to ensure that the person retrieving or generating information could interact with a ubiquitous and pervasive e-health system without any obstruction or adaptation of the normal workflow or style of working [18]. The most notable characteristic that such systems should exhibit are: (i) context and location awareness are to be smoothly integrated, i.e., the access and the visualization of health-related information always depend on the overall contexts of the patient and of the user [19], (ii) fault-tolerance, reliability, security and privacy-awareness are a must in order to accommodate the strict requirements of all healthcare applications [20], (iii) effective mobile devices are to be used to provide access to relevant health-related information independently of the current physical location and physical condition of the user [21], and (iv) unobtrusive sensor technology is needed to enable the gathering of physiological information from the patient without hampering his/her daily life [22].

3 Overview of Software for the Community-Care

The correct deployment of information and communication technologies plays a central role for the integration of health and social care services. The European Science Foundation has organized a workshop in 2010 [23], which provided some interesting results. In particular, it highlighted the following points of intersection between health and social care, which have to be considered for developing an integrated information system:

- Storage of all significant events of a specific patient, either related to health or social conditions;
- Coordination of planned activities;
- Memorization of referent and delegated persons, including consultants;
- Memorization of objectives and achieved goals, also in everyday life;
- Individuation of key points, challenges and menaces for wellness;
- Identification of causal events for health problems and abilities.

To realize an integrated and coordinated information system, with shared objectives among the domains of social assistance and health care, it is indispensable to have a common language and a terminology. This is necessary to evaluate, plan and provide services correctly, and to monitor activities. Thus, ontologies and metataxonomies have to be created, integrating health ontologies which are already in use [24].

Finally, the concluding document of the workshop underlines the importance of:

- Provision of harmonized health care and social assistance, to satisfy the extended needs of individuals, taking into account the differences in needs, preferences, capacities and support;
- Acknowledge the role of involved individuals as informal caregivers;
- Adaptation of services according to the profile of the individual recipient;

- Use of modern information and communication technologies to enable services as part of the larger system of health care and social assistance;
- Direct interpersonal interaction, which cannot be replaced by electronic services
- The possibility of citizens to move across European states and further abroad, also while supported by care services.

Moreover, some wider themes were highlighted:

- Availability and security of information;
- Preventive study of the users' needs;
- Support of software to respect the critical time-lines of the system;
- Training of final users.

In fact, just as the care services which have to be provided, also the supporting information systems should be developed according to a systematic analysis of priorities, preferences and constraints, using local-scale studies with a attentive and critical approach. Technology should provide support for planning, negotiation and resources management, also across different sectors, with adequate levels of availability and security [25, 26]. To be usable by a larger public, the system should be distributed also over mobile and user-friendly devices, exploiting for example touch screens and drag-and-drop gestures.

As an interesting sample of available commercial applications related to home and community care (HACC software), here the list provided in [27] will be considered, highlighting their various features. Our interest is mainly focused on the use cases which are covered by these applications. Thus, it is possible to list the features which users and organizations expect from this kind of software. The following applications are considered.

- ACA-Antares Meal Management System[1] supports the management of all aspects of meal provision into communities. It supports the choice of menus, management and orders delivery, payments and accounts. Orders can be configured starting from predefined patterns, in accordance to the main cultural and dietary requirements. Also deliveries can be differentiated, for example for cold and hot meals. Moreover, it allows to manage the work shifts of personnel, including paid workers and voluntary helpers. It generates configurable records and can interface with banks and lending institutions.
- AIM Community Care Solutions[2] is a modular system, with different functionalities mainly oriented to the care of elders. It supports the provision of assistance to clients, the management of invoicing and payroll. The system can be integrated with other software of AIM for managing the financial aspects.
- Carelink+ [3] is a care management software for handling clients, services and processes. It can manage the work shifts of the employers and volunteers,

---

[1]http://www.acalink.net/foodservices.html.

[2]http://www.aimsoftware.com.au/software.html.

[3]http://www.carelinkplus.com.au/.

allowing to select the best person for the necessities of any particular patient. It can manage personalized care plans, from which data can be extracted and organized in configurable reports. It can also handle financial data and payrolls. It uses various technologies, including maps, SMS, a web portal and possibly external services. A mobile app is also available. Through the web portal, assisted people and families can access their data, checking the status of requested services and their personal budget. Moreover, through the web portal, clients and service providers can keep continuously in touch.

- CIM[4] is focused on supporting the care of elders, together with the appropriate accounting. Available modules range from those dedicated to businesses, for the management of accounting and payroll, to those dedicated to communities, supporting services of social assistance and also sport activities.
- Xpedite CityManager[5] offers a rich set of specific modules, which can be used on their own, or integrated in a larger application. Access control can be configured to grant only the permissions needed to complete the assigned activity. Each module can generate appropriate reports. Available modules include specific support for: elders and disabled people; meal management; health of children and safeguard of maternity; management of preschool services; immunizations and vaccinations, including records of missed treatments; activities of daily living; reservation of resources and services; services dedicated to young people; needs of assistance centres; management of holiday periods for school children; administration of waiting lists. We have not found information about access to the system from the web or from mobile devices.
- GoldCare Home and Community Care Solution[6] is a suite of integrated applications for managing community services. It also provides a web-based work environment. It supports a fact-based approach to manage therapies, during the whole cycle of cares, integrating data of both social assistance and health care. It manages clinical data, in order to identify and monitor accidents, storing information about infection episodes and breeding grounds. Thus, it helps in containing the risk factors. A planning tool is available, together with an interactive web-based calendar, which allows users to easily monitor and change current appointments, and keep track of past skipped ones. With respect to the financial aspects, it manages accounting and payrolls. Notifications are sent to mobiles, thus the beginning and termination of services, or skipped appointments.
- HACCPAC[7] is presented as a complete information system, which supports the management of home care, including various aspects of domestic life and

---

[4]http://cimcare.com/.

[5]http://www.xpeditepro.com.au/products.html.

[6]http://www.goldcarehomes.com/.

[7]http://www.vada.net.au/products/haccpac.

transportation. The additional module MEALPAC manages the provision of meals. Various type of data can be handled for each client: required services, their frequency and priority, family background, medical data, etc. The relation between the client and the team is identified by the supplied services. Each service is associated with some team members and a determined state (occasional, cancelled, unproductive appointment, etc.). The security of a certain data is limited to three possible access levels: read and write, only read, no access. Various custom reports can be generated. The additional module LAPTOP SYNC allows to synchronize data when a worker returns to his office. HACCPAC MOBILE is a mobile app which can also be synchronized for offline use.

- HMS[8] is composed of a main part and additional modules. The scheduler module is used for managing the staff and services, with an agenda-style look. Multiple calendars can be used together, for managing appointments and wages. The transit module is quite atypical with respect to other programs: it allows to optimize transports, integrating GPS and map data to find optimal paths. It improves the management of bookings and plannings. A mobile app is also available.
- PJB Data Manager[9] supports various types of services, including home nursing and community care and related financial data. Data access can be restricted according to security policies. It also offers a number of customizable reports.
- Sharikat Community Services System[10] is a modular application. Each module supports the management of payments and can generate detailed reports. A module supports the management of home-care services, including relations with clients, caregivers and members of the assistance team. It also allows to manage work shifts. A module is dedicated to home maintenance, signaling required works and marking those already initiated or completed, or refused for a particular reason. It can handle requests and keep track of hours dedicated to each work. A module is dedicated to meal provision, from their preparation to their delivery, on the basis of the menu defined by the client. Demographic data of clients is maintained. A module manages transports for communities, and can be joined with a module for social assistance. A module manages accommodations and residences for elders, including their waiting list. Furthermore, there are other modules which are dedicated specifically for the needs of minors, veterans, etc.

---

[8]http://hms.com/.

[9]http://www.pjbaus.com/.

[10]http://www.sharikatkhoo.com.au/.

4 Identification of Common Use Cases

After having studied the requirements for community-care systems reported in the literature and after having analyzed a sample of available commercial applications, we have individuated some use cases which are apparently covered by most available systems. Given the complexity of a typical community-care system, the use cases have been divided into the following areas of management:

Financial management and accounting:

- Strategic management;
- Personal management;
- Customer management;
- Management of appointments, also including the management of waiting lists;
- Management of generic assistance services, which for example the meal delivery service.

Figure 1 shows the main actors that can be classified as: workers, suppliers and customers (or assisted). The workers, who may be salaried or not, are then divided according to the sectors in which they exercise their profession:

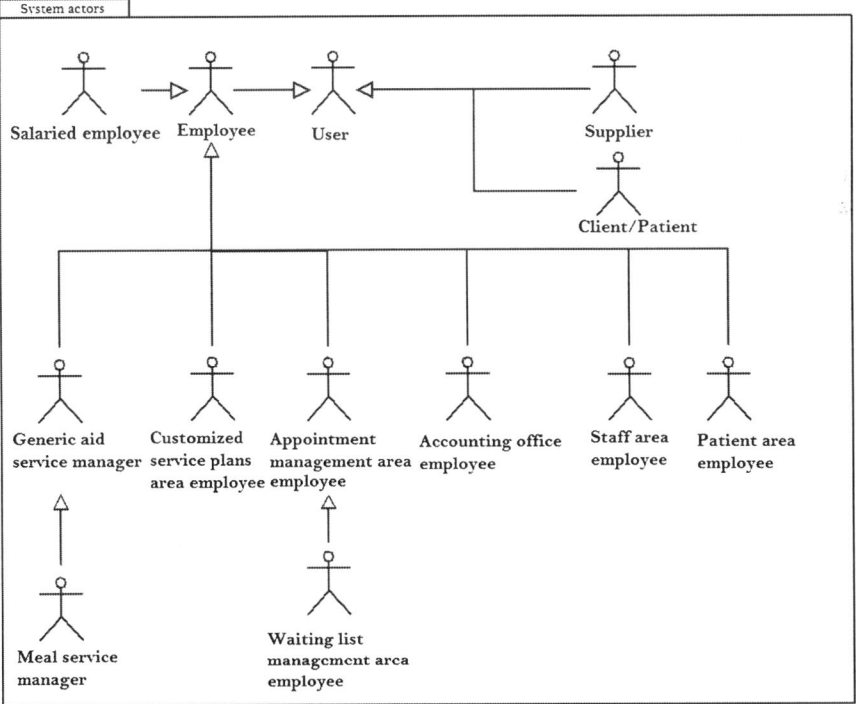

Fig. 1 Main actors of the system

- Worker who administers a generic service. A generic service lends itself very well to be extended to more specific services such as, for example, the meal service;
- Worker who manages the aspects concerning the management of customized service plans;
- Worker of the appointments service, particularly those employed to the management of waiting lists;
- Worker of the accounting and financial sector;
- Worker of the personal sector;
- Customer field worker.

In the following paragraphs, we will discuss the most specific use cases for community care.

Customer management. Customer management is quite complex. First of all, an employee working in this field should have the ability to manage service data and to record new customers, with all the expected information (such as identity records, health status, the required services and their level of priority). A special case of insertion is the recording of a customer who requests the meal delivery service: in addition to the general information, it is necessary to know special dietary needs, allergies and food intolerances. The priority level must also be visible to workers who deal with the appointment management, so as to give preference to customers having higher priority. The customer personal profile must be displayable by operators of the appointment service and, for example, by employees to the canteen service, in such a way that they can check the diet of a customer. It would also be appropriate to provide to patients and caregivers the ability to view their own profile, in order to be able to contact those involved in the management of customers, in case of errors or omissions. Due to the service nature, customers are not allowed to edit their personal profile. Use cases are represented graphically in Fig. 2.

Appointment management. The appointments management has to deal with all aspects of events organization. The waiting lists management is performed by a dedicated subset of workers. The use cases are showed in Fig. 3. Each worker in this sector must be able to record a new appointment on both the agenda of the involved workers and the agenda of the patient. The registered events can, at a later stage, be modified or canceled. The employees of this sector must be able to monitor the status of the events and, in particular, to check the justification for any canceled or skipped appointments. Those who deal with waiting lists need to have the ability to insert and remove clients from the lists. Waiting lists must be visible from all employees in the appointments sector, so that the availability of a service within the agenda can be assigned to customers with higher priority. Each worker or customer must be able to display his commitments, possibly via a web interface or a mobile application. It might also be helpful to have a reminding system via SMS.

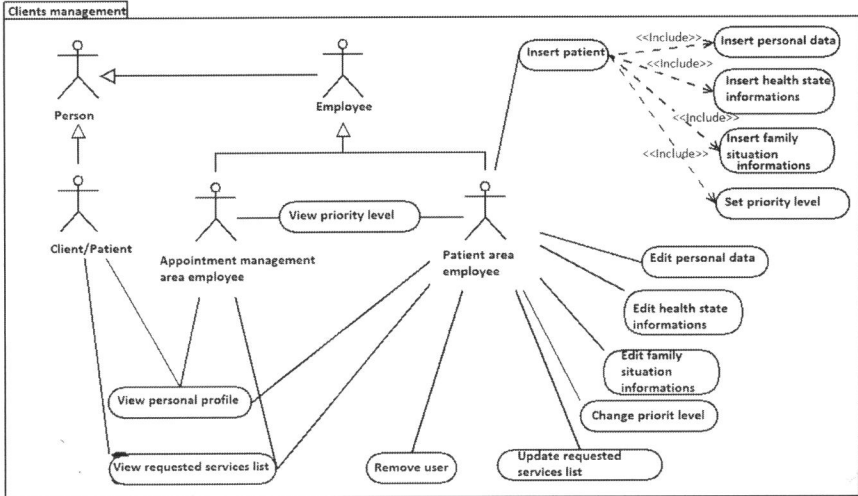

Fig. 2 Use case of customer management

Care service management. Care service management is designed in such a way as to be adapted to the administration of different services types. Services are viewed and managed as independent entities with respect to the needs of individual customers. The main use cases were extracted taking into account the common characteristics to all services. In the event that these cases were not sufficient to cover all aspects related to a service provided by the organization, it is possible to extend them at a later stage in order adapt them to more specific services. They are schematically described in Fig. 4. In the system, in addition to the standard service of home care, the meal delivery service has been introduced. The meals service differs from the other ones in that it requires a number of operations related to the menu management, from its compilation to the management of orders. In this sector, only the aspects related to a standard menu have been considered. Basic services can be managed from any employee of the meal sector, while the more specific ones are run by a subset of skilled workers in such services. So those who work in the meal sector are a specialization of the workers of the Administrative Services sector. Each worker who manages the services, must be able to: register a new service, upgrade the status of a service and, if necessary, delete the service from the system. Since the meal service is seen as an extension of a generic service, a worker involved in the management of this service can also enter a new meal service or change it. From the point of view of the marketing, it would be useful to show to any user some information about the services for promotional purposes; this information may be displayed by means of a web portal.

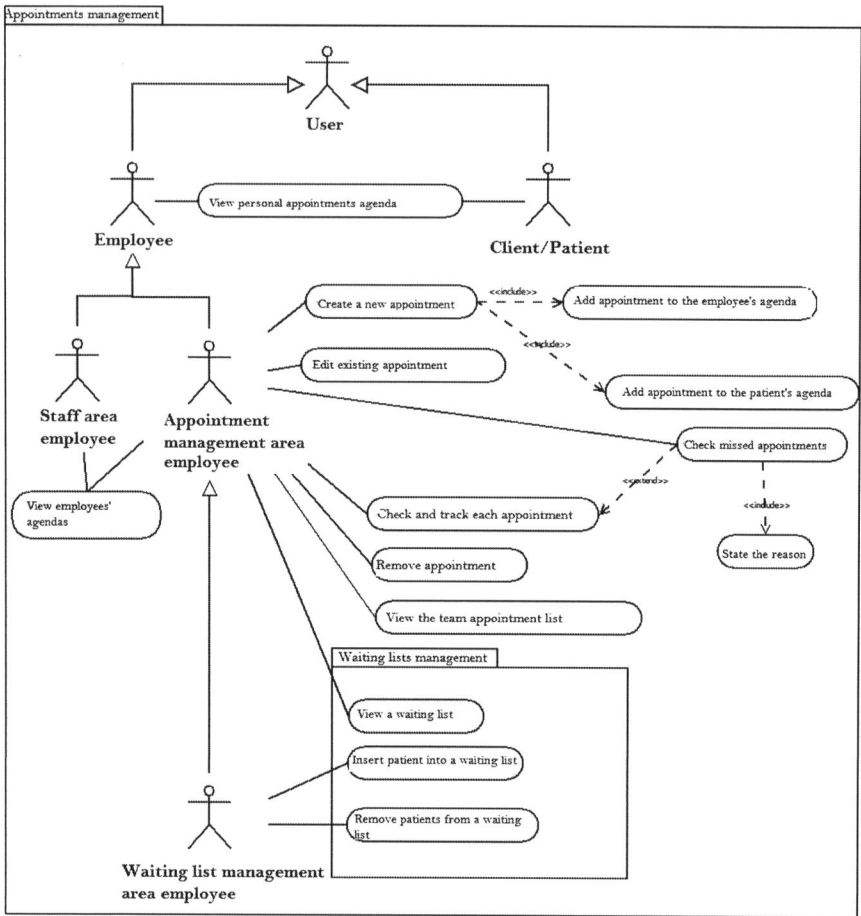

Fig. 3 Use case of appointment management

5 A Case Study on an Open-Source Platform

CiviCRM is a web-based, open-source platform, for the heterogeneous activities of organizations management, which may have different sizes and different purposes. To our knowledge, it is quite unique as an open source project in this application area. The software can be integrated with a number of CMSs, including Drupal, Joomla and Wordpress. The core module can handle contacts, membership, accounting, case management, events, email marketing, contributions, advocacy campaigns, peer-to-peer fundraisers, reports. It is highly customizable; it allows to organize contacts and members into groups; it allows to add multiple tags to each record; users need to be granted precise permissions, to access the various kinds of

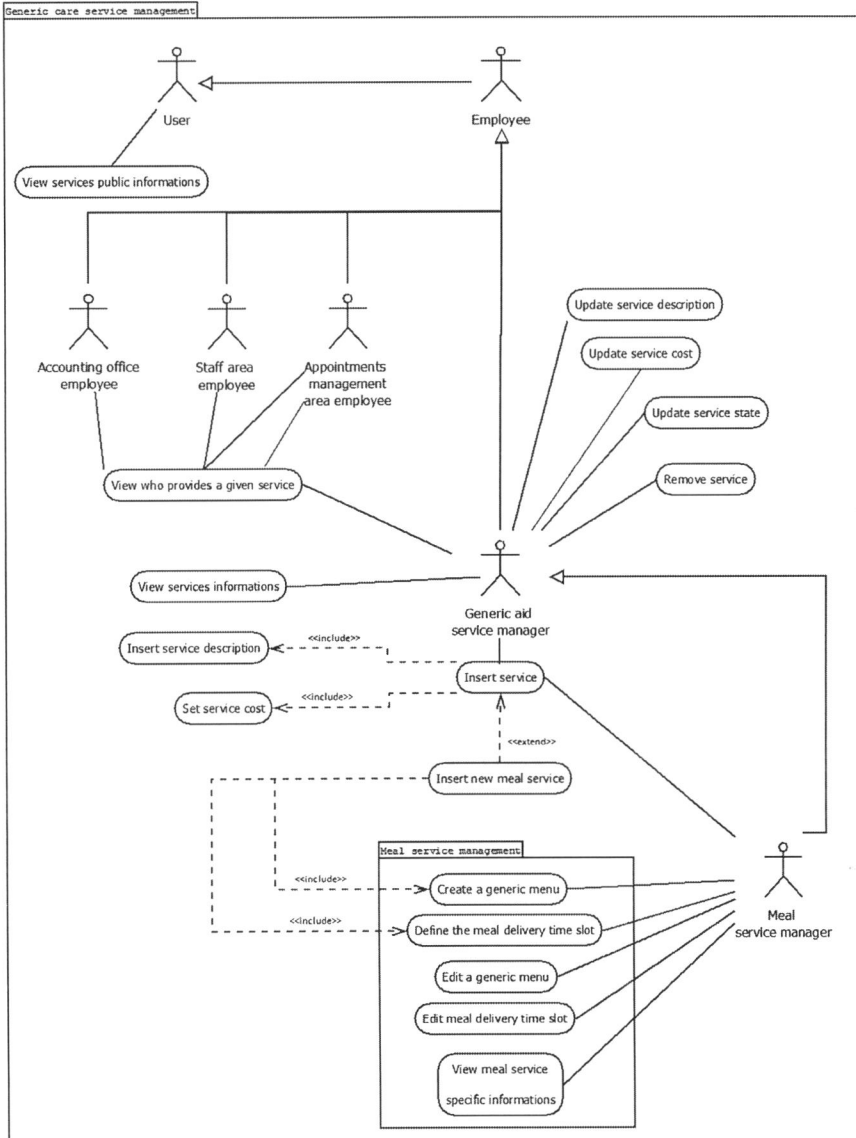

Fig. 4 Use case of care service management

stored information. CiviCRM can be adapted to specific cases thanks to its many personalization options. Mainly thanks to the possibility to define custom types of records, it allows users to model and store data of any particular application domain. We tested the system for the management of an hypothetical organization, offering three kinds of services for community care: domestic maintenance, personal hygiene and psychological support. Each client can ask for one or more services, either for periodic or episodic assistance, according to his own care plan.

In the system, there are two main types of **users**: caregivers and clients. Caregivers can be waged workers or volunteers, and they are further distinguished by means of a custom tag. For clients, a group of custom fields stores information related to their health status: swallowed drugs, allergies and intolerances, generic health information. Both clients and workers can belong to one or more of six specific groups, representing the requested or offered services and the played role: workers of domestic maintenance, personal hygiene, or psychological support; clients of the same three services.

Appointments are managed as three custom types of CiviActivity: domestic maintenance appointments, personal hygiene appointments, psychological support appointments. In fact, an activity is represented in the system as a record, which can be associated with various data, including: typology, participating subjects, manager of the activity, title, description, date and time, address, state (e.g. "scheduled", "cancelled", etc.) and priority level. Some custom fields have also been added for representing health data.

Events, such as workshops and meetings, can be handled as some types of CiviEvent. They are stored each as a record, containing all data related to the event. Thus, they allow to manage the definition of basic data, such as data, time and location, and also the participation choices. For each event, it is possible to decide if authenticated users of the system can register autonomously, or not.

Since the **user interfaces** are web-based, they are accessible by heterogeneous devices, from PC to tablet and smartphones. In particular, there are two types of user interfaces: the public user interface and the staff user interface. The public user interface provides generic informations about the organization. With this interface, customers are continuously updated about the organizations services, activities and events. The main goal of the staff user interface is to allow the management of the organization and of the public user interface. In fact, an authenticated staff user can add new contents to the public user interface and manage the existing ones. A staff user can also manage clients, appointments and events.

Thanks to a proper reporting feature, which is provided by the CiviReport module, staff users are able to create custom **reports**. Reports allow to extract and highlight interesting information from the CRM. Various kinds of reports can be generated. In particular, for the management of our hypothetical organization, we created reports for events and contacts. In this case, for example, it is possible to filter results for just volunteers, waged workers, or clients. The generated reports are printable and downloadable as a PDF or a CSV files.

The CiviCase module provides support for cases, and thus it is particularly important for our purposes. It enables the monitoring of interactions among individuals, e.g., caregivers and assisted people. The set of available tools realizes a kind of timeline, for the administration of services to provide to certain clients. CiviCase can thus manage personalized assistance plans. The CiviCase allows the creation of custom cases, and thus it is adaptable to various kinds of organizations with different requirements. Different types of cases can be defined, and each one is associated with a sequence of interactions, i.e., activities. Some types of cases are characterized by a standard timeline, i.e., a predictable sequence of activities. This is useful to measure the advancement level of a case. In any case, it is possible to add unforeseen activities, thus customizing the management of some specific case. Apart from the timeline, a case is characterized by a set of involved people, with their own particular role. This way, for example, all involved caregivers have a tool to share important information more easily. Additional people may be associated to the case, for any particular reason, also for episodic involvement. A dashboard is available with CiviCase, which provides an overview of all cases, highlighting the most imminent ones. Some predefined case include Housing Support, and Adult Care Referral.

A Drupal CivCRM module is available, for integrating CiviCRM functionalities into a Drupal site. Apart from the modules distributed by CiviCRM, a number of Drupal extension modules for integration with CiviCRM are available, including: Webform CiviCRM Integration, CiviCRM Cron, CiviCRM Entity, CiviCRM Events Calendar, CiviCRM Contact Form Integration, CiviCRM Multiday Event. In our tests, we used extensively the Views module of Drupal. In fact, the Views module can create dynamic and personalized views over any set of entities in the system. It is possible to customize both the list of entities, and the set of fields to show for each entity. We used it for visualizing the data of CiviCRM, in particular information about workers, services and events.

Being based on Drupal, the system can leverage its fine grained permission management, which is based on a traditional Role-Based Access Control (RBAC). Moreover, through available extension modules, it is also possible to grant specific permissions on the basis of local relationships. E.g., a caregiver can be granted access to some specific profile data, schedules etc., only about his own patients and not for all other users, even if they have the same role.

List and details of **people** are managed as a View of "CiviCRM Contact" entities (see Fig. 5). Other than waged workers and volunteers, also assisted persons are resent. The different groups can be separated through a filter. Each record in the list represent a link for showing details about the specific contact.

List and details of services are realized in a similar way, but for "CiviCRM Group" entities (see Fig. 6). The list of people working for a particular service is an

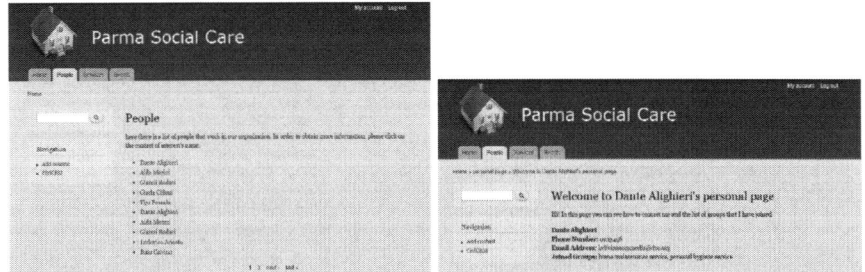

Fig. 5 List and details of people

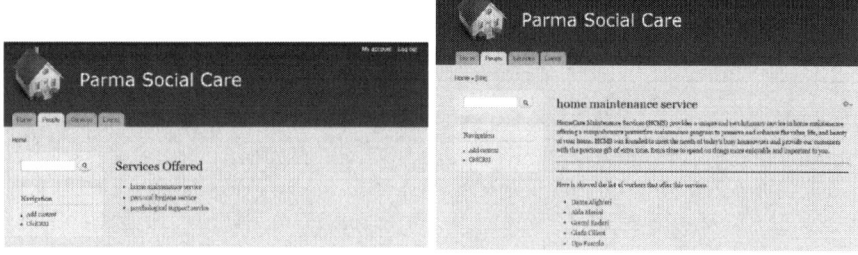

Fig. 6 List and details of services

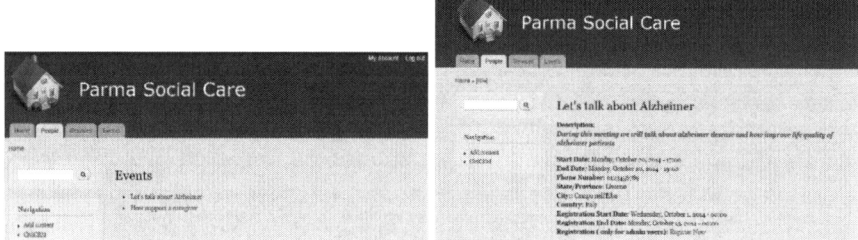

Fig. 7 List and details of events

associated view, included in the page footer. It applies a contextual filter based on the current group id. Online registration is enabled for the event and the operation id performed in the specified period.

List and details of **events** are also made of a View, which selects "CiviCRM Event" entities (see Fig. 7). Each event in the list is presented as a link that allows to access the details of the event. People registered for participation are associated with the event object. A form provided by CiviCRM can allow users to register for the event autonomously. However, it requires that the online registration is enabled for the event and the operation is performed by an authenticated user in the specified period.

6   Functional Evaluation of the Tested Open Source Platform

Thanks to its modular and customizable structure, CiviCRM is able to adapt to the main requirements of various organizations. The customization requires a preliminary study of the use cases for the organization. In its basic form, the software does not fit perfectly to some of the management areas identified in Sect. 4, in particular those regarding finance and payroll. In fact, despite allowing the dispatch of invoices via email, CiviCRM features related to finance and accounting appear to be limited. However, it offers many features matching a good part of the use cases identified. Some functionalities can be supported thanks to the reporting capabilities provided by the CiviReport module and the ability to customize its dashboard. The software does not directly support the management of meal delivery service. With some effort, however, it is possible to create a new type of record suitable for this purpose, with appropriate custom fields. The CiviCase module allows to manage customized care plans in a rather complete way, while no tool is specifically dedicated to the management of waiting lists for services. The management of people and contacts, except for the payment aspects, is permitted by the core module of CiviCRM. In principle, custom fields could be used to store information relating to payroll, but a dedicated tool would certainly be convenient. CiviEvent is a module for the management of public events in their various aspects, including user registration and management of waiting lists. Event management identifies a set of use cases not emerged from the preliminary analysis carried out in Sect. 4. The system has also the capabilities of mailing and sending mass SMS messages. A solution of this type appears to be good for small organizations, especially for non-profit ones. For more complex organizations, the definition of a team of people is essential. This requires to identify and study the use cases for the organizational reality under consideration. Quite obviously, in some very specific projects with rigid requirements, the customization effort of a generic software as CiviCRM and Drupal may be too cumbersome and nevertheless have a limited scope. For those projects, the possibility to create an ad hoc management software has to be carefully considered.

7   Conclusion

The creation of a unified system, being able to integrate data coming from the health system with those useful for community care, is an actual possibility and opportunity. Community care is the principal way to enable people with particular weaknesses to continue to live their own lives within their family background, without having to be transferred to hospitals or nursing homes. This fact is consistent with the definition of health given by World Health Organization.

Although the use of software in health care is becoming a well-established fact, the application of computer science to community care appears to be less common. Moreover, their integration, due to the heterogeneity of information to manage, turns out to be an expensive and problematic process. In this article, after an overview of existing software systems for community care, we extracted the main use cases to develop a case study on an open source platform. The functional evaluation of this software has demonstrated that it meets most of the previously analysed use cases, while a few gaps related to some specific tasks can be circumvented by creating custom record types. Therefore, this kind of solution should be particularly useful for small organizations, especially for non-profit organizations. For larger organizations, the high number of customizations makes the development of the system complex and expensive. Thus, whether starting from an open source platform or not, in these more complex cases, the management system needs to be designed carefully, comparing the various features of available solutions with all the specific requirements.

References

1. Stacey M (1976). The sociology of the national health service, no 22, 194. University of Keele, Keele
2. Bugge C, Alexander H, Hagen S (1999) Stroke patients informal caregivers patient, caregiver, and service factors that affect caregiver strain. Stroke 30(8):1517–1523
3. Franchi E, Poggi A, Tomaiuolo M (2015) Information and password attacks on social networks: an argument for cryptography. J Inf Technol Res 8(1):25–42
4. Franchi E, Tomaiuolo M (2013) Distributed social platforms for confidentiality and resilience. Social Netw Eng Secure Web Data Serv, 114–136. (IGI Global)
5. Poggi A, Tomaiuolo M (2010) Integrating peer-to-peer and multi-agent technologies for the realization of content sharing applications. Stud Comput Intell 324(2011):93–107. doi:10. 1007/978-3-642-16089-96
6. Moreno A, Valls A, Isern D, Sanchez D (2006) Applying agent technology to healthcare: the GruSMA experience. In: Intelligent systems, IEEE, vol 21, no 6, pp 63–67, Nov–Dec 2006
7. Jih W, Hsu JY, Tsai T (2006) Context-aware service integration for elderly care in a smart environment. AAAI workshop on modeling and retrieval of context retrieval of context. AAAI Press, Menlo Park, CA, pp 44–48
8. Franchi E, Poggi A, Tomaiuolo M (2016) Social media for online collaboration in firms and organizations. Int J Inf Syst Model Des (IJISMD), 7(1)
9. Bergenti F, Poggi A, Tomaiuolo M (2013) Using multi-agent systems to support e-health services. Handbook of research on ICTs for human-centered healthcare and social care services, pp 549–567
10. Hadzic M, Chang E, Ulieru M (2006) Soft computing agents for e-health applied to the research and control of unknown diseases. Inf Sci 176:1190–1214
11. Horling B, Lesser V (2005) A survey of multi-agent organizational paradigms. Knowl Eng Rev 19(4):281–316
12. Capgemini, Global Commerce Initiative (2008). Future supply chain 2016 report. Serving consumers in a sustainable way. Retrieved 29 Feb 2016, from http://www.futuresupplychain. com/downloads/
13. De Mola F, Cabri G, Muratori N, Quitadamo R, Zambonelli F (2006) The UbiMedic framework to support medical emergencies by ubiquitous computing. ITSSA 1(1):15–26
14. Fuhrer JP, Guinard D (2006) Building a smart hospital using RFID technologies. In: Proceedings of the 1st european conference on eHealth (ECEH06), pp 131–142, Fribourg, Switzerland
15. Cagnoni S, Matrella G, Mordonini M, Sassi F, Ascari L (2009) Sensor fusion-oriented fall detection for assistive technologies applications. In: ISDA 2009— 9th international conference on intelligent systems design and applications, 5365056, pp 673–678
16. Ugolotti R, Sassi F, Mordonini M, Cagnoni S (2013) Multi-sensor system for detection and classification of human activities. J Ambient Int Humanized Comput 4(1):27–41
17. Vittikh, V et al (2007) Multi-agent system of Samara region social services based on social passports and smart cards of citizens. In: Proceedings of the 6th international joint conference on Autonomous agents and multiagent systems (AAMAS '07). ACM, New York, NY, USA, Article 277, 7 pages

18. Croitoru M et al (2007) Conceptual graphs based information retrieval in HealthAgents. Comput-Based Med Syst 7(20–22):618–623
19. Bricon-Souf N, Newman C (2007) Context awareness in health care: a review. Int J Med Inf 76(1):2–12
20. Song X. et al. (2006) Understanding requirements for computer-aided healthcare workflows: experiences and challenges. In: Proceedings of the 28th international Conference on software engineering, pp 930–934. ACM Press, Shanghai, China
21. Gao T et al (2007) The advanced health and disaster aid network: a light-weight wireless medical system for triage. IEEE Trans Biomed Circ Syst 1(3):203–216
22. Amft O, Habetha J (2007) The MyHeart project. In: Langenhove L (ed) Smart textiles for medicine and healthcare. Woodhead Publishing, Cambridge, UK, pp 275–297
23. Rigby M (2010) The challenges of developing social care informatics as an essential part of holistic health care: report of an ESF exploratory workshop held at Keele University on 21–23 July 2010, Keele
24. Bicer V, Kilic O, Dogac A, Laleci GB (2005) Archetype-based semantic interoperability of web service messages in the health care domain. Int J Seman Web Inf Syst 1(4):1–23
25. Tomaiuolo M (2013) Trust management and delegation for the administration of web services. In: Organizational, legal, and technological dimensions of information system administration, pp 18–37
26. Tomaiuolo M (2013) dDelega: Trust management for web services. Int J Inf Secur Priv (IJISP) 7(3):53–67
27. Victoria Govt. (2015) Comparative guide to HACC MDS software products in Victoria 2012. 13 Aug 2015. Retrieved 29 Feb 2016, from https://www2.health.vic.gov.au/about/publications/policiesandguidelines/comparative-guide-to-hacc-mds-software-products-in-victoria-2012

Implementation of a Solution for the Remote Monitoring of Subjects Affected of Metabolic Diseases: The Metabolink Project

Daniele Sancarlo, Grazia D'Onofrio, Arcangela Matera, Anna Maria Mariani, Domenico Ladisa, Enrico Annese, Francesco Giuliani, Francesco Ricciardi, Antonio Mangiacotti and Antonio Greco

Abstract Diabetes represents one of most serious public health disease. The aim of the Metabolink project was to develop a smart solution for elderly people with diabetes and obesity, in order to promote a healthier style of life, improve diabetic control trying to reduce overall cost for the community. It consists of an app for smartphone linked to a system and a process of data collection based on bidimensional barcode (QRcode) and NFC-tag technologies. The system was accepted by all the patients and they learned efficaciously in a few hours how to use it. Unfortunately, we observed a drop-out of about 50% in the first month. Patients remaining in the study refers a slight improvement in the Quality of Life Enjoyment and Satisfaction Questionnaire (Q-LES-Q) and General Satisfaction Questionnaire (GSQ) and they decided to continue to use it after the end of the follow-up.

Keywords Diabetes · Obesity · ICT · Prevention program · Life style · Phone app

D. Sancarlo (✉) · G. D'Onofrio (✉) · A. Matera
U.O. Geriatria, IRCCS "Casa Sollievo della Sofferenza",
V.le Cappuccini 1, 71013 San Giovanni Rotondo, Italy
e-mail: d.sancarlo@operapadrepio.it

G. D'Onofrio
e-mail: g.donofrio@operapadrepio.it

A. Matera
e-mail: arcangelamatera@yahoo.it

A.M. Mariani · D. Ladisa · E. Annese
Exprivia S.p.a., Via Olivetti 1, Molfetta, Italy
e-mail: annamaria.mariani@exprivia.it

D. Ladisa
e-mail: domenico.ladisa@exprivia.it

© Springer International Publishing AG 2017
F. Cavallo et al. (eds.), *Ambient Assisted Living*, Lecture Notes
in Electrical Engineering 426, DOI 10.1007/978-3-319-54283-6_14

1   Introduction

The diabetes represents one of most serious public health disease for the planet [1]. The WHO estimated about 60 million of subjects are affected in Europe. In Italy the rough prevalence is 5.8% [2]. The prevalence of disease in the next years will grow both as a result of the aging of the population and to the increase of the risk factors such as overweight and obesity, sedentary lifestyle and lack of proper nutrition education. Milestone studies have shown that an intensive glycemic treatment significantly reduces microvascular complications [3, 4] with a moderate positive long-term effect on macrovascular complications [5]. The health care systems are called to face this disease that it has not only direct cost linked to pharmacological and complications treatment but also an indirect significant social cost [6]. It is therefore essential for the diabetic patient to carry out a continuous and accurate monitoring of clinically relevant parameters (as blood glucose, blood pressure) and to follow a health life style in order to reduce disease complications permitting to live better maintaining independence for much more longer time. Moreover the majority of patients with diabetes is older and frequently present significant comorbidity making the integrated management of the disease more complex. The aim of the Metabolink project was to develop a smart solution for elderly people with diabetes and obesity, in order to promote a healthier style of life, improve diabetic control (glycemic control, blood pressure, adherence to a specific diet and treatment) trying to reduce overall cost for the community.

E. Annese
e-mail: enrico.annese@exprivia.it

F. Giuliani · F. Ricciardi · A. Mangiacotti · A. Greco
ICT Department, IRCCS Casa Sollievo Della Sofferenza,
San Giovanni Rotondo, Italy
e-mail: f.giuliani@operapadrepio.it

F. Ricciardi
e-mail: f.ricciardi@operapadrepio.it

A. Mangiacotti
e-mail: a.mangiacotti@operapadrepio.it

A. Greco
e-mail: a.greco@operapadrepio.it

2 Materials and Methods

The Metabolink solution was developed to provide a continuous health monitoring to patients who suffer from metabolic disease such as obesity or diabetes. A secondary goal is the collection of a wide and well-structured database for a large-scale analysis about metabolic diseases and the evaluation of their medical and anthropometric features. Patients can be remotely and constantly monitored by their careers. In this project the methodology used to select the more appropriate technologies was the Analytic Hierarchy Process (AHP) technique [7, 8].

All made possible by the versatility offered in smartphones apps and technology such as qrcodes, wireless networking, non-intrusive sensors and MEMS (Micro Electro Mechanical Systems).

It consist of an app for smartphone linked to a system and a process of data collection based on bidimensional barcode (qrcode) and NFC-tag technologies. Entering into detail the app can:

- record the food, the drug therapy and physical activity; evaluate weight, blood pressure, pulsations, glycaemia using measurements devices wireless connected with the smartphone;
- show a diagram on patient's lifestyle trend;
- motivate patients in choosing a healthy lifestyle through periodic feedback from caregivers and the comparison of their own results with those anonymously published by the community;
- communication in real time to caregivers about recorded data and measured vitals;
- real time upgraded data about the Individual Plan (food, physical activity and drug therapy) provided by the caregiver;
- send alarms in case of "out of range" remote sensing.

In addition it is possible for the carers to access to the patients data to access in real time to the data through a connection to the DB and in this manner they can:

- manage their patients' database, medical history and Individual Plan;
- refer to diagrams about their patients' lifestyle trend (real time);
- receive warnings about patient's health;
- communication to the patient and review the diet, the physical activity or the therapy at any time;
- report and summarize data, providing statistics and exporting files for epidemiological survey.

Technological features:

- smartphone integration with measurement devices available (such as NFC, Bluetooth) to simplify taking and communicating vital signs;
- physical activity intensity measurement using GPS and accelerometer sensor on smartphone.

2.1 Overall View

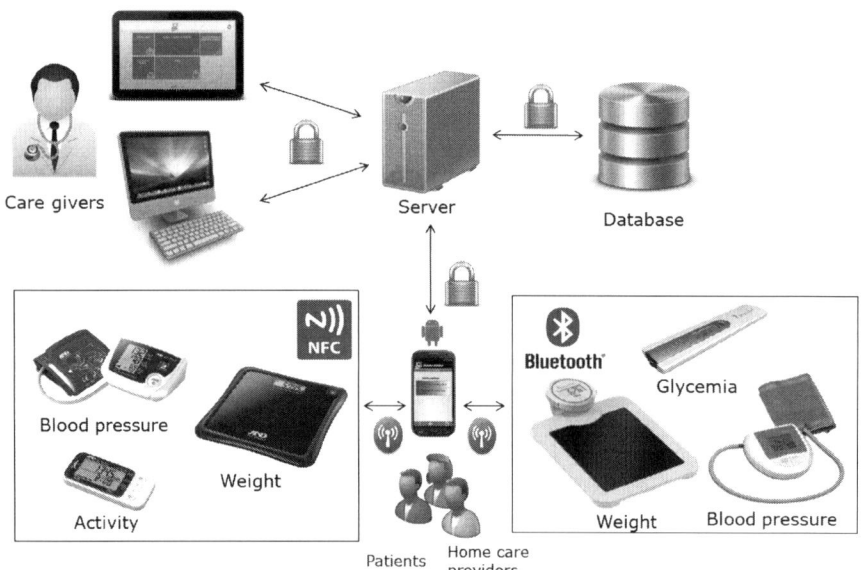

We started the enrollment of patients at the outpatients department of the Geriatrics Unit to validate the solution from October 2015 to December 2015 using the following inclusion criteria: (1) age $\geq$ 60 years, (2) diagnosis of diabetes, and (3) ability to provide informed consent. Two cohorts of 20 patients were included: (1) Cohort treated with Metabolink support in addition to the standard care. (2) Cohort treated with standard care. Each patient of the first cohort were adequately informed and they was provided by a kit comprising a glucose meter, a scale, a blood pressure monitor, a count steps and a mobile-phone all with NFC interface. The follow-up lasts 2 months. Every patient received at the beginning and at the end of the study a complete clinical assessment including a standardized comprehensive geriatric assessment (CGA) [7]. We choice to administer CGA to better define the cohort characteristics and to improve the outcomes in this kind of patients as largely documented in literature. To define our standardized CGA be have chosen tools validated and widely diffused worldwide in order to improve reproducibility and objectivity of the data presented. Multidimensional Prognostic Index (MPI) based on a CGA for predicting mortality risk in older patients were performed.

In this evaluation we included the following domains: (1) functional status assessed by the Activities of Daily Living scale (ADL) [8]; (2) the Instrumental od Activities of Daily Living Scale (IADL) [9] scales; (3) cognitive status assessed by the Short Portable Mental Status Questionnaire (SPMSQ) [10]; (4) comorbidity as assessed by the Cumulative Illness Rating Scale (CIRS) [11]; (5) nutritional status according to the Mini Nutritional Assessment (MNA) [12]; (6) the risk of developing pressure sores assessed by the Exton Smith Scale (ESS) [13]; (7) the number of drugs taken by patients at admission; (8) co-habitation status, i.e. alone, in family or in institution; (9) Evaluation of quality of life using the Quality of Life Enjoyment and Satisfaction Questionnaire (Q-LES-Q) [14]. The satisfaction were measured though the use of the General Satisfaction Questionnaire (GSQ) [15] at the end of the study.

3   Results and Discussion

The involved subjects predominantly male (53%) with a mean age of 70 years old, almost completely autonomous in the basal activity (mean = 5 ADL) and instrumental activity (IADL = 7) of daily life. The average level of education was 5 years. They had a good nutritional status (MNA = 27), lived autonomously at their home and showed a mean co morbidity score of 4 with a mean Multidimensional Prognostic Index of 0.3. No statistically significant differences are present between cohorts at baseline and after 2 months.

After experimental period, from a subjective point of view patients in cohort 1 have appreciated the possibilities offered by the system and felt them more secure, showing an improvement (even if not significatively) of 1.4% on the MPI.

In addition we have observed a trend with a slight improvement in Q-LES-Q and in the General Satisfaction Questionnaire in patients of cohort 1 versus cohort 2. Cohort 1 have shown an improvement of 3.89% on the Q-LES-Q score and 3.77% on the GSQ score. Unfortunately the results were not significant different from a statistical point of view for the extremely small sample size but the trend are promising. The drop-out after one month of experimentation was 50%.

4   Conclusion

This study explored the application of the Metabolink system in the treatment of diabetes elderly patients. The system was accepted by all the patients and they learned efficaciously in a few hours to use it. Unfortunately we observed a drop-out of about 50% in the first month mainly due to the NFC implementation and complexity of diet module. Patients remaining in the study refers a slight improvement in the Q-LES-Q and GSQ and they decided to continue to use it after the end of the follow-up. The study presents several limitation: the relatively small sample size, the short follow-up and the relatively high percentage of drop-out determining an important bias to consider in the data extrapolation in other context. Clearly the diabetes is a chronic disease that requires a multidisciplinary approach to be appropriately faced. It's clear that more work has to be done to produce a solution more suitable to the elderly population and validated with a consistent sample size but we think that this will be mandatory considering the demographic change, the associated increasing health cost and sustainability of the health and social national systems.

Acknowledgments The project Metabolink was funded by the Apulia Region through the PCP program.

References

1. Wild S, Roglic G, Green A et al (2004) Prevalence of diabetes: estimates for the year 2000 and projections for 2030 diabetes care 27:1047–1053
2. Osservatorio ARNO Diabete, Il profilo assistenziale della popolazione con diabete, Bologna
3. Intensive blood-glucose control with sulphonylureas or insulin compared with conventional treatment and risk of complications in patients with type 2 diabetes (UKPDS 33). UK prospective diabetes study (UKPDS) group. Lancet, 1998. 352(9131): 837–853
4. Group AC et al (2008) Intensive blood glucose control and vascular outcomes in patients with type 2 diabetes. N Engl J Med 358(24):2560–2572
5. Ray KK et al (2009) Effect of intensive control of glucose on cardiovascular outcomes and death in patients with diabetes mellitus: a meta-analysis of randomised controlled trials. Lancet 373(9677):1765–1772
6. Kanavos P, van den Aardweg S., Schurer W (2012) Diabetes expenditure, burden of disease and management in 5 EU countries. LSE Health, London School of Economics
7. Saaty TL (1977) A scaling method for priorities in hierarchical structures. J Math Psychol 15:234–281
8. Saaty TL (1980) The analytic hierarchy process: planning, priority setting, resource allocation
9. Pilotto A, Ferrucci L, Franceschi M et al (2008) Development and validation of a multidimensional prognostic index for one-year mortality from comprehensive geriatric assessment in hospitalized older patients. Rejuvenation Res. 11:151–161
10. Katz S, Downs TD, Cash HR et al (1970) Progress in the development of an index of ADL. Gerontologist 10:20–30
11. Lawton MP, Brody EM (1969) Assessment of older people: self-maintaining and instrumental activities of daily living. Gerontologist 9:179–186
12. Pfeiffer E (1975) A short portable mental status questionnaire for the assessment of organic brain deficit in elderly patients. J Am Geriatr Soc 23:433–441
13. Linn B, Linn M, Gurel L (1968) The cumulative illness rating scale. J Am Geriatr Soc 16:622–626
14. Guigoz Y, Vellas B (1999) The mini nutritional assessment (MNA) for grading the nutritional state of elderly patients: presentation of the MNA, history and validation. Nestle Nutr Workshop Ser Clin Perform Progr. 1:3–11
15. Bliss MR, McLaren R, Exton-Smith AN (1966) Mattresses for preventing pressure sores in geriatric patients. Mon Bull Minist Health Public Health Lab Serv 25:238–268

MuSA: A Smart Wearable Sensor for Active Assisted Living

V. Bianchi, A. Losardo, F. Grossi, C. Guerra, N. Mora, G. Matrella,
I. De Munari and P. Ciampolini

Abstract This paper focuses at features introduced in the wearable sensor MuSA, to support behavioral analysis within the context of the HELICOPTER project, funded in the AAL European joint program. In particular, the wearable device performs two key function: on one hand it is used as a behavioral data source, continuously monitoring the quantity of user physical activity (through the energy expenditure index evaluation), location and posture; on the other hand, MuSA enables fusion of data coming from the environmental sensors, properly attributing actions on a particular sensor to a specific user in a multi-user environment. These function are carried out without the need of external devices (RFID tags etc.), but only relying on sensors embedded on the wearable device and its communication capabilities. Some sample results coming from pilot studies are shown.

Keywords Active assisted living · Wireless sensors network · Wearable device · Behavioral analysis · Physical activity estimation · Identification · Localization

1 Introduction

Wearable sensors are becoming more and more diffused in many application scenarios, and most notably in Ambient and Active Assisted Living [1, 2] contexts. Wearable devices brings into the AAL picture many valuable, subjective insights, allowing for accurate evaluation of physical activity, localization and inherently carrying user identification information.

In the framework of Ambient and Active Assisted Living, strategies for prevention and early discovery of age-related diseases, based on effective interaction among different sensing technologies, are of great importance. Wearable devices

V. Bianchi (✉) · A. Losardo · F. Grossi · C. Guerra · N. Mora ·
G. Matrella · I. De Munari · P. Ciampolini
Dipartimento di Ingegneria e Architettura, Università degli Studi di Parma,
Parco Area delle Scienze 181/a, 43124 Parma, Italy
e-mail: valentina.bianchi@unipr.it

© Springer International Publishing AG 2017
F. Cavallo et al. (eds.), *Ambient Assisted Living*, Lecture Notes
in Electrical Engineering 426, DOI 10.1007/978-3-319-54283-6_15

play a pivot role in such a scenario, as assumed in the framework of the HELICOPTER project (Healthy lifestyle support through comprehensive tracking of individual and environmental behaviors [4], funded by European AAL Joint Programme), where data coming from clinical, environmental and wearable sensors are fused together for health-monitoring and prevention purpose. In this paper, besides introducing the HELICOPTER architecture, we focus on some new features which have been introduced in the wearable Multi-Sensor Assistant [3, 4] device, to exploit its potential in a behavioral analysis context based on fusion of data coming from a heterogeneous set of sensors.

The project view is introduced in Sect. 2 below, whereas details on wearable device design and role are given in Sect. 3. Preliminary results, coming from living-lab tests, are discussed in Sect. 4, and conclusions are eventually drawn in Sect. 5.

2   The HELICOPTER Project

Wearable sensors are becoming more and more diffused in many application scenarios, and most notably in Ambient and Active Assisted Living [1, 2] contexts. Wearable devices bring into the AAL picture many valuable, subjective insights, allowing for accurate evaluation of physical activity, localization and inherently carrying user identification information.

Many chronic diseases, endemic among elderly population, could be more effectively treated (or even prevented) by accounting for frequent monitoring of suitable indicators: clinical sensors have thus been developed, suitable for home use.

Connectivity of such sensors enables telemedicine services, providing a link toward caregivers and the healthcare system: however, the monitoring quality fully relies on end-user scrupulousness in complying with the given schedule. This is, of course, adequate when a specific medical condition occurs. However, in a prevention-oriented daily routine this may be perceived as a boring, intrusive task, possibly jeopardized by cognitive or memory issues. Also, the clinical view provided by telemedicine practices is constrained by the availability of self-manageable devices (which inherently yields a low dimensional view) and by the time-discrete intervals of the assessment. Increasing both dimensionality and continuity can be achieved by complementing telemedicine services with AAL components: in fact, many health issues may be inferred from "behavioral symptoms" (such as changes in feeding or sleeping patterns, physical activity, toilet frequency, etc.) which can be assessed by means of indirect indicators, using the information coming from wearable and environmental sensors. They are, of course, not reliable enough for actual clinical diagnosis, but may provide early detection of anomalies that we call "diagnostic suspicion" and may address the user, or the caregivers, toward more accurate assessment, based on clinical evaluation [6].

The overall HELICOPTER architecture is hence composed by a heterogeneous layer of sensing devices, which includes:

- **clinical sensors**, which provide the system with accurate data about physiological parameters, implying user awareness and collaboration.
  In the current implementation, a bodyweight scale, a blood pressure monitor, a pulsoxymeter and a glucose meter have been included. Commercial, off-the-shelf devices have been selected, the overall system being open to further addition or different suppliers.
- **environmental sensors**, providing data related to the user interaction with the home environment, linked to behavioral meaningful patterns. This includes: room presence sensors, bed or chair occupancy sensors, fridge and cupboard sensors (to monitor feeding habits), toilet sensors, power meters (to monitor appliances usage; e.g., TV set). In this case, no user awareness or activation is required.
- **wearable devices**, which provide information about individual physical ac-tivity, also enabling emergency button services.

The HELICOPTER service consists in the continuous scan of the overall sensors picture, aimed at early detection of "diagnostic suspicions": this would help the caregivers in better and earlier assessment of professional care needs, and provide the end-user with an increased safety feeling, coming from the awareness of being continuously watched over.

All sensors are seamlessly connected in a virtual network: however, different wireless protocols are exploited at the physical level. Namely, clinical sensors exploit standard Bluetooth communication technology, following telemedicine mainstream technologies, whereas environmental and wearable sensors exploit the ZigBee communication protocol, in compliance with the "Home automation" ZigBee profiles [7].

Data coming from all the wireless sensors are gathered by a home gateway device, consisting of a tiny/embedded PC [8], which runs a supervision process and takes care of data storage. Data coming from the peripheral devices are abstracted, making them independent of the actual physical feature of the given sensor. The HELICOPTER database enables communication among different system modules: in particular, behavioral analysis and anomaly detection are carried out by dedicated modules, periodically querying the database. Similarly, a variety of interfaces can be implemented (aimed at end-users or caregivers) which exploit the database contents for providing appropriate feedbacks [8]. The database is at the crossroads among different subsystems (sensing, processing, inter-faces) and thus supports system modularity; a suitable data structure has been devised and implemented, exploiting a MySQL open-source architecture.

A simple example, related to the heart failure diagnostic suspicion, helps in illustrating the concept: Congestive Heart Failure (CHF) is among the primary causes of hospitalization in elderly population, and regular lifestyle monitoring is recommended to control it and minimize its impact on quality of life. People suffering from CHF tend to develop one or more among the following behavioral indicators:

- Increased urinary frequency and/or nocturia;
- Sudden changes of body weight;
- Decrease of physical activity, due to tiredness and fatigue;
- Discomfort in sleeping lying in bed, due to edema.

Such indicators, in turn, can be detected by means of "non clinical" sensors:

- Toilet sensor;
- Bodyweight scale;
- Wearable motion sensor;
- Bed and chair occupancy sensors.

Based on outcomes of such sensors, a reasoning engine may evaluate the likeliness of the heart failure condition. Once a possible CHF crisis is inferred, the user may be asked to self-check relevant physiologic parameters by using networked clinical devices. In the example at hand, these include blood pressure and blood oxygen concentration measurement, which are then fed back to the behavioral model, to confirm or reject the diagnostic suspicion.

On the same guidelines, a set of age-related diseases has been selected in the current HELICOPTER development stage, shaping related behavioral models. The model list includes:

- Hypoglycaemia;
- Hyperglycaemia;
- Cystitis;
- Heart failure;
- Depression;
- Reduced physical autonomy;
- Prostatic hypertrophy;
- Bladder prolapse.

Although each model may actually involve a different set of sensors, the overall hierarchy is similar, exploiting the environmental and wearable sensors for inferring potentially troublesome situations, to be confirmed by involving clinical devices into the evaluation.

Discussion of data analytics strategies goes beyond the scope of this paper, and will be presented elsewhere. Here we shall content ourselves by mentioning that a two-phases strategy is implemented: first, data coming from the home monitoring are continuously scanned for relative anomalies (i.e., meaningful changes in behavioral patterns, assessed in a relative, non supervised fashion). Then, all detected anomalies are forwarded to an expert system, which combines anomalies to assess the probability of a diagnostic suspicion. The reasoning engine consists of several Bayesian Belief Networks [10] (one per each diagnostic suspicion the

HELICOPTER system currently accounts for) built upon medical knowledge. The DS models are arranged in a hierarchical fashion: simpler analysis can be based on behavioral monitoring only, and more accurate information can be extracted by including clinical parameters as well.

Based on the estimated probability, different feedbacks are given to the end-user, his caregivers and the professional carers.

3 The MuSA Wearable Sensor

Wearable sensors are a key component in the HELICOPTER scenario and exploit the wireless sensor platform MuSA [3, 4], specifically designed with assistive purposes and shown in Fig. 1. Internal MuSA architecture features a CC2531 SoC [11], which fully manages wireless communication as well as local data processing.

MuSA embeds an Inertial Measurement Unit (IMU, ST device LSM9DS0-iNEMO [12]), featuring a 3D digital linear acceleration sensor, a 3D digital angular rate sensor and a 3D digital magnetic sensor within the same chip. The IMU is exploited to evaluate human body position and orientation information, primarily aimed at fall detection purposes [13, 14]. Within the HELICOPTER scenario, MuSA is exploited for additional key functions: (i) estimating physical activity and (ii) supporting user identification and localization.

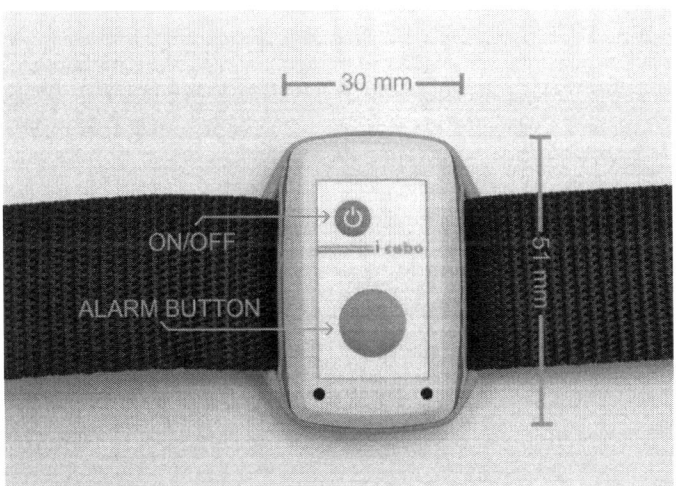

Fig. 1 MuSA wearable device

3.1   Physical Activity Estimation

Physical activity (PA) is a meaningful health indicator [15], which enters many "diagnostic suspicion" scenarios. To evaluate PA, some specific features of the motion pattern need to be identified: walking velocity is often regarded as an expressive indicator [16]. Accurate evaluation of the walking velocity, based on body-worn accelerometer, however, is a demanding task [17], due to noisy acceleration patterns and integration drift errors. On the other hand, in the underpinned behavioral assessment, relative changes are mostly relevant to infer anomalies. In fact, referring to absolute velocity thresholds is unpractical: due to large variability in human behavior, this would yield either too a coarse resolution in anomaly detection (suitable for detecting major safety issues only) or unacceptable false-alarm rates.

We therefore selected a less overtaxing approach, by referring to the "energy expenditure" (EE) calculation introduced in [18]. According to such approach, EE can be estimated by the simple relationship:

$$EE = k_1 + k_2 I_{A,tot}, \tag{1}$$

where k_1 and k_2 are suitable constants (empirically characterized) and $I_{A,tot}$ depends on the acceleration components (a_x, a_y, a_z):

$$I_{A,tot} = \int_{T_W} a_x dt + \int_{T_W} a_y dt + \int_{T_W} a_z dt \tag{2}$$

Since each component is independently integrated over a short time window (T_W), uncertainties related to noise and to integration drift error are minimized. The overall computation burden is therefore greatly reduced, allowing for implementing the algorithm in the MuSA firmware and thus enabling daylong monitoring.

The acceleration components (a_x, a_y, a_z) are sampled at a 60 Hz rate. Then a high-pass filter (Butterworth, 4th order) is applied, to eliminate frequency components at baseband and numerical integration is carried out. The radio-link is exploited to communicate synthesized EE data only, with no need of real-time transfer of large data streams, thus optimizing battery lifetime.

Despite its overall simplicity, such an approach still retains basic information about the intensity of physical activity, as shown in Fig. 2.

The figure reports the estimated EE for eight (healthy) subjects walking on a motorized treadmill, the speed of which was incremented at 1 km/h per minute intervals. A good repeatability of measurement is obtained across different subjects, and the ability of discriminating among different walking velocities and patterns is shown. In the example, when switching from 5 to 6 km/h, users started to run, thus exhibiting an abrupt increase in the EE value. Other tests have been carried out involving eight subjects over 55 years old and two over 80 years old, walking both

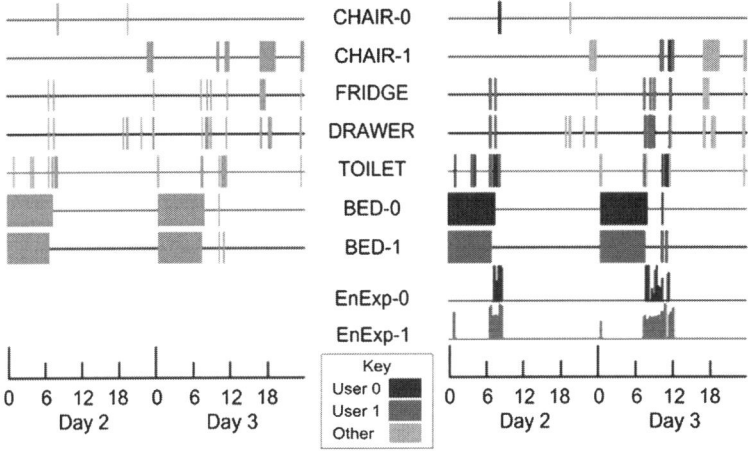

Fig. 2 Tagged sensor activity data: *Left* environmental sensors only, *Right* EE calculation, sensor data tagging

on a treadmill and down a hallway, and have shown similar results, i.e. the EE values where consistent and repeatable.

Within the behavioral assessment scheme, EE is therefore assumed as both a quantitative (i.e., measuring PA intensity) and a qualitative indicator, by discriminating physically "active" and "inactive" periods during the daily activities.

3.2 User Identification and Localization

A further concern, with reference to the assessment of user behavioral profiles, comes from multi-user environments: if more than one single person lives in the monitored environment, information coming from non-personal devices becomes not univocal and further qualifiers are needed to associate such information with the actual user performing the action. In principle, knowing the exact location of the user and of environmental devices in the home space would allow to straightforwardly perform such tagging. Indoor localization is a lively research field: many solutions have been proposed, based on various methods or technologies, ranging from RSSI [19] or time of flight [20] to geo-magnetic field [21] and Mutually Coupled Resonating Circuits [22].

In this case too, however, precise indoor localization can be regarded as an overkilling task, and a simpler, topological association may better match peculiar constraints on implementation intrusiveness and costs. We therefore adopt a proximity-based approach, which exploits MuSA wearable sensors (inherently carrying identification information) and native features of the radio communication protocols. In particular, the Received Signal Strength Index (RSSI) can be evaluated for every communication message; according to [23], RSSI can be correlated to the distance $d_{i,j}$ between a given transceiver couple (i, j):

$$d_{i,j} = k * 10^{-RSSI_{i,j}} \tag{3}$$

where k is a constant involving signal propagation features, related to the actual signal path. Hence, a first tagging mechanism can be devised: every time an environmental sensor is activated, it polls all wearable devices within the home, and compares RSS indexes. The user wearing the device which features the highest RSSI (and thus the lower distance) is then identified as the one actually interacting. This does involve neither additional hardware components nor any prior knowledge about the sensor network and home physical features. It can therefore be regarded as a "plug and play" approach, requiring no home-specific calibration or training.

The above method relies on a few assumptions: first, the propagation constant k is assumed not to significantly vary among compared paths: while not holding in the general case, such assumption is reasonable when comparing path in the close nearby of the fixed-position environmental sensor. Second, the sensor activation is attributed to the closest user, which again seems to be acceptable in most real-life situation. Of course propagation noise and crowded conditions may possibly limit accuracy: nevertheless, identification feature does not trigger any "mission-critical" activity and simply supports building of behavioural profiles, on a statistical basis. Hence, some errors possibly occurring in trickiest situations can be tolerated, just resulting in statistical noise and not jeopardizing the whole picture. Accuracy in the order of 90% was evaluated over a wide range of situations, in a multi-user, multiple-sensors lab emulating a living environment [24]. Sample identification data are reported in Fig. 2, where data coming from environmental sensors are fused, according to the strategy described above, with wearable sensor data to provide identification. Grey data on the left refers to raw outputs of environmental sensors, while corresponding "tagged" data are reported on the right, along with EE estimates. Red ticks are marked when wearable sensors are inactive (thus preventing identification) or when the action is carried out by a third person (family member, caregivers).

4 Preliminary Results

The HELICOPTER system is currently being tested within a living-lab approach, availing itself of nearly 35 pilot homes implemented in the Netherlands and in Sweden. About 50 (65+) end-users are involved, both living alone or in couples.

In Fig. 3 are shown data coming from environmental (as listed in Sect. 2) and wearable sensors, as sampled for a week period in a dwelling where a couple lives: as within all the HELICOPTER pilot homes, the data represent a real-life scenario, since no instructions or particular tasks were assigned to users, besides remembering to wear the MuSA during the day. When a sensor detects an activity a bar is

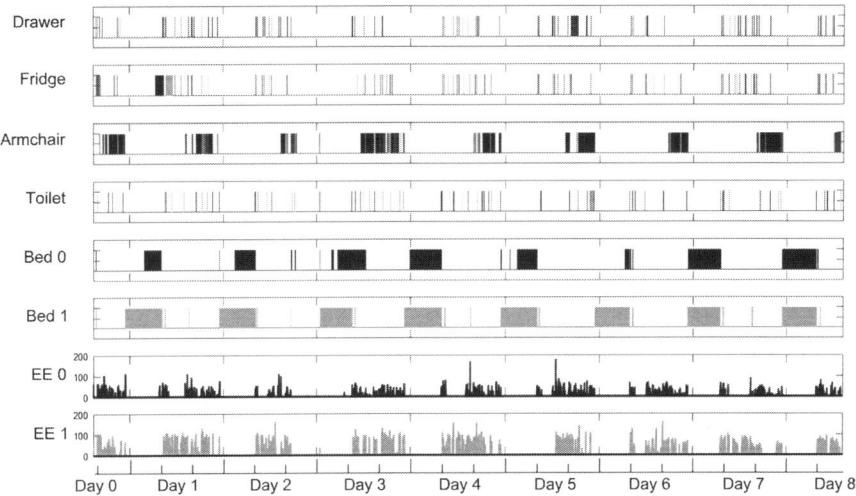

Fig. 3 Activity log from the HELICOPTER sensor network. (NL_01 pilot, 2 persons)

shown on the graph, colored blue or green if the consequent identification process selected user 0 or 1 respectively, or colored red if the identification gave no results (i.e. the action was carried on by a third person or the user was not wearing the MuSA). The identification strategy allows for effectively tag most of the sensor data, allowing to build the knowledge base upon which anomaly detection can be carried out.

Consistent views of user's daily life routines can be gained from such a plot. For instance, quite different users' sleeping patterns can be appreciated.

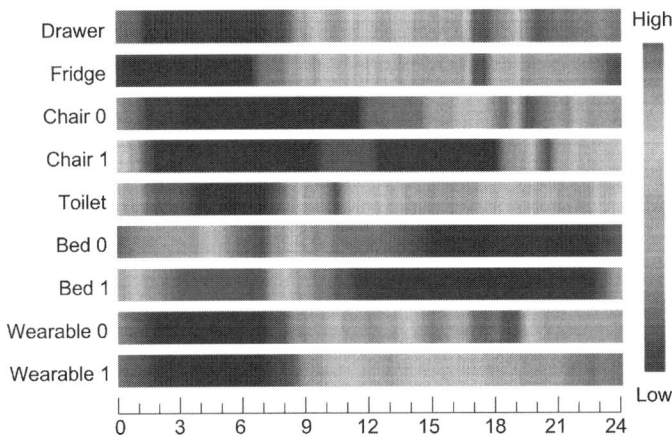

Fig. 4 Normalized average activity profiles for environmental sensors (NL_01 pilot, 2 persons)

In Fig. 4, a "heatmap" showing average distribution of sensors events along the daytime is shown, making such a difference more clearly visible.

The current setup logs about 20,000 events/day/home, on the average. Pilots are expected to run for several months continuously, thus providing a rich knowledge base for testing Diagnostic Suspicion models. Besides the current experiment, this will provide a valuable benchmark for testing further data fusion and behavioral analysis approaches.

5 Conclusions

In this document, the home infrastructure supporting HELICOPTER services is described. More specifically, clinical, wearable and environmental sensors have been selected and implemented, aiming at early detection of symptoms of age-related diseases. The approach exploits indirect behavioural indicators, coming from environmental sensors. Attributing information coming from environmental sensors to a specific user (within the family members set, for instance) is of paramount importance. Hence, specific identification features have been studied, with the aim of finding general solution and of trading off among performance, cost and system intrusiveness.

The wearable device MuSA contributes to the behavioural profile in many different ways. On the one hand, it provides subjective information about posture, intensity and duration of physical activity throughout the day; on the other one, it enables sensor data tagging. To this purpose, a proximity-based identification mechanism has been implemented, which requires no calibration or training and is therefore suitable for a "plug and play" approach.

Data are currently being accumulated exploiting a living lab environment, which involves nearly 50 elderly users in two different European countries. Behavioral models (based on anomaly detection and probabilistic estimation of diagnostic suspicion risks) are to be applied to such data, as soon as enough data will be collected to support a reliable assessment of customary activity patterns.

Acknowledgements This work has been supported by the Ambient Assisted Living Joint Program (HELICOPTER project, AAL-2012-5-150). Also, contributions by Claudia Bertoletti, Francesco Corradini, Giulia Ferretti and Nicola Garulli are gratefully acknowledged.

References

1. Grossi F, Bianchi V, Matrella G, De Munari I, Ciampolini P (2009) Internet-based home monitoring and control. Assistive Technol Res Ser 25:309–313. doi:10.3233/978-1-60750-042-1-309
2. Matrella G, Grossi F, Bianchi V, De Munari I, Ciampolini P (2008) An environmental control hw/sw framework for daily living of elderly and disabled people. In: proceedings of the 4th

IASTED international conference on telehealth and assistive technologies, Telehealth/AT, pp 87–92

3. Bianchi V, Grossi F, De Munari I, Ciampolini P (2011) MuSA: a multisensor wearable device for AAL. In: proceedings of 2011 federated conference on computer science and information systems, FedCSIS 2011:375–380

4. Bianchi, V, Guerra, C, De Munari, I, Ciampolini, P (2016) A wearable sensor for AAL-based continuous monitoring. In: Lecture notes in computer science (including subseries lecture notes in artificial intelligence and lecture notes in bioinformatics), 9677: 383–394. doi:10.1007/978-3-319-39601-9_34

5. Losardo A, Grossi F, Matrella G, De Munari I, Ciampolini P (2013) Exploiting AAL environment for behavioral analysis. Assistive Technol Res Ser 33:1121–1125. doi:10.3233/978-1-61499-304-9-1121

6. ZigBee Alliance website. Available at http://www.zigbee.org

7. Grossi F, Bianchi V, Losardo A, Matrella G, De Munari I, Ciampolini P (2012) A flexible framework for ambient assisted living applications. In: proceedings of the IASTED international conference on assistive technologies, AT 2012:817-824. doi:10.2316/P.2012.766-007

8. Steinhauer HJ, Mellin J (2015) Automatic early risk detection of possible medical conditions for usage within an AMI-system. In: Ambient Intelligence-Software and Applications, pp 13–21. doi:10.1007/978-3-319-19695-4_2

9. Losardo A, Bianchi V, Grossi F, Matrella G, De Munari I, Ciampolini P (2011) Web-enabled home assistive tools. Assistive Technol Res Ser 29(448):455. doi:10.3233/978-1-60750-814-4-448

10. CC2531 datasheet. Available online at http://www.ti.com/product/cc2531

11. LSM9DS0-iNEMO datasheet. Available online at http://www.st.com

12. Bianchi V, Grossi F, Matrella G, De Munari I, Ciampolini P (2008) A wireless sensor platform for assistive technology applications. In: Proceedings of the 11th EUROMICRO conference on digital system design architectures, methods and tools, DSD 2008:809–816. doi:10.1109/DSD.2008.131

13. Montalto F, Bianchi V, De Munari I, Ciampolini P (2014) Detection of elderly activity by the wearable sensor MuSA. Gerontechnology 13(2):264. doi:10.4017/gt.2014.13.02.354.00

14. Bianchi V, Grossi F, De Munari I, Ciampolini P (2009) Integrating fall detection into a home control system. Assistive Technol Res Ser 25:322–326. doi:10.3233/978-1-60750-042-1-322

15. Studenski S, Perera S et al (2011) Gait speed and survival in older adults. JAMA 305(1):50–58. doi:10.1001/jama.2010.1923

16. Yang S, Li Q (2012) Inertial sensor-based methods in walking speed estimation: a systematic review. Sensors 12:6102–6116. doi:10.3390/s120506102

17. Bouten C (1994) Assesment of energy expenditure for physical activity using a triaxial accelerometer. Med Sci Sports Exerc 26(12):1516–1523

18. Tian Y, Denby B, Ahriz I, Roussel P (2013) Practical indoor localization using ambient RF. In: IEEE instrumentation and measurement technology conference, pp 1125–1129. doi:10.1109/I2MTC.2013.6555589

19. Santinelli G, Giglietti R, Moschitta A (2009) Self-calibrating indoor positioning system based on ZigBee devices. IEEE Instrum Measur Technol Conf: 1205–1210. doi:10.1109/IMTC.2009.5168638

20. Saxena A, Zawodniok M (2014) Indoor positioning system using geo-magnetic field. IEEE Instrum Measur Technol Conf: 572–577. doi:10.1109/IPIN.2012.6418947

21. De Angelis G, De Angelis A, Dionigi M, Mongiardo M, Moschitta A, Carbone P (2014) An accurate indoor positioning-measurement system using mutually coupled resonating circuits. IEEE Instrum Measur Technol Conf: 844–849. doi:10.1109/I2MTC.2014.6860862

22. Wilson J, Patwari N (2010) Radio tomographic imaging with wireless networks. IEEE Trans Mob Comput 9(10):621–632. doi:10.1109/TMC.2009.174
23. Guerra C, Bianchi V, De Munari I, Ciampolini P (2015) Action tagging in an indoor environment for behavioural analysis purposes. In: proceedings of 37th annual international conference of the IEEE engineering in medicine and biology society, EMBC 2015: 5036–5039. doi:10.1109/EMBC.2015.7319523
24. Guerra C, Bianchi V, De Munari I, Ciampolini P (2015) CARDEAGate: Low-cost, ZigBee-based localization and identification for AAL purposes. In 2015 IEEE international instrumentation and measurement technology conference, I2MTC 2015: 245–249. doi:10.1109/I2MTC.2015.7151273

How to Help Elderly in Indoor Evacuation Wayfinding: Design and Test of a Not-Invasive Solution for Reducing Fire Egress Time in Building Heritage Scenarios

Gabriele Bernardini, Enrico Quagliarini,
Marco D'Orazio and Silvia Santarelli

Abstract Population aging increases the importance of emergency safety for elderly, especially in complex and unfamiliar spaces. Individuals who can autonomously move should be encouraged to evacuate by themselves, and adequate help should be provided to them. To this aim, a "behavioral design" approach of these elderly facilities is proposed: understanding behaviors and needs in emergency; designing systems for interacting with them during an emergency; testing solutions in real environment or by using validated simulators. Wayfinding tasks are fundamental aspects in evacuation: elderly have to receive proper information about paths to be used, in the simplest, clearest and most unequivocal way, so as to reduce wrong behavioral choices and building egress time as much as possible. This work proposes a robust wayfinding system based on photoluminescent material (PLM) tiles with continuous applications along paths. Tests concerning a significant case study (an historical theatre) evidence how the proposed system allow to significantly increase elderly evacuation speed (more than 20%) in respect to the traditional system. It could be introduced in other buildings for increasing elderly safety and data are useful to define man-wayfinding systems interactions.

Keywords Elderly safety · Elderly emergency evacuation · Risk-reduction building components for elderly · Wayfinding systems · Historical building safety · Fire evacuation

G. Bernardini (✉) · E. Quagliarini · M. D'Orazio (✉) · S. Santarelli
Department of DICEA, Università Politecnica delle Marche,
via Brecce Bianche, 60131 Ancona, Italy
e-mail: g.bernardini@univpm.it

M. D'Orazio
e-mail: m.dorazio@staff.univpm.it

E. Quagliarini
e-mail: e.quagliarini@univpm.it

F. Cavallo et al. (eds.), *Ambient Assisted Living*, Lecture Notes
in Electrical Engineering 426, DOI 10.1007/978-3-319-54283-6_16

1 Introduction

Population aging is going to radically change needs, requirements and scopes of many fields in our society. Only in Italy, more than the 30% of population will be composed by over 65 population in 2065, according to the recent 2015 ISTAT estimations [1]. They will be surely more active and involved in the society than today. For this reason, the environment they will join should be able to host them in an accessible, comfortable and safe way. Solutions for their free use of spaces should be urgently provided, especially for individuals who can autonomously move.

A particular attention should be posed to elderly safety in emergency conditions, such as in case of fire, earthquake, flooding. Elderly represents one of the most vulnerable categories in emergency conditions [2], especially since they move in spaces that are unfamiliar to them or that are not designed to be easy used by them also in ordinary (because, e.g., for the building layout) [3, 4]. In these cases, their safety level could suffer critical choices about what to do and where to move during the evacuation process [5]. Therefore, this occupants' category can suffer secondary higher risks in respect to the other individuals, because of increased egress time and possible interferences with hazardous environmental modifications (e.g.: exposure to smoke or flames in building fire) [2, 3, 6].

Since occupants' safety depends on a rapid building evacuation [7, 8], all occupants should be properly guided during their emergency motion towards proper paths and exits. In particular, people with motion autonomy (and so many of the hosted elderly) should exit the building by themselves: they do not need the intervention of an assistant, but they can be simply helped by proper evacuation facilities, such as wayfinding systems [9].

Our research is aimed at reaching this goal by designing systems that can help these occupants during the whole evacuation procedure, by taking advantages of a "behavioral" point of view [10, 11]. Needed activities are:

1. understanding human behaviors and their needs during the emergency process, and then define behavioral models for representing evacuation interactions;
2. designing systems (mainly, wayfinding systems) for interacting with them during the evacuation;
3. testing the proposed solutions through experiments or behavioral models (and related simulation tools).

Each designed element should be tested about both technological requirements and influence in space perceptions and motion.

Literature demonstrates how wayfinding systems are effectively able to suggest people the evacuation path and then reducing the egress time [12, 13]. However, they should guarantee an immediate identification of directional information in different environmental situations [14]. Wayfinding systems include: reflective signs [15], photoluminescent (PLM) signs [16, 17], electrically-illumined signs [15], interactive systems and portable devices [10, 18, 19]. Their effectiveness is influenced by pedestrians' perception depending on both individuals' characteristics and environmental conditions [13, 20]. According to the interaction level, they can be "active" [21] or "passive" since they are able to suggest the evacuation direction depending on the surrounding environment conditions (e.g.: presence of fire [22] along paths), or not (e.g.: fix arrow direction [12, 23]).

PLM signs systems [24–26] are the most robust ones because they do not need any supply (no interventions on building structure), are easy-to-apply and remove, need a low level of maintenance and are efficient also in black-out or smoke conditions. Identification distances [14, 27], influence on evacuation time and speed [25, 28] and appreciation questionnaires on the involved individuals [12, 23, 29] are performed for system effectiveness assessment. Evacuation drills in different buildings are performed [8, 29, 30], but few studies involve high occupants' number [31, 32]. Current literature generally evidences how the design of the facilities seems to be not properly based on human evacuation needs and behaviors. At the same time, a lack of data about interactions with older adults and most vulnerable people [2], especially in critical environment, is verified.

For these reasons, this study proposes a PLM system (which requirements are based on these occupants' behaviors) and then test it in a critical scenario for elderly safety. Historical buildings [33–35] represents an important location because they are generally characterized by high risk level (because of, e.g., wooden structures), complex layout (with usual difficulties in access by elderly), and contemporary use leading high occupants' densities (such as for cultural activities, e.g.: museums, theatres, concert halls). Related current fire safety regulations are mainly based on dimensional requirements (width, length) of evacuation paths and exits [36–38], but denote a schematic approach in relation to effective human behaviors at all [3], especially about the ones of disabled people and elderly [33]. Hence, these spaces are often unable to supply an adequate safety level to them. Finally, the increasing number of elderly (only for Italy, over the 20% [1] of over 65 usually frequent these spaces) who spends free time in related places suggest the pressing need to provide them a useful help in emergency. In particular, an Italian-style historical theatre is chosen for experiments about the designed PLM guidance system. We evaluate the system effectiveness in terms of evacuation time reduction by focusing on autonomous Elderly evacuation experiments. Our system could be used as a useful support for older adults evacuation in many emergency situations and buildings.

2 Materials and Methods

The work is organized in two phases according to the adopted "behavioral design" approach. The first one involves the definition of the wayfinding system by understanding human behaviors in evacuation and taking advantages of previous literature results. The second phase concerns experimental drills in an historical Italian-style theatre, in order to verify the effectiveness of the system in terms of evacuation speed and egress time.

2.1   Rules for Wayfinding System Definition on Behavioral Bases

The definition of an "efficient" passive wayfinding system is performed by take advantages of main results of previous studies on man-wayfinding systems and man-fire interactions [3, 6, 12]. In particular, limits of current systems and results of previous tests allows to define essential requirements (given the "correct" directional information in a "clear" and "unequivocal" way, especially for vulnerable individuals), in each environmental condition (normal, emergency lightning, smoke and blackout conditions). Regulations about technical requirements and materials characterization are considered [16, 17, 39], by mainly considering Italian regulations and guidelines are because of the application to an Italian case-study. Finally, proposing an easy-to-apply and easy-to-remove system would increase the wayfinding system attractiveness for particular scenarios, such as the historical ones.

2.2   Evacuation Drills

The Italian-style "Gentile da Fabriano" theatre (Fabriano, AN, Italy), built during the second half of the XIX century, was chosen as critical environment. It is a typical horseshoe-shaped theatre with 721 seats (4 tiers and a gallery), as shown by Fig. 1. It respects current Italian regulations about fire safety [38] and a punctual

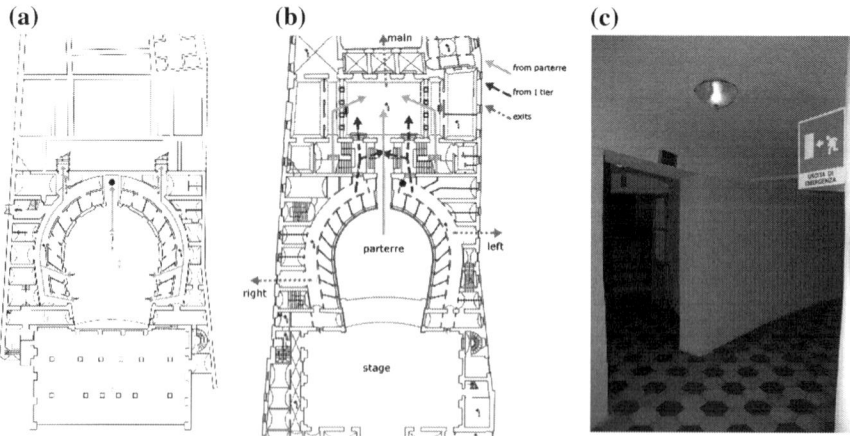

Fig. 1 Theatre layout and actual emergency wayfinding system: **a** the parterre plan with evacuation paths; **b** first order plan including main entrance hall spaces and view of the parterre, including evacuation exits identification; **c** a view of the current punctual wayfinding system placed in the theatre

PLM wayfinding signs system is actually placed in the theatre, as shown by Fig. 1. The existing traditional punctual is composed by standard directional signs (a person running and a triangle with tail) [16, 40], hung at the wall (minimum height from the floor: ≈200 cm) placed at directional intersections. However, it can be useless in case of fire because of smoke rising at the ceiling.

In order to evaluate the system effectiveness by mainly focusing on elderly, individual's and collective drills are performed. 97 individuals take part in experiments; about the 50% of the whole sample was composed by over 55 individuals, while over 65 where about the 20% of it (about the other individuals: 10–25 years-old = 15%; 26–40 years-old = 25%; 40–55 years-old = 10%). No people with motion impairments are involved in the tests. All people confirmed having normal or corrected-to-normal vision. All people confirmed to be unfamiliar with the architectural spaces (or rather, they had no previous experience of the theatre spaces, especially in emergency conditions). Two tests were performed.

2.2.1 Individual's Evacuation

16 individuals in the overall sample is randomly selected, by obtaining a sub-sample with the same age characteristics of the global one. One by one, each person is placed in a theatre box, then he/she is asked to evacuate the building by using the identified evacuation path in emergency (simulated black-out, smoke) conditions. No previous information about the path configuration is given to them. All individuals tested the two escape systems in a random order, so as to avoid errors due to the influences of order of tests. Hence, for 8 individuals, the first test involved the current punctual wayfinding system, and for others by our proposed system. Fixed cameras were placed along the path (at the box door, at directional changes in path configuration, at the emergency exit) in order to evaluate the evacuation time, according to previous studies [23]. Then, speeds were calculated as the ratio between the evacuation path length and the occurred evacuation time.

Average evacuation speeds were analyzed with a particular attention to older adults. In addition, a linear interpolation on experimental data is performed in order to define the tendency of speed against individual's age for each used system. Percentages differences between the two systems, about an evacuation motion quantity dy (e.g.: evacuation time [s], speed [m/s]), are offered according to the following Eq. 1:

$$dy = \frac{y_{trad} - y_{prop}}{y_{trad}} (\%) \tag{1}$$

where *trad* subscript refers to the traditional punctual system, while *prop* to the proposed one. Adopted approximations were 1 s for evacuation times and 0.1 m for path length estimation.

2.2.2   Collective Drill

The proposed evacuation wayfinding system was applied along path on the left part of theatre according to Fig. 1, while the current punctual one involves the right part of it.

The whole sample entered the theatre and occupies seated at the parterre and I tier. Individuals' positions were randomly choices by taking account a homogenous distribution for the two sides (by having similar positions in specular parts).[1] The test was performed during a show in order to reproduce real cases conditions as soon as possible. No previous information about evacuation paths was given to them. Emergency lighting started working, while the fire alarm rang and the voice alarm announced: "Please, the evacuation drill is started. Staff members are invited to activate safety procedures, while the audience is invited to not hurry and to exit the theatre by following the wayfinding systems". The evacuation drill ended when the last occupant exited the theatre. At the end, persons were asked to fill out a questionnaire including aspects on evacuation wayfinding system appreciation (the question is: "Did you find the system helpful in evacuation choices?"). According to Sect. 2.2.1, video cameras were placed at the starting point (one camera on the stage for the parterre; two cameras along the I tier corridor, one for each tier side), at each significant intermediate door and exit. Evacuation path choices, speeds and times were retrieved by videotapes analysis, with a particular attention to older adults, and percentage differences were calculated. The drill was useful in order to quantify both overall evacuation values and data concerning elderly evacuation.

3   Results

Results demonstrates the capabilities of a "behavioral approach" for elderly evacuation facilities.

3.1   Wayfinding System Definition on Behavioral Bases

The first man-environment interaction to be considered while defining this wayfinding system is connected to smoke interferences and signs visibility. Reflective signs could be not visible in case of poor environmental lightning, such as in case of smoke or black-out. Moreover, when PLM signs are placed near to the ceiling (as in current application), they could become useless in a fire, because of the possible rising smoke. On the contrary, PLM floor elements are always visible

---

[1]In particular, for the parterre, individuals' positions are shown by Fig. 4.

Table 1 PLM characterization according to current guidelines (ISO 16069:2004)

Tested element	Luminance (mcd/m^2) after 2 min	Luminance (mcd/m^2) after 10 min
directional signs	600	400
stripes	500	300

[3, 6, 12]. Hence, PLM are chosen and applied on the floor. Table 1 resumes the characterization of photopic luminance of components according to regulations procedures [17, 41]: luminance conditions are chosen by considering the ideal duration of each test (≤ 10 min). The guidelines minimum value is 20 mcd/m^2 [41].

Wayfinding systems composed by continuous elements seem to increase the evacuation motion [42] and also seem to allow a better perception of architectural spaces where occupants are moving [12], especially when strips are placed at plano-altimetric variations of the path (stair-steps markers, wall corners, handles, doors). A similar requirement is especially needed by vulnerable individuals, including elderly, and when people are not familiar with the architectural spaces.

The dimension of directional elements should be suitable for both occupants' visual features and architectural spaces dimensions: in indoor conditions, a chevron (width: 5.0 cm) can be generally seen from an average distance of about 18 m [14]. Colors of signs should be green for the background and white for the directional symbol [14, 16], so as to guarantee a clearer directional indication. According to these behavioral analysis, shows the proposed continuous PLM wayfinding system, composed by: adhesive round tiles (diameter: 10.0 cm) with directional arrow (chevron with tail, width: 5.0 cm), with 70.0 cm between them, and placed on the floor, at the middle of the evacuation path; adhesive stripes (dimension: 2.5 cm 60.0 cm) placed at each stair-steps. This system is not yet used in buildings and so people, especially older adults, could be not familiar with related signs and information. For this reason, real world evacuation experiments are essential while assessing their effectiveness.

Finally, the system should have a low impact level on the building in terms of application (easy-to-apply and to-remove) and maintenance: hence, adhesive tiles and strips are chosen. In this way, the solution maintains not-invasive features in relation to the application scenario while is able to help people in a more efficient way in respect to current solutions. At the same time, in respect to "active" wayfinding solutions, it does not need any external supply (e.g.: electrical) and could be fully used by occupants also during power outage (Fig. 2).

3.2 Evacuation Drills Results

Individual's and collective drills demonstrates the efficiency of the wayfinding system in helping occupants' during the egress process.

(a)   (b)   (c)

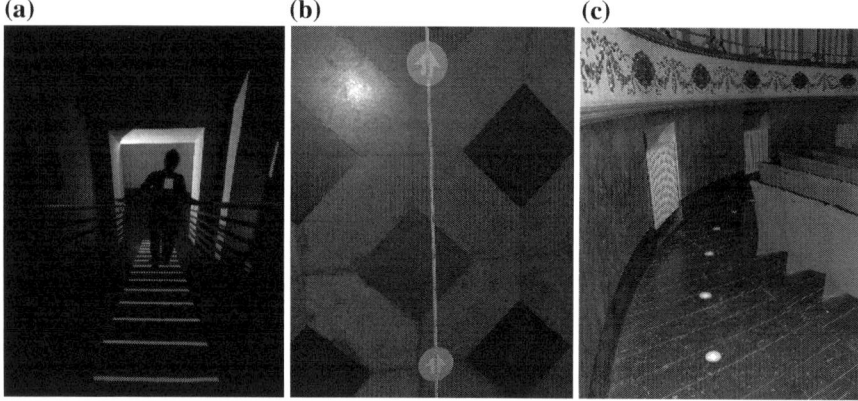

Fig. 2 The proposed system: **a** PLM adhesive strips along the stairs, guarantying the visibility in black-out conditions; **b** the *directional arrows* on the floor; **c** a view of the parterre by focusing on the *directional arrows*

3.2.1 Individual's Evacuation Results

In particular, an overall increasing of evacuation speed for single moving pedestrians is retrieved by individual's tests. In these conditions, people seem to be influenced only by the wayfinding system, because any additional interference due to surrounding individuals is introduced. Then, emergency environmental conditions being equal, percentage differences in motion speeds effectively demonstrate the effectiveness of our system in respect to the traditional punctual one.

While using the traditional wayfinding system, average speed in the sample is about 0.85 m/s with a standard deviation of 0.28 m/s. In particular way, average elderly speed is about 0.51 m/s. On the contrary, while using the proposed wayfinding system, average sample speed is about 0.98 m/s, with 0.28 m/s standard deviation. For elderly, average value is about 0.79 m/s. Our data confirm speeds found in literature by other experiments about PLM systems, by evidencing the same speed ranges (0.64–0.96 m/s) [26, 28].

An increasing of evacuation speeds equal to +15% is obtained for the whole sample. These data demonstrate how the proposed system can effectively increase the individual's safety level in evacuation: the traditional system seems to introduce behavioral hesitation while moving along spaces, while the proposed one clearly address the correct motion direction and support people in spaces perception also in critical (e.g. smoke) conditions [3, 12]. A similar issue is really relevant for older people, who could generally suffer of these problems while autonomously moving. In fact, elderly evacuation speeds connected to the proposed continuous system grow of about +54%.

Finally, Fig. 3 resumes these evacuation tests results by offering their interpolation (individual's age versus motion speed). Linear regressions show an $R^2 > 0.7$ and then seem to demonstrate a valuable data fitting. Figure 3 also shows

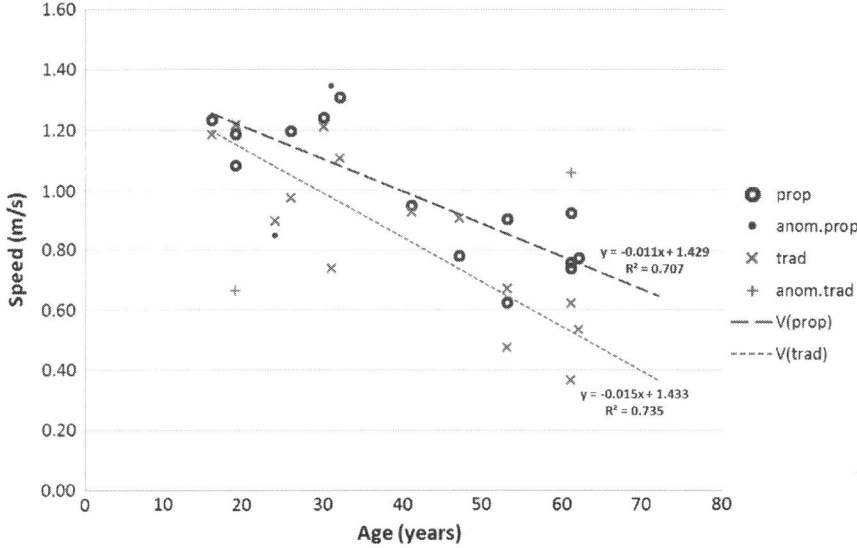

Fig. 3 Individuals' age versus evacuation speed: *prop* refers to the proposed system, while *trad* to the punctual traditional one. Anomalous data are also evidenced (*anom*) and tendency lines (*V*) are shown

the linear regression equations: they could be useful in order to quickly estimate building egress times for single pedestrians.

3.2.2 Collective Drill Results

Collective drills are able to evidence if individuals in "perturbed" conditions (including additional man-man interactions) can correctly perceive the wayfinding system and are able to take advantages of its directional information.

Table 2 resumes an overview of the drill results. In particular, evacuation times for the two samples (using the traditional and the proposed system) demonstrates how the proposed system is able to hasten the egress process (about −26% for the maximum egress time). Reasons are essentially due to the increased use of secondary paths, as also graphically shown by Fig. 4. People using the traditional system generally moves towards the main exit (because of herding behaviors and memory effects [43]). On the contrary, individuals using our proposed system (left theatre side) trust in using secondary path addressed by the continuous PLM signs. They are visible and their information is clearly perceived by occupants, as demonstrated by percentages to related questionnaires answers in Table 2. Thanking to secondary path use, people (and especially elderly), take advantages of avoiding overcrowding conditions along the theatre corridors and could increase their speed of about +30% (+26% for over 65 individuals).

Table 2 Collective drill results distinguished by the used system, and including egress maximum time, evacuation speeds and questionnaire answer about perceived effectiveness of wayfinding systems

Quantity	Traditional	Proposed	Percentage difference (%)
Maximum egress time [s]	167	122	−25
Average egress time [s]			
Overall sample	91	68	−26
Over 65	107	81	−24
Average speed [m/s]			
Overall sample	0.28	0.37	+30
Over 65	0.28	0.35	+25
Signs were useful for path identification [%]			
Overall sample	31	87	+180
Over 65	12	65	+440

Data for elderly are evidenced

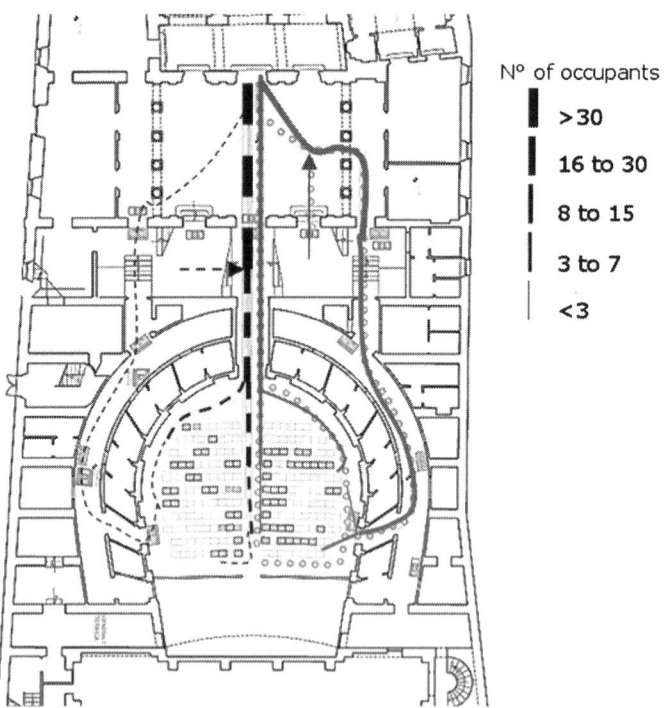

N° of occupants
- > 30
- 16 to 30
- 8 to 15
- 3 to 7
- < 3

Fig. 4 Individuals' evacuation path during the drill: *dashed lines* refer to the traditional system, while continuous to the proposed one. *Lines thickness* expresses the number of people using the path

4 Conclusion

In case of fire evacuation, people carry out wayfinding activities in order to egress the building. Wayfinding actions are fundamental for individuals who can autonomously reach the building exits. A correct identification of proper evacuation path is able to diminish overall time and so to prevent hazardous conditions to occupants (e.g.: prolonged exposure to toxic smokes; structural failures). This is really relevant in case of vulnerable people, such as elderly. A possible solution is the introduction of efficient wayfinding systems, especially when occupants are not familiar with architectural spaces.

Historical buildings surely represent one of the riskiest environment for elderly, because of the buildings features, their layout, high occupants' density, level of familiarity of people with the spaces. In these scenarios, wayfinding systems should guarantee: a low impact on the original building; an high level of effectiveness on human evacuation behaviors; a clear perception of motion paths; a successful help to all people categories, in all the possible environmental conditions. This study proposes a robust wayfinding system by taking advantages of a "behavioral design" approach: understanding individuals' needs; developing solution to accomplish their requests; testing the solutions by validations activities; defining rules for describing human interactions with the proposed solution, so as to also develop models for their simulation.

The proposed system is based on continuous (placed close to each other along the path) photoluminescent (PLM) signs, because they could give an efficient support to evacuating pedestrians also in low visibility conditions (black-out, smoke presence). The proposed system is also easy-to-apply and remove because composed by adhesive elements. An Italian-style historical theatre is chosen as a representative case study within historical buildings in order to verify the proposed system effectiveness in respect to current punctual exit signs. Results show how evacuation speeds significantly increase in both individuals' and collective drills (up to +50% for over 65) while occupants are guided by the proposed system. Advantages are essentially due to the clear path and spaces identification given by the short distances between two consecutive signs. The same results descend from both motion quantities evaluation and analyses on questionnaires to attendees. Study outcomes suggest how wayfinding systems on existing building should involves a smaller distance between signs in order to help occupants during the evacuation (especially autonomous older ones).

Moreover, relations about evacuation speeds and individuals' age are traced by using experimental values, depending on the tested wayfinding system (traditional or proposed ones). However, further studies should extend the results validity, especially for silver age individuals. At the same time, some possible adaptation of similar systems (in terms of technological requirements and operative definition) could be proposed by adopting requirement analysis coming from some interview with older people. Final outcomes would be useful in defining models for man-environment interactions in emergency conditions, by including specific aspects such as the ones connected to elderly characterization.

The proposed system can be easily introduced in historical building in order to decrease the total evacuation time, and so to increase of the occupants' safety level. At the same time, this system could be extended to all other building characterized by autonomously elderly presence and need of low-impact and reversible interventions. In fact, it does need no supply or physical building modifications for the application.

Future researches should investigate the systems optimization by a deeper analysing the human perception of the wayfinding elements, in order to minimize the signs number. Innovative techniques that directly measure typical individual's quantities about perceptual attention in reference to the signs (e.g.: brain activities, pupils motion) should be employed.

Finally, this study underlines the capabilities of the "behavioural design" approach for elderly safety in critical environment. In this case, we focus the definition on low-impact and passive wayfinding technologies, but they could be enhanced by combining signs systems and sensors-based technologies (both about occupants' behaviours and building response to fire).

Acknowledgements Authors would thank the Municipality of Fabriano (AN, Italy) for drills authorization in the "Gentile da Fabriano" theatre, and the theatre staff, the Croce Azzurra and the Civil Protection volunteers, the City Fire Department of Fabriano for their support during the tests.

References

1. Italian Institute of Statistics (ISTAT) (2015) Italia in cifre
2. Tancogne-Dejean M, Laclémence P (2016) Fire risk perception and building evacuation by vulnerable persons: points of view of laypersons, fire victims and experts. Fire Saf J 80:9–19
3. Kobes M, Helsloot I, de Vries B, Post JG (2010) Building safety and human behaviour in fire: a literature review. Fire Saf J 45(1):1–11
4. Bernardini G, Quagliarini E, D'Orazio M (2016) Towards creating a combined database for earthquake pedestrians' evacuation models. Saf Sci 82:77–94
5. D'Orazio M, Spalazzi L, Quagliarini E, Bernardini G (2014) Multi-agent simulation model for evacuation of care homes and hospitals for elderly and people with disabilities in motion. In: Longhi S, Siciliano P, Germani M, Monteriù A (eds) Ambient assisted living—Italian forum 2013. Springer International Publishing, New York City, pp 197–204
6. Proulx G (2008) Human behavior and evacuation movement in Smoke. ASHRAE Transac 14 (2):159–165
7. Babrauskas V, Fleming J, Russell BD (2010) RSET/ASET, a flawed concept for fire safety assessment. Fire Mat, 341–355
8. Proulx G (2002) Movement of people: the evacuation timing. In: SFPE handbook of fire protection engineering, pp 342–366
9. Zanut S, Carattin E (2010) Wayfinding ed emergenza. In: Sicurezza accessibile. Disabilità visiva: accorgimenti e strategie per migliorare la leggibilità e la comunicabilità ambientale, EUT Edizio., Trieste, pp 138–154

10. D'Orazio M, Bernardini G, Longhi S, Olivetti P (2014) Evacuation aid for elderly in care homes and hospitals: an interactive system for reducing pre-movement time in case of fire, in Atti del convengo FORITAAL2014
11. Bernardini G, D'Orazio M, Quagliarini E (2016) Towards a 'behavioural design' approach for seismic risk reduction strategies of buildings and their environment. Safety Sci
12. Jeon G-Y, Hong W-H (2009) An experimental study on how phosphorescent guidance equipment influences on evacuation in impaired visibility. J Loss Prev Process Ind 22(6): 934–942
13. Kobes M, Helsloot I, de Vries B, Post J (2010) Exit choice, (pre-)movement time and (pre-) evacuation behaviour in hotel fire evacuation—behavioural analysis and validation of the use of serious gaming in experimental research. Procedia Eng 3:37–51
14. Wong LT, Lo KC (2007) Experimental study on visibility of exit signs in buildings. Build Environ 42(4):1836–1842
15. British Standards Institution (2000) BS 5499-4:2000—safety signs, including fire safety signs. Code of practice for escape route signing
16. Italian Organization for Standardization (UNI) (2004) UNI 7543:2004—safety colours and safety signs
17. DIN (2009) DIN 67510, Photoluminescent pigments and products
18. Ran H, Sun L, Gao X (2014) Influences of intelligent evacuation guidance system on crowd evacuation in building fire. Autom Constr 41:78–82
19. Pu S, Zlatanova S (2005) Evacuation route calculation of inner buildings. In Research book chapter in geo-information for disaster management. Springer, Berlin, pp 1143–1161
20. Kobes M, Helsloot I, de Vries B, Post JG, Oberijé N, Groenewegen K (2010) Way finding during fire evacuation; an analysis of unannounced fire drills in a hotel at night. Build Environ 45(3):537–548
21. Ibrahim AM, Venkat I, Subramanian KG, Khader AT, De Wilde P (2016) Intelligent evacuation management systems. ACM Transac Intell Syst Technol 7(3):1–27
22. Wang S-H, Wang W-C, Wang K-C, Shih S-Y (2015) Applying building information modeling to support fire safety management. Autom Constr 59:158–167
23. D'Orazio M, Longhi S, Olivetti P, Bernardini G (2015) Design and experimental evaluation of an interactive system for pre-movement time reduction in case of fire. Autom Constr 52:16–28
24. Proulx G, Tiller DK, Kyle BR, Creak J (1999) Assessment of photoluminescent material during office occupant evacuation. National Research Council of Canada, Institute for Research in Construction
25. Proulx G, Bénichou N (2009) Photoluminescent stairway installation for evacuation in office buildings. Fire Technol 46(3):471–495
26. Proulx G, Kyle B, Creak J (2000) Effectiveness of a photoluminescent wayguidance system. Fire Technol 36(4):236–248
27. Tuomisaari M (1997) Visibility of exit signs and low-location lighting in smoky conditions. VTT Building Technology
28. Jeon G-Y, Kim J-Y, Hong W-H, Augenbroe G (2011) Evacuation performance of individuals in different visibility conditions. Build Environ 46(5):1094–1103
29. Fahy RF, Proulx G (2001) Toward creating a database on delay times to start evacuation and walking speeds for use in evacuation modeling.In: 2nd international symposium on human behaviour in fire, pp 175–183
30. Gwynne SMV (2007) Optimizing fire alarm notification for high risk groups research project. Notification effectiveness for large groups
31. Purser DA, Bensilum M (2001) Quantification of behaviour for engineering design standards and escape time calculations. Saf Sci 38:157–182
32. Xudong C, Heping Z, Qiyuan X, Yong Z, Hongjiang Z, Chenjie Z (2009) Study of announced evacuation drill from a retail store. Build Environ 44(5):864–870

33. Lena K, Kristin A, Staffan B, Sara W, Elena S (2010) How do people with disabilities consider fire safety and evacuation possibilities in historical buildings?—A Swedish case study. Fire Technol 48(1):27–41
34. Santos C, Ferreira TM, Vicente R, Mendes da Silva JR (2013) Building typologies identification to support risk mitigation at the urban scale—Case study of the old city centre of Seixal, Portugal. J Cult Heritage 14(6):449–463
35. Elsorady DA (2013) Assessment of the compatibility of new uses for heritage buildings: the example of Alexandria National Museum, Alexandria, Egypt. J Cult Heritage 15(5):511–521
36. Ministry of Interior (Italy) (1992) D.M. 20-05-1992 n. 569—fire safety in historical buildings used as museum and art galleries
37. Confederation of Fire Protection Associations Europe (2013) Managing fire protection of historic buildings
38. Italian Government (1996) DM 19/08/1996: fire safety criteria for entertainment public spaces (Regola tecnica di prevenzione incendi per la progettazione, costruzione ed esercizio dei locali di intrattenimento e di pubblico spettacolo)
39. ISO (2011) ISO 3864-1, Annex A, relationship between dimensions of safety signs and distance of observation
40. Italian Government (2008) DLgs 9/4/2008 n. 81: Annex XXV—general requirements for emergency signs (allegato XXV, Prescrizioni generali per i cartelli segnaletici)
41. ISO (2004) ISO 16069, Graphical symbols—safety signs—S afety way guidance systems (SWGS)
42. IMO Organization International Maritime (2002) Interim guidelines for evacuation analyses for new and existing passenger ships
43. Lakoba TI, Kaup DJ, Finkelstein NM (2005) Modifications of the Helbing-Molnar-Farkas-Vicsek social force model for pedestrian evolution. Simulation 81(5):339–352

The A.I.zeta Framework: An Ontological Approach for AAL Systems Control

Guido Matrella, Monica Mordonini, Roberto Zanichelli
and Riccardo Zini

Abstract The AAL Systems have been devised to monitor the life of persons in their home, in order to infer information on their state of health and to support their wellbeing. The achievement of this purpose is possible by means of various technologies and systems (such as, for instance, home environment sensors, personal sensors and clinical devices). This article describes the design and early development of a software tool, that allows to control an AAL System, completely based on an ontological approach. From this innovative point of view, an ontological formalization is used to describe a domain and to implement an automatic reason. This approach provides a dynamic model that can change its state and expand accordingly to rules that are also a part of the model. Such a description is continually updated with information provided by the AAL System database that reports the significant events recorded by the sensors. Then, exploiting the potential of an OWL-DL reasoner, decisions about the feedbacks that the System have to activate, are inferred.

Keywords AAL system · Ontology · Smart environment · Context aware system

---

Guido Matrella—Macro-areas of interest: well-being and active ageing, prevention and lifestyles

---

G. Matrella (✉) · M. Mordonini · R. Zanichelli · R. Zini
Dip. di Ingegneria dell'informazione, Parco Area delle Scienze 181/a, Parma, Italy
e-mail: guido.matrella@unipr.it

M. Mordonini
e-mail: monica.mordonini@unipr.it

R. Zanichelli
e-mail: roberto.zanichelli@studenti.unipr.it

R. Zini
e-mail: riccardo.zini@studenti.unipr.it

© Springer International Publishing AG 2017
F. Cavallo et al. (eds.), *Ambient Assisted Living*, Lecture Notes
in Electrical Engineering 426, DOI 10.1007/978-3-319-54283-6_17

223

1 Introduction

The AAL (Active and Assisted Living) Systems are technologies devised to monitor the well-being of elderly, disabled people, or people with impairments, with a particular focus on the activities of daily living performed in the home environment. Such systems can help to motivate users to adopt a healthier lifestyle. In addition, they can support the caregivers providing them information on users' behaviours. The use of an AAL system can allow users to remain in their own home for a longer period, living in autonomy and security, improving the quality of their life.

To be useful (and so be accepted), AAL Systems must ensure real benefits for users in everyday activities. Therefore, versatility and configurability are crucial features for such systems in order to fit the needs of the pathologies of the users, in harmony with their specific habits. In [1] a semantic context modeling the reasoning was taken into account to make an assistive solution that is able to adapt to the changing needs of the end-users.

Furthermore, information provided by sensors networks to detect the users' behaviour need to be contextualized in order to implement the most appropriate response. In [2] the anticipation of health hazards was provided by an ontology-based domotic environment in which the system was able to act in a contextualized environment, which enabled it to recognize the user's actions. In [3] the behaviours of inhabitants in smart homes were modeled by the process of the data coming from the sensors through a set of rules that described the relationship between sensor events that were typical for the inhabitant's way of life. The issues of ontology and context aware systems were often dealt in smart environments for eHealth: for example, in [4] ontology was used to context modeling, while in [5] a common knowledge ontology is employed to guide high-level context reasoning to achieve various proactive services in an elderly health-monitoring system. In [6] only the basic reasoning mechanisms of description logic are used to detect patterns of events in smart environments.

The ontological descriptions represent an effective approach to model a complex domain such as that AAL, in [7] the authors proposed the use of high-level context ontologies to create a reference architecture for building AAL systems. The ontologies are useful for context-server applications, that are most flexible because heterogeneous clients and sensors can be integrate. In [8] the results of a simulated AAL environment using a knowledge driven approach are described: AAL environment was be modeled by ontologies and different semantic reasoners were used to infer knowledge about the underlying context.

Furthermore, the functions of an AAL System must take in account the needs of informal and formal caregivers, to provide them with a suitable support. To relate various points of view and different skills, a design effort to define the semantics of the involved domains (medical, technical, social) is required. In order to facilitate the interoperability and the integration of heterogeneous systems, different works have been devoted to the definition of ontologies for the AAL context and several approaches have been proposed.

For example, in [9], the authors' solution to accommodate dynamic behaviour of AAL system needs and diversity of system requirements is to use higher level of system abstraction by using ontology. This work was partially supported by Project eWall that is the outcome of a EC-funded project that contributes to the prolongation of independent living of various patients' types and senior citizens. Unlike traditional eHealth/eCare solutions, eWall [10] offers a new experience to the users by creating Caring Home Environments based on advances sensing and reasoning in an unobtrusive way. In this work the developed ontology serves not only as a conceptual model for representing the AAL domain concepts, but also as an effective basis for the development, maintenance, configuration, and execution of AAL services and applications. This idea is very stimulating in the develop of a AAL system control in order to facilitate its customization and its evolution in time, and in the following we try to exploit the property of consistency, validation and inference of a description logic to detect significant events and then behaviours of a particular system.

In [11], authors proposed an event-based human activity recognition through an ontology-based methodology to perform semantic queries on a data repository, where records originated from networks of heterogeneous sources. In this work the domain ontology was described in OWL and a DL-reasoner was chosen to introduce new knowledge in the ontology, but the described methodology combines an ontological approach with a Complex Event Processing (CEP) engine which has the task temporally manage the events. The attempt described below is to develop a tool based only on an ontological description of a domain together to an inference engine to obtain the complete control of an AAL system.

The work described in the following is a development of the research in the use of ontologies in AAL Systems carried out in a previous work [12], in which the focus was on the design of an ontology for an AAL system able to monitor the behaviour of the persons, aiming to recording their feeding habits.

The main idea of the present work is the development of a software framework that exploits the logical inference to handle useful information through a flexible set of rules on which consistency is validated as a result of the logical reasoning.

Ontologies enable the definition of a high-level model of a complex domain: the definitions of basic concepts and the relations among them can be described by the means of a standard and machine-interpretable language while formal ontologies models can support the logical inference and the possibility of recognizing the equivalence of two concepts. This is essential to provide the AAL system with an automatic reasoner in order to check the consistency between different domains and the state of the environment detected by sensors networks.

These features have a key role in the harmonization of different aspects of the domain: clinical user's model, bad habits, event recognition from a pattern of alarmed sensors. So the framework, called A.I.zeta, can be also used to define, validate and recognize a set of contexts for each instance (i.e. specific user's behaviours). When someone of these contexts are detected, the framework estimates a degree of importance for the occurred event, automatically generating appropriate feedbacks.

The work was carried out using, as a reference domain, the AAL System developed in the HELICOPTER Project. The goal of the HELICOPTER Project (funded in the framework of the European AAL Joint Programme [13]) is to exploit ambient-assisted living techniques to provide older adults and their informal caregivers with support, motivation and guidance in pursuing a healthy and safe lifestyle. The HELICOPTER AAL System implements a platform to acquire data from home, personal and clinical sensors. In particular, for the HELICOPTER project, a wearable sensor (called MuSA—Multi Sensors Assistant [14]), conceived for personal activity recognition, users' identification and fall detection, was used.

In Sect. 2, the idea that underlies the work is explained; in Sect. 3, the A.I.zeta framework is illustrated; some first results are presented in Sect. 4; Conclusions and future developments close the paper.

2   An Ontological Inference Approach to Control an AAL System

In this work, the main goal was to realize a software that can take advantage of the ontological inference and modeling to provide supervising and control to an AAL system.

AAL systems are examples of supervisory control system. The traditional approach in this kind of systems is the development of an expert software in which the logic of the control is coded inside the application. Some of these software use "knowledge-based" tools for modeling purposes, but at the end of these processes the knowledge and the query are assembled in a single block as shown in the top of Fig. 1. The approach discussed in this paper tries to keep, even at runtime, separate the conceptual model from the operational level and proposes a solution in which "knowledge-based" tools can effectively use the inference process for automatic reasoning and not only for modeling, as shown in the bottom of Fig. 1. This allows more flexibility to the system, and a better control of the complex system being able to explain and highlight the interaction between the variables into play.

In this context, the description provided by the ontological approach is very effective as consequence of the generality of the ontology, that consist in open universe in which infinite elements can be added with infinite level of specialization through the set theory.

Given an ontological model of the AAL domain, defining the appropriate sets and intersections (that describe, for example, the type of sensors, the physical location in the home environment, the definition of time, the definitions of alarms conditions, etc.), the ontological inference allows to understand if the state of the system (so the values measured by sensors) is consistent with the

TRADITIONAL APPROACH

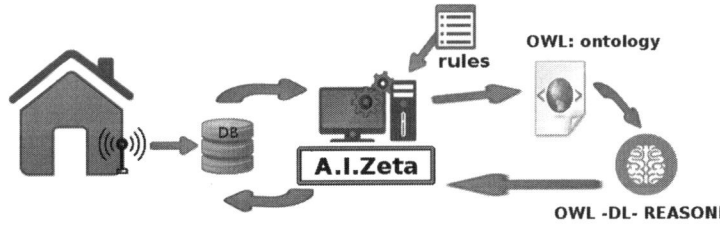

ONTOLOGY DRIVEN APPROACH

Fig. 1 Difference between generic traditional system (*top figure*) and the proposed approach (*bottom figure*)

system-knowledge about the user (which it is also modeled using an ontology) and provide new information that is automatically inferred from the raw data.

As reference for this work, the HELICOPTER AAL System was chosen; it uses a data fusion approach mixing data provided by: home, personal and clinical sensors. All data are stored in a MySQL Database.

In the approach proposed in this work, through the periodic monitoring of the DB (structured as the one used in HELICOPTER AAL project) and by the interpretation of stored data by means of the configurable interface with the database that parse the data, the production of "new knowledge" for a properly structured ontology is possible. Changes in the state of the sensors imply an update in the ontology description through the configurable interface with the database. Then, an automatic reasoner processes the ontology, performing an automatic inference of situations of emergency or anomalies detection in the user's behaviour. The "new knowledge" consist in axioms added to the ontology by the reasoner (Figs. 2, 3, 4, 5, 6 and 7).

In these cases, the System must generate alarms to the caregivers or produce feedback to the end users accordingly to the generated axioms that states defined conditions.

A.I.zeta works as a sort of broker between the data stored in the DB and the description of the domain realized by a specific ontology:

1. each update of the status of sensors stored in the DB is immediately read;
2. by specially described rules, changes in DB become changes in the ontological description; A.I.zeta "map" the physical events detected by the sensors to appropriate formal OWL descriptions; to simplify the writing of the rules, a

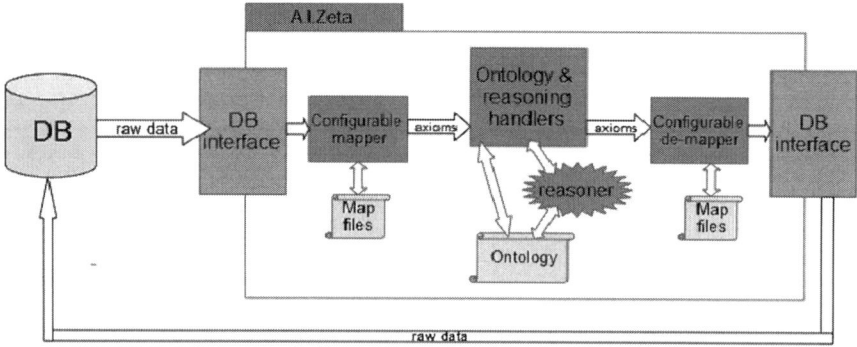

Fig. 2 A.I. zeta system overview

Fig. 3 Representation of part
of the ontology domain

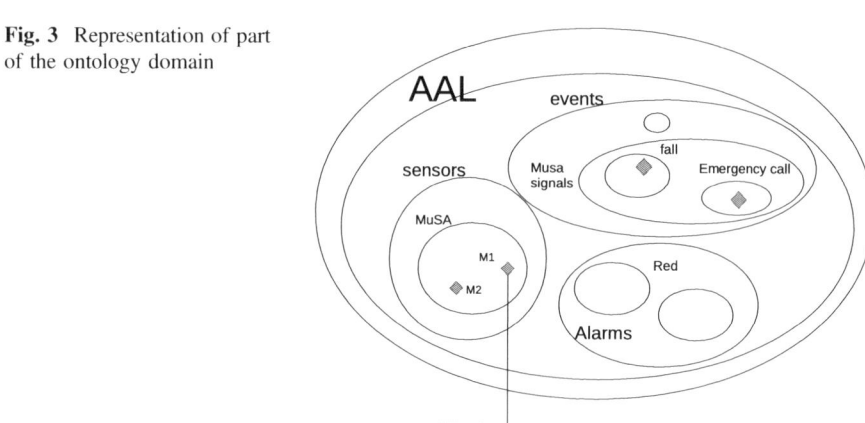

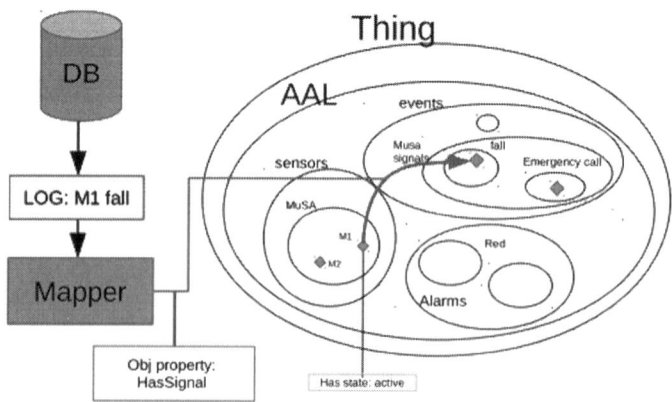

Fig. 4 Data-flow from database to ontology model

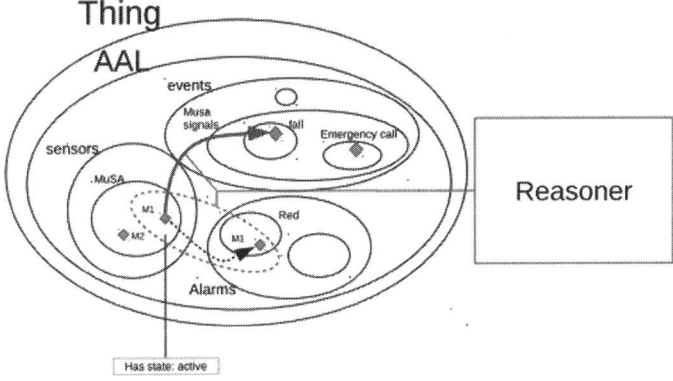

Fig. 5 Representation of the reasoning effects

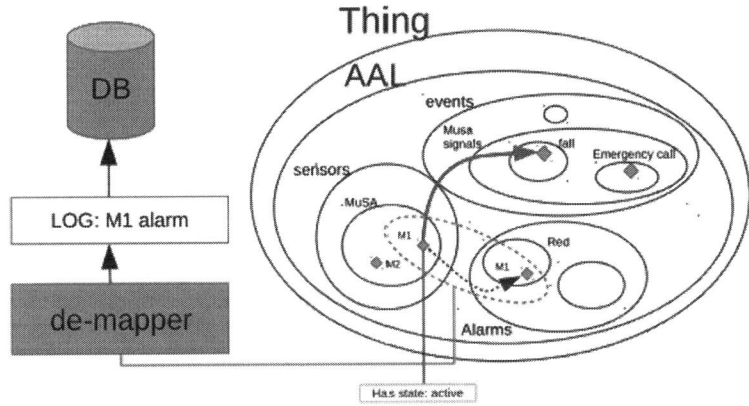

Fig. 6 Data-flow from ontology to database

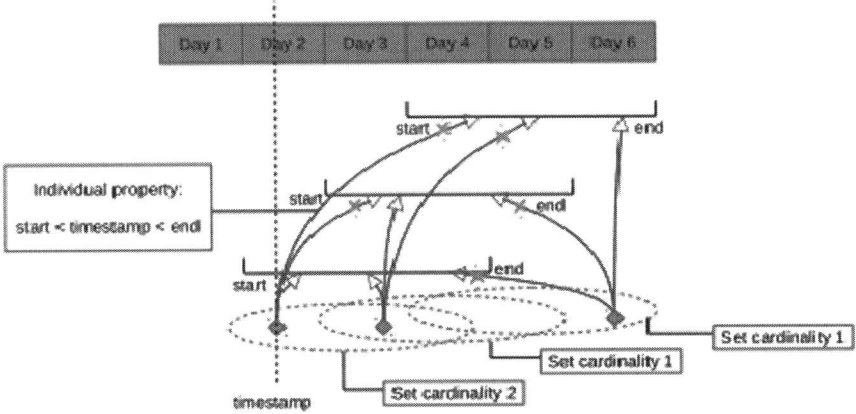

Fig. 7 Time windows concept

structured and dedicated editor was developed. This activity is called "mapping";

3. an automatic reasoner processes the OWL ontology and produces a new OWL description, inferring the detection of anomalies in the user's behaviour;
4. A.I.zeta transforms the automatic inferences produced by the reasoner in new records for the System DB; this activity is called "de-mapping" and uses the same rules editor, previously mentioned.

Exploiting a rules-based approach, A.I.zeta can ensure a high level of flexibility; every generic AAL System DB can be mapped and de-mapped in a suitable ontology description. The ontology can be managed and designed with various tools, like one of the most known "Protégé" that uses the same API present in A.I.zeta.

3   The A.I.zeta Framework

The A.I.zeta is a software that acts as intermediate between a source of raw data and an ontology based reasoning system based on OWL-API [15] and Hermit [16] reasoner API.

The weak point of knowledge-based systems has always been the ability to use the reasoning capabilities in a more automatic and natural way. The actual solutions are often based on static query embedded in the programs code and it is still difficult to interpret the reasoning output in way that is more dynamic.

To obtain a flexible system that is capable of fully benefit of the reasoning process that can be integrated in a data based system, two principles are taken into consideration:

1. The interface mapping;
2. An ontology design approach that can aid the inference process.

At the moment of this writing, the framework manly focuses on realizing this two tasks, but the design of this application is intended to provide a tool able to manage ontologies and their reasoning capabilities without the need of writing ad hoc programs, and provide interface to be able of handle interactions with the extern. The only part that is hard coded in the program is the database interface, because there are different database technologies and every implementation of database relays on its drivers and instruction set.

The A.I.zeta framework acquire the raw data through the external interface, the incoming data triggers the application's automatic handling process that interprets the raw information translating it in meta-information using the configurable mapping mechanism. Then try to infer "new knowledge" on those and at the end eventual new knowledge using the reasoner capabilities. The "new knowledge" is parsed into raw data through the inverse mapping mechanism and sent back to the database.

To understand the process, a simple example will be explained. This example refers to the detection of an alarm from the wearable sensor Musa. This sensor send logs to the database about its state (active or not responding) and can signal two types of events: an emergency call and a fall by the person who wear it.

This situation is modeled in the ontology in which are: a class representing the MuSA sensors present in the AAL environment, a subclass of MuSA that is reporting, corresponding to the group of signals that the sensor can send, and in reporting there are two subclasses identifying the type of signal: fall and emergency call. Classes are intended as synonym of set.

Then a "red alarm" subclass of MuSA represent the dangerous situation that has to be detected. This subclass id defined as equivalent class of a MuSA sensor related to some fall event through a certain object property, which relate MuSA individuals to fall individuals and a data property that relate the sensor to its active state.

The detection of this alarm can be divided in three steps:

1. During the periodic data polling, a log corresponding to a fall event is gathered by the framework. All logs are compared to the patterns stored in the maps collection. The fall signal pattern match the properly defined map, so the framework add some specific axiom to the ontology that states a fall individual in the fall-class under reporting and a property that relate the MuSA individual to the fall individual.

2. After the processing of the new logs the software triggers a reasoning process, inferring that the MuSA individual, with the property axiom, that relate it with the fall individual and has an active state, is equivalent to the "red alarm" class definition. The inferred ontology will then contain a new axiom that states that the particular MuSA individual also belong to the "red alarm" class because it satisfies the logic equivalence axiom.

3. This new axiom is parsed like the new logs though the de-mapping that compares it to the axiom patterns in the maps collection. The inferred axiom, when match the map, automatically trigger the translation to a log that is defined in the map and then the log, that represent the "red alarm", is sent to the database.

4 Interface Between AAL System DB and A.I.zeta

In this case, the DB is a MySQL type, and the interface is built upon the java library MySQL-connector.

The database interface acts only as a channel to gather and store data, from and into the database. The interface periodically query for new data and forwards it to the application. It also forwards the data coming from the de-mapping system.

Referring to the example this is the part of the software, which handle the instruction to read and write logs on the database.

5 Reconfigurable Mapping Through the Interface

The interface mapping mechanism provide, through an editor, the ability of defining some masks that pairs raw data patterns and axioms present in the ontology. Those masks pairs database's string, representing raw sensors data, into individuals and axioms present in the ontology model.

There are two types of masks, input and output, the first are used to translate data into axioms and the second type translate axioms to raw data.

This mechanism is used to automatically handle reasoning: the raw data goes in input to the framework, raw data is translated into ontology axioms, every input provided trigger the reasoning process, then the framework translate the inferred axioms that match the output masks into raw data and send them back to the source according to the provided data pattern.

The main goal of this mechanism is to simplify the use of ontologies in order to explicit the natural language forms.

Referring to the example, this framework part convert the signal log to the axiom relationship between the MuSA individual and the fall individual, also do the reverse operation on the inferred axiom producing a custom output log containing the new data produced after the reasoning.

6 Interface Between A.I.zeta and OWL-Based Ontology

The A.I.zeta framework automatically handles the ontology and the reasoner thanks to the integration of the OWL and Hermit APIs [15, 16]. Inside the application, there are packages that provide ontology handling and manipulation and other packages that handle the reasoning process and results.

Through the configurable mapping system and the editors that manage the masks, the software can be adapted to ontologies without rewriting the code of the application methods.

The inference process also benefits of this mechanism because inferred knowledge is automatically translated and externalized by the application.

All these processes are triggered by dataflow in order to make the entire system like a black-box that has the ontology model as internal parameter, raw-data as input while outputs are data derived from reasoning on the model.

7 Ontology Inference Based Design Approach

To use the framework to fully benefits of its reasoning capabilities is fundamental to understand how the inference process works and keep it in mind during the design the ontology. First, you have to do some closures on your domain and be sure that the thing you want to infer are totally characterized in your model, because the reasoner works in open-world assumption and cannot discriminate things that are in ambiguous domains.

For closures on domain is intended the definition of a hierarchical system of sets related with properties that has its own and precise identity and cannot be confused with any other classes even if defined in other domains. The cardinality relations inference process is funded on this sentence. With a banal example, if we say that we have an object with four legs we cannot understand, only with information, if that object is a table or a chair. But when someone adds the information that the legs that belong to that object are chair legs, and chair legs can belong only to chairs then we know that the object can only be a chair and this is the inference process that a reasoner can do. The additional information provided about the identity of the legs of the object are the closure on the domain because those information assures from a logical point of view that our deduction is correct.

Second, you have to design the rules of your domain in order to infer axioms that you can discern from others, like class equivalence or subclass inheritance.

The second rule is more a suggestion, because the accuracy of the model do not interfere with the reasoning capabilities, but the more accurate the model is, more accurate are the information you can infer.

One of the techniques mainly used in this first approach is the definition of categories like sensors and alarm and the creating a deeper subclass chain to define the closure on the domain. Then through equivalent classes axioms define the object that is related to a certain rule, for example a sensor became an engaged sensor when it is related with at least one signaling. Then when the property became true, the reasoner can infer an axiom that declares that the sensor is engaged and we can map this axiom in our system. Adding more rules and classes we can discern more kind of events. This is the approach used in the explained example, but as the reader can understand, the flexibility of the ontological model allows a great degree of freedom in the modeling choices.

Rules that can be modeled in the ontological domain can also include cardinality and logical operation allowing the representation of more complex contexts.

More complex examples will not be explained in detail as did for the previous one because the possible relations are n-dimensional, so it is very difficult to represent with graphs and schemes. As mentioned before this work focuses on how to handle inference in complex model rather than the model description itself.

In order to give a deeper insight of the model design a significant example will be presented in the next section.

8   The Time Model

In order to test the capability of the inference process a model with time concept has been developed even if it is not still integrated in the framework. Using a timestamp (a reference from the epoch) every event registered inside the software can be placed in a specific interval of time. A more detailed model could also include concept like day, month and year.

The proposed time model relays on time windows that could be opened on events or periodically with a defined expiration interval that depends on the behaviour that has to be observed. Then every event can be linked to all the interested time windows with a property that is satisfied if its timestamp is between the begin and the end of the window. With this model, properties based on cardinality of the relation could effectively count elements that satisfies the belonging to a window, also it is possible to count windows that are linked with some properties. A further mechanism is needed to detect no more relevant windows to remove them from the model (not presented to avoid excessive complexity).

From a more ontological point of view a set representation is schematized in the following picture.

In the proposed example there are groups of classes that represents the windows and multiple event detection on a window and a set containing the events. Every window has a set that contains an instance (individual) of the window, a set that define the interval through the ranges on the "hasTimestamp" data property that links an individual with a primitive data type, in this case an integer, an equivalence class for the multi events, defined has equivalence with the real set, plus two object properties, that links individuals and sets.

The set containing the range allow inferring that individuals, which have timestamp inside the interval, belong to that set.

When the window instance is linked to the event individuals through the object property hasEvent, the multi-event equivalent class allow inferring that when there are at least two elements, that belong to this windows interval, that are linked to the windows instance, the window individual belong to multi event class window as shown in Fig. 8. The two events individual classified as belonging to that window still belong to the event set also.

This example is very significant because it illustrates how time- related concept can be modeled inside an ontology and not less important, how to use this model to benefit of the reasoning capabilities of those instruments. Another very interesting feature of the ontological model is that those concepts can be easily extended, in fact causal relation could be easily added with other properties on timestamps. Similarly, to what is already presented various representation of time-related concept could coexist in the same domain if logical consistency is maintained (Fig. 9).

The example also show a way to handle cardinality inference as mentioned in chapter 3, of course, extending the hierarchy and the relations, different concept can be automatically inferred.

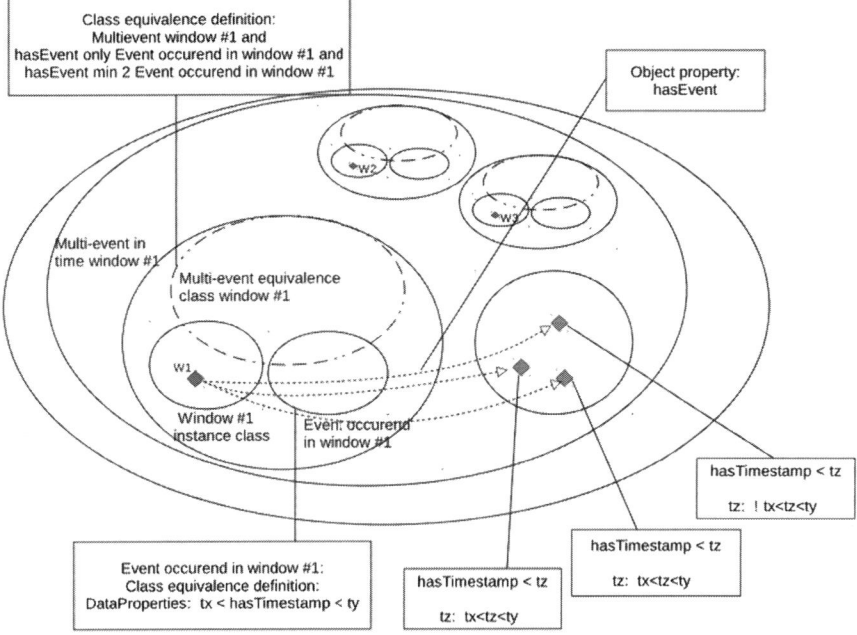

Fig. 8 Time window ontology model

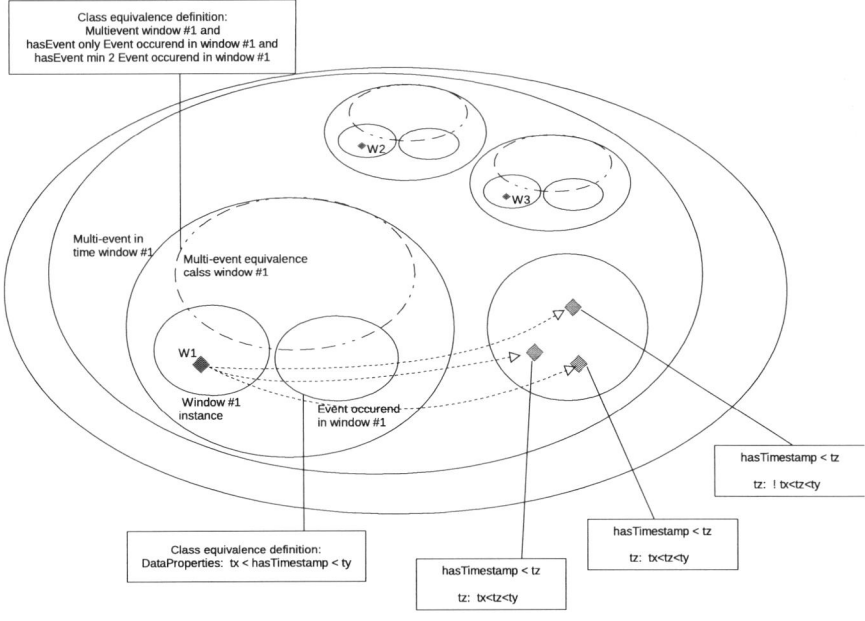

Fig. 9 Inference with time window

9   Results

Purpose of this work is demonstrate that an ontology-based approach to control an AAL system is possible. A such approach ensure a better flexibility, avoiding change in the control software and allowing for a high level description of functions (using the rules editor provided in the framework). No particular performance measurement are provided in this phase of the framework development. Although A.I.zeta is at his first steps, it is able to model part of an AAL ambient, sensors and rules and infer various kind of alarms accordingly to types and quantities of events occurrences. Currently the main difficulties consist in the integration of the time model patterns in the software, but successful inferences on time relations are a good starting point.

The system is able to map sensor events into the ontology model in total autonomy after having configured the map pattern and of inferring alarms related to those events, automatically generating feedbacks.

The first ontology designed is quite primitive, having the main purpose of verifying the reasoning capabilities of the system, and working like a sort of training example in writing rules useful for inferring knowledge.

However, the proposed examples have successfully shown the framework capabilities of handling data, reasoning and feedbacks.

Only one type of sensor was modeled into the system but it can be easily extended defining classes and individuals in the ontology through API or external editing tools like the most known Protégé [17] that is the currently used.

The time concept based on the event timestamp that is associated with properties to events, even if not integrated in the dataflow, allowed to verify the cardinality inference and proposed a functional way to handle time relations inside the ontological context.

Actually the windowed time model can classify when multiple events occurs in a certain period, and even if the framework need further develops to infer these situations in total autonomy, this example shows the effectiveness of the ontology design for the reasoning purposes.

10   Conclusions

Ontological descriptions are often used to model complex domain, also in the case of AAL Systems. The goal of this work was to conceive an innovative approach that, exploiting the possibilities offered by an automatic reasoner, enable an AAL System to infer complex autonomous decisions, using the semantic reasoning tool not only for model consistency but also to use the inference capabilities.

To this purpose a software framework, called A.I.zeta, has been created.

The inference made on cardinality relations and time models can be considered a good example of complex inference.

All this process was automatically driven by A.I.zeta, that:

- queries the AAL System DB to monitor the status of the sensors of the system;
- updates the status of ontology based on programmable rules (called maps);
- performs the ontology analysis by the use of an automatic reasoner;
- processes the results of inferences and returns the appropriate feedback at the DB, also in this case on the basis of programmable rules.

From this point of view, the preliminary results of this work are quite interesting.

Besides of the actual results, further improvements are necessary to make map editors works in a way that can explicit natural language forms and now this mechanism is ready, further efforts are to be spent on modeling AAL ambient and rules to extend the possible inference.

Time model need to be extended with causality relations (A occurred before B and other before/after relations) and concepts like night, day and seasons. In part, these concepts can be modeled on the basis of how we shaped them in our previous work.

As future develop there's the idea of integrating ontology models into the simulator to benefit of reason's consistency checking methods and to model complex behavior through axioms to take advance of the flexibility of the ontologies.

Acknowledgements The framework described in this article has used the AAL System developed in the context of the HELICOPTER AAL Project [18, 19] as a reference. In particular, the simulations carried out during the test of the A.I.zeta software, have exploited a database format, modeled on the specifications of the HELICOPTER Project.

References

1. Aloulou H, Mokhtari M, Tiberghien T, Biswas J, Yap P (2014) An adaptable and flexible framework for assistive living of cognitively impaired people. IEEE J Biomed Health Inform 18(1):353–360
2. Miori V, Russo D (2012) Anticipating health hazards through an ontology-based. In: IoT domotic environment. In 6th International Conference on IMIS, Ubiquitous Computing
3. Rodner T, Litz L (2013) Data-driven generation of rule-based behavior models for an Ambient assisted living system. In: IEEE Third international conference on consumer electronics, pp 35–38, vol 5
4. Kwang-Eun K, Kwee-Bo S (2008) Development of context aware system based on Bayesian network driven context reasoning method and ontology context modelling. In: Control, automation and systems
5. Yuanyuan C, Linmi T, Guangyou X (2009) An event-driven context model in elderly health monitoring. In: Ubiquitous, autonomic and trusted computing
6. Scalmato A, Sgorbissa A, Zaccaria R (2013) Describing and recognizing patterns of events in smart environments with description logic. Cybern IEEE Transac 43(6):1882–1897
7. Kurschl W, Mitsch S, Schoenboeck J (2008) An engineering toolbox to build situation aware ambient assisted living systems. Broadband communications, information technology & biomedical applications, 2008 third international conference on, Gauteng, pp 110–116

8. Ausín D, Castanedo F, López-de-Ipiña D (2012) On the measurement of semantic reasoners in Ambient Assisted Living environments. Intelligent Systems (IS), 2012 6th IEEE international conference, Sofia, pp 082–087

9. Grguric A, Huljenic D, Mosmondor M (2015) AAL ontology: from design to validation. Communication workshop (ICCW), 2015 IEEE international conference on, London, pp 234–239

10. http://ewallproject.eu/

11. Culmone R et al (2014) AAL domain ontology for event-based human activity recognition. Mechatronic and Embedded Systems and Applications (MESA), 2014 IEEE/ASME 10th International Conference on, Senigallia, pp 1–6

12. Mordonini M, Matrella G, Mancin M, Pesci M (2015) An ontology designed for supporting an AAL experience in the framework of the FOOD project. In: Ambient assisted living; biosystems & biorobotics, vol 11, pp 253–263, Springer International Publishing, New York city

13. http://www.aal-europe.eu

14. Bianchi V, Grossi F, De Munari I, Ciampolini P (2012) Multi sensor assistant: a multisensor wearable device for ambient assisted living. J Med Imaging Health Inf 2(1):70–75

15. https://www.w3.org/TR/owl2-overview/

16. http://www.hermit-reasoner.com/

17. http://protege.stanford.edu/

18. http://www.HELICOPTER-aal.eu/

19. http://www.aal-europe.eu/projects/HELICOPTER

Human Indoor Localization for AAL Applications: An RSSI Based Approach

**L. Ciabattoni, F. Ferracuti, A. Freddi, G. Ippoliti,
S. Longhi, A. Monteriù and L. Pepa**

Abstract Ambient intelligence technologies have the objective to improve the quality of life of people in daily living, by providing user-oriented services and functionalities. Many of the services and functionalities provided in Ambient Assisted Living (AAL) require the user position and identity to be known, and thus user localization and identification are two prerequisites of utmost importance. In this work we focus our attention on human indoor localization. Our aim is to investigate how Received Signal Strength (RSS) based localization can be performed in an easy way by exploiting common Internet of Things (IoT) communication networks, which could easily integrate with custom networks for AAL purposes. We thus propose a plug and play solution where the Beacon Nodes (BNs) are represented by smart objects located in the house, while the Unknown Node (UN) can be any smart object held by the user. By using real data from different environments (i.e., with different disturbances), we provide a one-slope model and test localization performances of three different algorithms.

L. Ciabattoni (✉) · F. Ferracuti · G. Ippoliti · S. Longhi · A. Monteriù · L. Pepa
Dipartimento di Ingegneria dell'Informazione, Università Politecnica
delle Marche, Via Brecce Bianche, 60131 Ancona, Italy
e-mail: l.ciabattoni@univpm.it

F. Ferracuti
e-mail: f.ferracuti@univpm.it

G. Ippoliti
e-mail: g.ippoliti@univpm.it

S. Longhi
e-mail: s.longhi@univpm.it

A. Monteriù
e-mail: a.monteriu@univpm.it

L. Pepa
e-mail: l.pepa@univpm.it

A. Freddi
SMARTEST Research Centre, Università degli Studi eCampus,
Via Isimbardi 10, 22060 Novedrate, CO, Italy
e-mail: alessandro.freddi@uniecampus.it

© Springer International Publishing AG 2017
F. Cavallo et al. (eds.), *Ambient Assisted Living*, Lecture Notes
in Electrical Engineering 426, DOI 10.1007/978-3-319-54283-6_18

Keywords Human indoor localization · Ambient assisted living · Internet of things · Smart home

1 Introduction

Ambient Assisted Living (AAL) is typically classified according to the targeted functional domain, and might include safety systems, medical devices, telemedicine platforms, assistive robots and many others [9]. Regardless of the assistive functionality or service provided, AAL technologies typically require the user position and/or identity to be known. While indoor localization (and mapping) of artificial systems (e.g. robots) is an already mature research field [4, 11, 13, 16], indoor user localization has started to attract a lot of interest in the AAL research community only in the last years, and it is still one of the open challenges to solve [29]. In 2011, the Evaluating AAL Systems through Competitive Benchmarking (EvAAL) was established, which aims at establishing benchmarks and evaluation metrics for comparing Ambient Assisted Living solutions [7]. Since then several localization solutions for AAL have been proposed, such as the RESIMA architecture for assisting people with sensory disability in indoor environments [2], and CARDEAGate for providing an inexpensive and scarcely intrusive way for user localization and identification [14].

Most of the times, however, localization systems for AAL applications are based on custom solutions, and thus are difficult to integrate with other systems and require an extensive calibration during the deployment phase [10]. In this work we focus our attention on indoor human localization based on the Internet of Things (IoT) paradigm, seen as the interconnection of devices within the existing internet infrastructure to offer advanced connectivity of devices, systems, and services. The proposed localization is thus performed without the use of ad hoc sensors, i.e., using wireless networks already installed at home, like those required by smart objects to operate. Among the available localization methods, those based on Received Signal Strength Indicator (RSSI) are probably the most suitable for localizing a person indoor, since they are low-cost, present low-complexity and exploit already existing networks without the use of further hardware. RSSI is an indicator which can be used in many applications, such as the implementation of message routing or self-healing strategies for sensor networks, the detection of obstacles crossing the radio-links and especially the localization of nodes. RSSI-based localization techniques rely on two different types of nodes: an Unknown Node (UN), which acts as a receiver and whose position has to be estimated, and Beacon Nodes (BNs), which act as transmitters and whose positions are known. Two types of localization schemes are mainly documented in the literature for RSSI-based localization [30]: fingerprinting [21, 32] and path loss model [1, 5, 6, 34]. The *RSSI-fingerprinting algorithm* consists in the calibration and online tracking processes. One of the main drawbacks of the RSSI based locating methodologies is the extensive calibration phase for building a fingerprint database. As an alternative, *path loss models* can effectively predict the signal strength [12, 17]. Existing prediction models may fall into two categories: the deterministic and empirical models [33]. The deterministic model is accurate and site-specific, but demands a heavy computational load, while the empirical approach can be easily computed but is less accurate. Once the distance of the UN from the nearest BNs has been calculated, then it is possible to estimate the UN position by using different estimation algorithms, such as Min-Max, Multilateration and Maximum Likelihood [22, 24]. RSSI, however, is susceptible to several disturbances, such as noise, interference, multi-path fading, dilution of precision, which greatly affect the signal received power [23]. A poor ranging usually determines poor position estimates and, hence, unsatisfactory localization performances: this limit depends on the ranging errors and cannot be overcome by the use of more sophisticated estimation algorithms. The recent RSSI literature is mainly focused in finding solutions to improve the localization accuracy [18, 33], to deal with dynamic environments [27] and to minimize the power consumption of the localization system [31]. These solutions, however, are oriented towards the world of wireless sensor networks, where accuracy, robustness and optimized results are obtained at the cost of high complexity algorithms and time consuming setup phases, and are often limited to heavily structured environments. On the other hand, commercial solutions typically require the use of ad hoc devices and do not exploit the already existing wi-fi network (such as the iBeacon from Apple [15]).

In the proposed work, instead, we focus our attention on the world of IoT and smart homes for AAL, and want to investigate how RSSI localization can be performed in an easy way by exploiting common IoT communication networks. We thus propose a plug and play solution where the BNs are represented by smart objects located in the house, while the UN can be any smart object held by the user. By using real data from different environments (i.e., with different disturbances), it is then possible to provide an empirical model, based on the one-slope model introduced by Panjwani and Abbott [25] and recently used in [21], which provides an acceptable localization accuracy for many services in smart homes, but retaining at the same time the simplicity of a real plug and play solution. At the same time, we compare this approach with the classical one: a path loss model trained and validated on the same testbed. Three different and well-known localization algorithms are tested and their results are presented. The work is organized as follows. Section 2 provides the description of the used hardware and software platforms. Section 3 contains a brief presentation of the experimental test environments, together with the considered test protocol. In Sect. 4 we describe the model and its training in two different scenarios as well as an introduction of the considered localization algorithms. Section 5 deals with the presentation of the experimental results obtained in the two scenarios. Conclusions and future works end the work.

2 Experimental Setup

The whole system is composed by different real-world smart objects, each one equipped with an *Apio General* [3] (in detail two lamps, an ambient monitoring device and a loudspeaker). The Apio General is actually a USB stick that integrates an Atmel microcontroller with a Lightweight Mesh communication module able to create a mesh network among these objects. The gateway node is the ambient monitoring device (namely *ComfortBox*) and is composed by a Raspberry PI, an *Apio Dongle* and different sensors (temperature, humidity, indoor air quality, noise and brightness). The Apio Dongle has the same hardware specs of the Apio General but a different firmware and acts as a concentrator node. The gateway node has the task to elaborate, store and synchronize the data with the cloud (see Fig. 1).

In the presented setup, the Apio General devices which transmit data from the smart objects are the BNs (see Fig. 2), while the UN is a temperature sensor (see

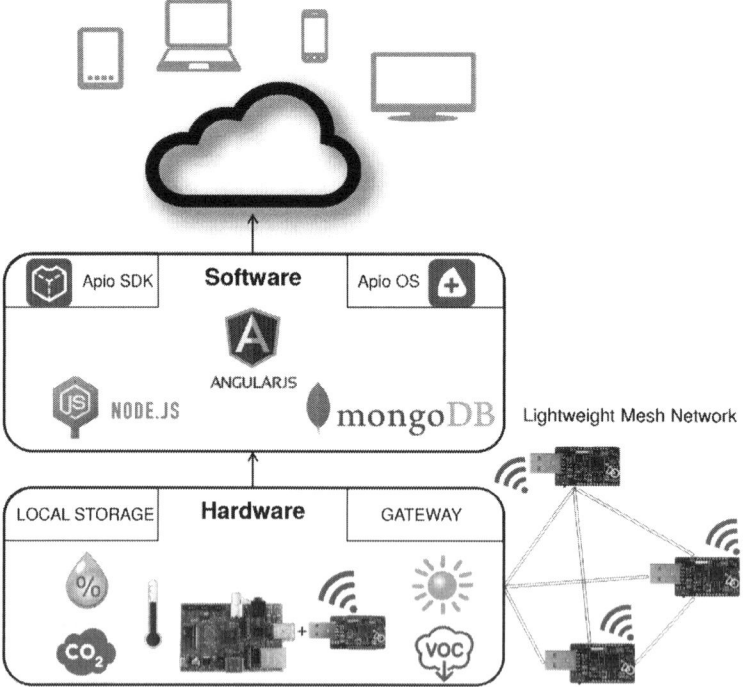

Fig. 1 The system architecture

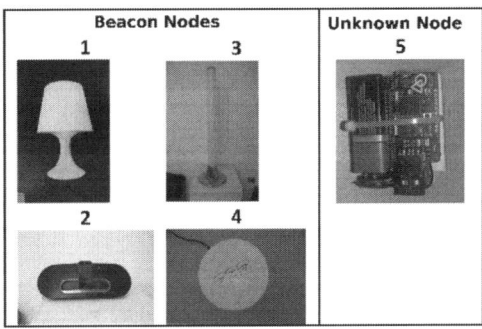
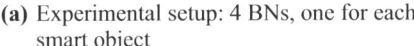
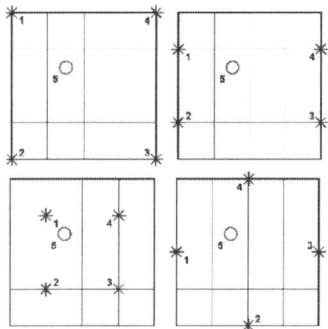

(a) Experimental setup: 4 BNs, one for each smart object

(b) Beacons positioning

Fig. 2 Experimental setup and beacons positioning

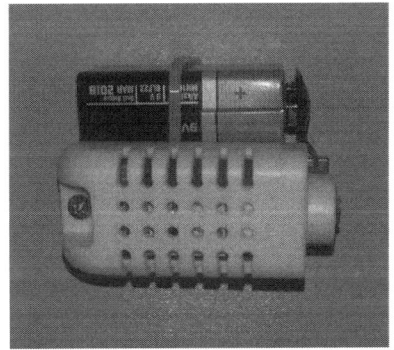
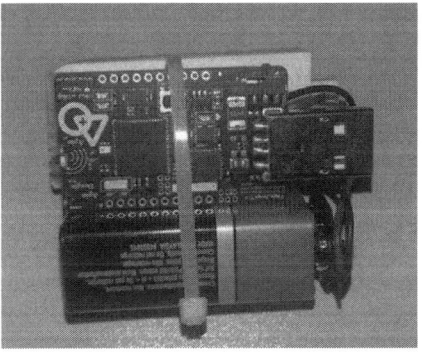

(a) A DHT22 sensor and a 9 V battery (front view)

(b) An Apio General equipped with the Atmel microcontroller and the Lightweight Mesh module (rear view).

Fig. 3 Unknown Node to localize

Fig. 3) held by the user and equipped with an Apio General. The software platform is built using *Node.js* for what regards the server side and cloud synchronization. The client side is based on *Angular.js* and the non-relational database is built using MongoDB. Thanks to the communication module, objects create a mesh network and each one can receive the RSSI value of each other. The source code of the whole OS, USB sticks firmware, server and client modules as well as web applications are available for free on GitHub [26].

3   Experimental Tests

Experiments were performed by considering an area of 36 m^2 out of the total surface of five different test environments: a college lab and an office within the campus of the Polytechnic University of Marche (Ancona, Italy), a garage, a dwelling's living room and a gym in the city of Senigallia (in the province of Ancona). Each test environment is composed by 16 squares with a 1.5 m side (see Fig. 2), 4 BNs (blue dots) in 4 different configurations and 1 UN (red dot). Sixteen sampled locations were identified within each environment, and their position marked on the floor. The average beacon density was 0.11 beacon nodes per square meter.

RSSI values from beacons, placed at 0.75 m from the floor, were gathered at each sampled location while the receiver was in the pocket of the user approximately at the same height of the beacons. Sixteen different tests have been performed in each test environment (four for each beacon configuration). For each test we collected over 200 readings at each sampled location with a sampling frequency of 10 Hz. Over 250,000 readings were collected from the physical test beds.

4   Indoor Localization Algorithms

We first considered a one-slope model [25] and then used it to test three different localization algorithms, namely Min-Max, Trilateration and Maximum Likelihood. The one-slope model considers a parametric equation of the RSSI-distance (x) function as reported in Eq. (1):

$$\text{RSSI} = A \log(x) + B \tag{1}$$

where RSSI is measured in power ratio dBm and x, the distance between the beacon node and the receiver node, is expressed in meters. To find the values of A and B parameters, the least squares method has been considered (see Table 1). In particular, two different testing scenarios have been used to validate the data.

Scenario I We performed the training of the model by considering eight tests recorded for only one environment (namely the college laboratory) and the localization performances have been evaluated on the remaining eight tests.

Scenario II We trained the model with the readings collected in eight tests for all the five test environment, while the performances of the localization have been evaluated on the remaining tests.

Table 1 One-slope model parameters computed in two different scenarios [see Eq. (1)]

	Scenario I	Scenario II
A	−12.193	−14.3
B	−51.67	−53.54

4.1 Min-Max

Min-Max is the most used localization algorithm, whose success is mainly due to its extreme implementation simplicity [33]. Inverting the nominal distance-power loss law [see Eq. (1)], the unknown nodes estimate their distance from each beacon. Then, each unknown node draws a pair of longitudinal lines and a pair of lateral lines around each beacon to create a bounding box given by $[(x_i - r_i), (y_i - r_i)]$ $[(x_i + r_i), (y_i + r_i)]$. $(x_i - y_i)$ is the center of the beacon node while r_i is the distance computed by the model. The location of the unknown node is then approximated by the centre of the intersection box computed by the following equation:

$$\left[\max_{i \le 1 \le N}(x_i - r_i), \max_{i \le 1 \le N}(y_i - r_i)\right] \times \left[\min_{i \le 1 \le N}(x_i + r_i), \min_{i \le 1 \le N}(y_i + r_i)\right] \quad (2)$$

where N is the total number of beacons (4 in our algorithm). Intuitively, the smaller the intersection area the better the localization.

4.2 Trilateration

Trilateration is a decentralized localization algorithm based on geometry principles. As usual, the unknown node collects the beacon messages and estimate their distance to each beacon through the model. Then, any strayed node computes its own position by intersecting the circles centered on the positions occupied by three beacons and having radius equal to the estimated distance between the beacons and the node itself. The intersection should be ideally a single point on a surface. Due to several reasons this intersection is an area where the node is likely to be found. Since we have four beacon nodes, Trilateration is performed each time among three beacon nodes, thus obtaining four potential areas. The node is then positioned in the center of the intersection between these areas. Trilateration is more complex than Min-Max but, at least in principle, it provides better performance, implementing a more sophisticated localization technique.

4.3 Maximum Likelihood

The Maximum Likelihood (ML) localization technique is based on classical statistical inference theory. Given the vector of RSSI values $r = [r_1 \ r_2 \ldots r_n]^T$ obtained from n beacons with coordinates $[x_{B1}, x_{B2}, \ldots, x_{Bn}]$ and $[y_{B1}, y_{B2}, \ldots, y_{Bn}]$, the algorithm computes the a priori probability of receiving r for each potential position $[x, y]$ of the unknown node. The position that maximizes the probability is then selected as the estimated node position. The Maximum Likelihood method is more complex than the others, but it tries to minimize the variance of the estimation error as the number of observations, i.e., of beacon nodes, grows to infinity. In most of the test scenarios the number of beacons is limited, so that the ML performance can be rather unsatisfactory.

5 Experimental Results

According to past researches [20], we use the Cumulative Distribution Function (CDF) of localization error as well as basic statistical metrics (mean value, average value and standard deviation) of localization error to measure the localization performance. The CDF $F(e)$ of localization error e is defined in term of a probability density function $f(e)$ as follows:

$$F(e) = \int_0^e f(x)dx \quad (x > 0) \tag{3}$$

From the CDF of localization error, it is possible to establish the localization error at a given confidence level (e.g., 50, 90%). Figures 4 and 5 show the cumulative probability function of the error computed for both considered scenarios.

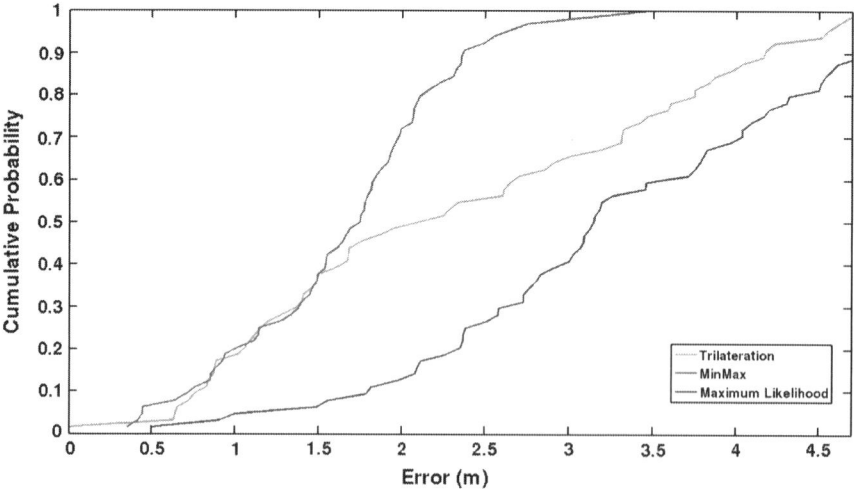

Fig. 4 Cumulative probability computed on the validation set in Scenario I

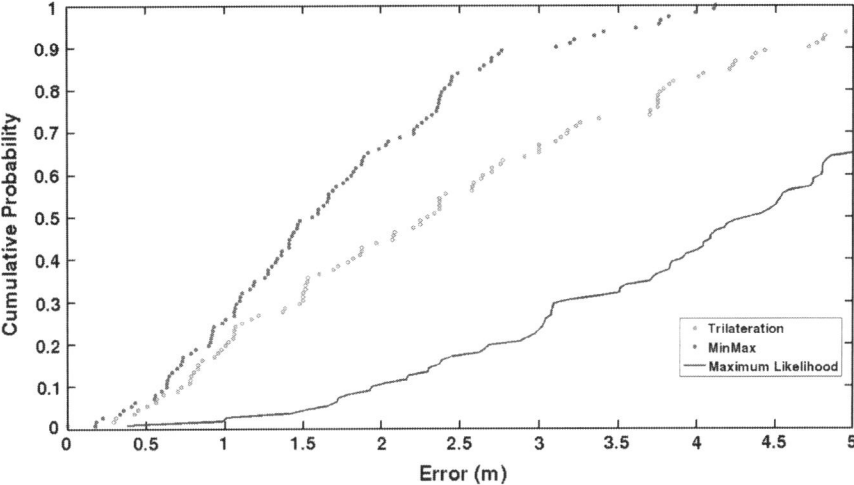

Fig. 5 Cumulative probability computed on the validation set in Scenario II

Table 2 summarize the mean value, standard deviation and median value of the error for the three algorithms considered. Results obtained are coherent with the previous literature works, as in [8, 19, 20, 28]. The research results indicate that the MinMax algorithm has the best accuracy among the three localization algorithms tested in both scenarios. Furthermore, the MinMax algorithm has other advantages over the other algorithms: it is easier to implement, the running time and data storage is linear with the number of beacons. These features bring more convenience to deploy the MinMax algorithm on resource constrained smart objects and mobile networks. The second important result of this research is that the modeling of five different real environments (Scenario II) does not strongly affect the localization results. Indeed, as it is possible to notice in Table 2, the average

Table 2 Accuracy performance comparison of the localization algorithms in the two different modeling scenarios (errors in meters)

Scenario I	Algorithm	Mean value	Std. deviation	Median
	Min-Max	1.5295	0.5937	1.7515
	Trilateration	2.2622	1.3221	2.1733
	Maximum likelihood	3.1504	1.1011	3.1504
Scenario II	Algorithm	Mean value	Std. deviation	Median
	Min-Max	1.7084	0.9412	1.5805
	Trilateration	2.4678	1.4790	2.3149
	Maximum likelihood	4.1766	1.5076	4.3752

performances of MinMax in Scenario II are only 0.18 m worse than those of Scenario I, when a single environment is used to train and validate the RSSI one-slope model.

6 Conclusions

In this work we present an RSSI based approach for human indoor localization in AAL applications. Localization is performed without the use of ad hoc sensors, but exploits the wireless networks already installed at home, like those required by smart objects to operate. Three algorithms were evaluated: MinMax, ML, and Trilateration. To evaluate the algorithms, over 250,000 readings were collected from five physical test beds. A one-slope model has been created in two different scenarios: by considering a single test bed both for training and validation (Scenario I) and by considering all the test beds (Scenario II). Results are coherent with the literature for what concern Scenario I and seems to be promising for Scenario II. When training a model for five scenarios the performances obtained are only 11.8% worse than those obtained in Scenario I. In particular, the MinMax algorithm shows the best performances and can have the potential for a future adoption in AAL applications. The results presented in the work are still preliminary, and the authors are currently testing different RSS models and custom algorithms for localization, together with different hardware solutions.

Acknowledgements This work was supported by the company Apio srl that provided the hardware components and the IoT objects. Thanks to the students Andrea Generosi, Andrea Marchetti and Giammarco Righi for their support during the experiments.

References

1. Ahn HS, Yu W (2009) Environmental-adaptive RSSI-based indoor localization. IEEE Trans Autom Sci Eng 6(4):626–633
2. Andò B, Baglio S, Lombardo CO (2014) RESIMA: an assistive paradigm to support weak people in indoor environments. IEEE Trans Instrum Meas 63:2522–2528
3. APIO (2015) APIO srl official website. https://www.apio.cc. Last access 15 July 2015
4. Armesto L, Ippoliti G, Longhi S, Tornero J (2008) Probabilistic self-localization and mapping—an asynchronous multirate approach. IEEE Robot Autom Mag 15(2):77–88
5. Baldini A, Ciabattoni L, Felicetti R, Ferracuti F, Freddi A, Longhi S, Monteriù A (2016) Room occupancy detection: combining RSS analysis and fuzzy logic. In: International conference on consumer electronics (ICCE), Berlin, Germany
6. Baldini A, Ciabattoni L, Felicetti R, Ferracuti F, Freddi A, Longhi S, Monteriù A (2016) A novel RSSI based approach for human indoor localization: the fuzzy discrete multilateration. In: International conference on consumer electronics (ICCE), Berlin, Germany
7. Barsocchi P, Chessa S, Furfari F, Potortì F (2013) Evaluating ambient assisted living solutions: the localization competition. IEEE Pervasive Comput 12:72–79

8. Barsocchi P, Lenzi S, Chessa S, Giunta G (2009) A novel approach to indoor RSSI localization by automatic calibration of the wireless propagation model. In: IEEE 69th vehicular technology conference (VTC), pp 1–5
9. Benetazzo F, Ferracuti F, Freddi A, Giantomassi A, Iarlori S, Longhi S, Monteriù A, Ortenzi D (2015) AAL technologies for independent life of elderly people. In: Ambient assisted living: Italian forum 2014, vol 11. Biosystems and biorobotics. Springer International Publishing, pp 329–343
10. Ciabattoni L, Freddi A, Longhi S, Monteriù A, Pepa L, Prist M (2015) An open and modular hardware node for wireless sensor and body area networks. J Sens, p 16, Article ID 2978703
11. Conte G, Longhi S, Zulli R (1996) Motion planning for unicycle and car-like robots. Int J Syst Sci 27(8):791–798
12. Fang SH, Lin T-N, Lee K-C (2008) A novel algorithm for multipath fingerprinting in indoor wlan environments. IEEE Trans Wireless Commun 7(9):3579–3588
13. Fulgenzi C, Ippoliti G, Longhi S (2009) Experimental validation of FastSLAM algorithm integrated with a linear features based map. Mechatronics 19(5):609–616
14. Guerra C, Bianchi V, De Munari I, Ciampolini P (2015) CARDEAGate: low-cost, ZigBee—based localization and identification for AAL purposes. In: IEEE international instrumentation and measurement technology conference (I2MTC), Pisa, Italy, pp 245–249
15. iBeacon (2015) iBeacon for developers official website. https://developer.apple.com/ibeacon/. Last access 25 May 2016
16. Ippoliti G, Jetto L, Longhi S (2005) Localization of mobile robots: development and comparative evaluation of algorithms based on odometric and inertial sensors. J Robotic Syst 22(12):725–735
17. Lassabe F, Canalda P, Chatonnay P, Spies F (2009) Indoor Wi-Fi positioning: techniques and systems. Ann Telecommun 64(9–10):651–664
18. Li L, Wu Y, Ren Y, Yu N (2013) A RSSI localization algorithm based on interval analysis for indoor wireless sensor networks. In: IEEE cyber, physical and social computing, pp 434–437
19. Lin TH, Ng IH, Lau SY, Chen KM, Huang P (2008) A microscopic examination of an RSSI-signature-based indoor localization system. In: The fifth workshop on embedded networked sensors (HotEmNets), Charlottesville, Virginia, pp 2–6
20. Luo X, OBrien WJ, Julien CL (2011) Comparative evaluation of received signal-strength index (RSSI) based indoor localization techniques for construction jobsites. Adv Eng Inf 25 (2):355–363
21. Narzullaev A, Park Y, Yoo K, Yu J (2011) A fast and accurate calibration algorithm for real-time locating systems based on the received signal strength indication. AEU-Int J Electr Commun 65(4):305–311
22. Nguyen X, Rattentbury T (2003) Localization algorithms for sensor networks using RF signal strength CS 252 class project. Citeseer, Tech. Rep., 2003
23. Patwari N, Ash JN, Kyperountas S, Hero AO, Moses RL, Correal NS (2005) Locating the nodes: cooperative localization in wireless sensor networks. IEEE Signal Process Mag 22 (4):54–69
24. Patwari N, Dea R, Wang Y (2001) Relative location in wireless networks. In: IEEE 53rd vehicular technology conference (VTC), vol 2, pp 1149–1153
25. Panjwani M, Abbott A (1996) Interactive computation of coverage regions for wireless communication in multifloored indoor environments. IEEE J Sel Areas Commun 14:420–430
26. Repository (2015) Anchor nodes and unknown node open source code from GitHub. https://github.com/ApioLab/. Last access 8 July 2015
27. Sahu P, Wu E-K, Sahoo J (2013) DURT: dual RSSI trend based localization for wireless sensor networks. IEEE Sens J 13(8):3115–3123
28. Sugano M (2006) Indoor localization system using RSSI measurement of wireless sensor network based on ZigBee standard. In: Wireless and optical communications, pp 1–6
29. Sun H, De Florio V, Gui N, Blondia C (2009) Promises and challenges of ambient assisted living systems. In: Sixth international conference on information technology: new generations (ITNG), Las Vegas, USA, pp 1201–1207

30. Wang X, Qiu J, Ye S, Dai G (2014) An advanced fingerprint-based indoor localization scheme for WSNs. In: 9th IEEE conference on industrial electronics and applications, Hangzhou, China, pp 2164–2169
31. Yaghoubi F, Abbasfar A, Maham B (2014) Energy-efficient RSSI-based localization for wireless sensor networks. IEEE Commun Lett 18(6):973–976
32. Yin J, Yang Q, Ni LM (2008) Learning adaptive temporal radio maps for signal-strength-based location estimation. IEEE Trans Mob Comput 7(7):869–883
33. Zanca G, Zorzi F, Zanella A, Zorzi M (2008) Experimental comparison of RSSI-based localization algorithms for indoor wireless sensor networks. In: Proceedings of the workshop on real-world wireless sensor networks, ACM, pp 1–5
34. Zhang B, Yu F (2010) LSWD: localization scheme for wireless sensor networks using directional antenna. IEEE Trans Consum Electron 56(4):2208–2216

User Indoor Localisation System Enhances Activity Recognition: A Proof of Concept

Laura Fiorini, Manuele Bonaccorsi, Stefano Betti, Paolo Dario and Filippo Cavallo

Abstract Older people would like to live independently in their home as long as possible. They want to reduce the risk of domestic accidents because of polypharmacy, physical weakness and other mental illnesses, which could increase the risks of domestic accidents (i.e. a fall). Changes in the behaviour of healthy older people could be correlated with cognitive disorders; consequently, early intervention could delay the deterioration of the disease. Over the last few years, activity recognition systems have been developed to support the management of senior citizens' daily life. In this context, this paper aims to go beyond the state-of-the-art presenting a proof of concept where information on body movement, vital signs and user's indoor locations are aggregated to improve the activity recognition task. The presented system has been tested in a realistic environment with three users in order to assess the feasibility of the proposed method. These results encouraged the use of this approach in activity recognition applications; indeed, the overall accuracy values, amongst others, are satisfactory increased (+2.67% DT, +7.39% SVM, +147.37% NN).

Keywords Activity recognition · User indoor localisation · Independent living · Wearable sensors

1 Introduction

One of the main challenges of AAL is to provide socially sustainable home care services for senior citizens and to reduce the caregiver's work burden, thus increasing their quality of work.

Older people prefer to live independently in their home as long as possible. In particular, they want to reduce the risk of domestic accidents because of

L. Fiorini (✉) · M. Bonaccorsi · S. Betti · P. Dario · F. Cavallo
The BioRobotics Institute Scuola Superiore Sant'Anna,
Viale Rinaldo Piaggio 34, 56025 Pontedera, PI, Italy
e-mail: laura.fiorini@santannapisa.it

© Springer International Publishing AG 2017
F. Cavallo et al. (eds.), *Ambient Assisted Living*, Lecture Notes
in Electrical Engineering 426, DOI 10.1007/978-3-319-54283-6_19

polypharmacy, physical weakness and other cognitive disorders which can increase the risks of accidents (i.e. a fall). Sometimes, cognitive decline is associated with the onset of difficulties with transportation, cooking, medication, management, and prospective memory tasks like remembering appointments and grocery lists [1].

Literature evidence underlines how ICT technology can help to prevent a decline in the quality of life and support senior citizens during daily activities [2]. In particular, information on which type of activity and how users spend their time at home could prevent the deterioration of cognitive disorders, support the management of their life and lead to target interventions from family and caregivers [3].

The rise of mobile phones, the Internet of Things and smart devices has facilitated the process of measuring individual activities and his/her surroundings. However, most AAL applications require more than the simple collection of measurements from a variable of interest: they require complex algorithms and sometimes a huge set of sensors involved. In this context, accurate information on the user's activity and behaviour represents one of the main challenges of pervasive computing in AAL fields [4]. Users with cognitive disorders (i.e. dementia, Alzheimer's disease) could be monitored to prevent undesirable consequences [5]. In this sense, changes in the behaviour of healthy older people could be correlated with cognitive disorders; in this sense, an early intervention could delay the complications of the cognitive disorders [6].

The first scientific work on activity recognition systems dates back to the late 1990s [7]. However, there are still many challenges and motivations that will stimulate research in this field [8]. Some of these challenges mainly regard the selection of sensors and, consequently, the choice of attributes to measure. It is also important to design a portable, unobtrusive and inexpensive data acquisition system. Additionally, due to the complex and real operative conditions, it is worth mentioning that it is essential to find an optimal balance between the type of intrusive sensors used, the measured attributes, the complexity of the algorithm, and the system accuracy.

In this context, we focus on the use of wearable sensors in order to measure attributes related to the body movement (using an accelerometer), physiological signal (using an electrocardiogram—ECG) and user's location inside the home in order to improve the accuracy of the activity recognition system.

1.1   Related Works

Analysing the state-of-the-art, according to Lara and Labrador [4] it is evident that activity recognition systems can be based mainly on two different approaches. In the first approach, i.e. "*external*", the sensors are placed on a fixed point of interest, and the information on the activity depends on the voluntary interaction of the user. The second approach envisages the use of "*wearable*" sensors placed on the human body. This type of sensor could provide information on four groups of categories: environmental context, body movement, user location and physiological signal.

1.1.1 External Sensors

This first approach envisages the use of "*external sensors*"; smart homes and cameras.

Over the last few years, Smart Home systems [9, 10] have been developed in order to support senior citizens improve their home safety. Recently, commercial IoT solutions [11, 12], have been commercialised to provide service of home remote monitoring. The idea behind this kind of system is to measure the user's interaction with everyday objects to understand their behaviour and activities. However, the accuracy and precision of the activity recognition systems depend on the number of sensors installed in the environment and on the target objects with which the user has to interact [13–15].

Cameras are mainly used for security and surveillance tasks. They are used for posture and gesture recognition, as well as the localisation of multiple users in indoor environments. People detection can be performed by detecting faces or human bodies, while more complex processing is needed to distinguish different users. Nevertheless, there are some issues regarding privacy, pervasiveness and complexity of video process that could limit the use of camera systems [16]. Over the last few years, user indoor localisation systems based on cameras have been developed; so these systems are considered as too invasive and too complex [17, 18]. For instance, Zhu and Sheng [19] present an activity recognition system that fuses together information on user location and human motion. However, they use the Vicon[1] motion capture system to estimate the user's location, which is not easy to install in a real house. Within the Robot-Era project, a user localisation system based on a sensor fusion approach was implemented, exploiting both range-free and range-based localisation methods [20].

1.1.2 Wearable Sensors

The second approach includes the use of "*wearable sensors,*" which could provide information on human movement, physiological signal, context and user location.

Human movement can be estimated by means of inertial sensors. For instance, tri-axial accelerometers, gyroscopes and magnetometers are the most broadly used sensors to recognise daily activity. They are used to estimate indoor and outdoor atomic actions (like walking, lying, descending/ascending stairs) [4], human gestures [21], and fall detection [22]. A recent study has highlighted how an accelerometer placed on a smartphone and smartwatches could be used to estimate daily activity, avoiding forcing the user to wear external sensors [23].

Vital sign data (i.e. heart rate, respiration rate, skin temperature, skin conductivity) could provide information on the user's physiological status and performed activity [24, 25].

---

[1]Vicon Motion Capture; official website: http://www.vicon.com/.

Other research groups have investigated how different typologies of wearable sensors could be fused to improve the efficacy of recognition tasks. For instance, Pärkkä et al. [26] aggregated a total of 22 signals including an accelerometer, vital signs and environmental sensors. Nevertheless, the presented system is very obtrusive because it requires a high number of sensors to be placed on the person. Lara et al. [27] present Centinela, a system that combines acceleration data with vital signs to achieve highly accurate activity recognition.

Mobile phones and portable devices are equipped with Global Positioning System (GPS), which represents a portable system that could provide information on the user's location, enhancing activity recognition tasks. This GPS system is able to locate the person in outdoor environments but does not work well in indoor environments.

1.2 Objective

In this context, this study aims to go beyond the state-of-the-art, presenting a proof of concept where information on body movement, vital signs and user's indoor location are aggregated to improve the activity recognition task (Fig. 1).

The presented solution includes two accelerometers placed on the human body: one on the chest and one on the lower back. These two positions are chosen because, in the future, these sensors could be integrated into "smart fashionable accessories" like a necklace or a fashion belt. Moreover, a commercial chest-bend monitors cardiac activity (electrocardiogram—ECG), and an unobtrusive user indoor localisation system provides information on the user's location [20].

In order to achieve the proposed goal, a strict methodology based on five main phases has been applied. The goal of this proof of concept is to demonstrate how information on user location can improve the recognition of eight common daily

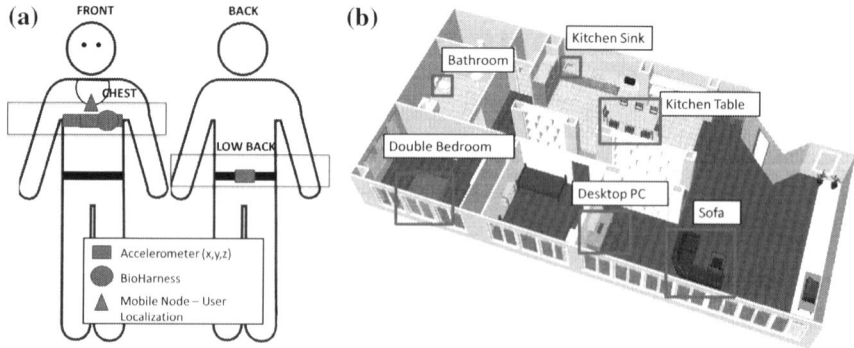

Fig. 1 Proof of concept experimental settings. **a** Wearable sensor distribution on the human body; **b** Selected locations where the selected activities are performed

activities. Then, two different recognition models (with or without the information on user location) were built to compare the performance.

The remainder of the paper is organised as follows. Section 2 presents the methodology used in this work. Section 3 describes and discusses the results, while finally Sect. 4 concludes the paper.

2 Materials and Methods

In this section, the methodology chosen for the data analysis is described in detail. It includes the experimental protocol definitions, a description of the experimental settings and the data analysis. The adopted methodology follows five main phases, which are listed below and described in detail in the following paragraphs:

Phase I This phase includes the definition of the experimental protocol, the optimal choice of sensors and their software integration.

Phase II This phase includes the preparation of the test-bed (Domocasa Lab), the recruitment of testers and the data acquisition according to the protocol defined in Phase I.

Phase III This phase includes the preparation of data and the feature extraction for each participant. The included features were chosen according to the state-of-the-art and the aims of the paper.

Phase IV In this phase, a classification analysis based on three supervised machine learning algorithms [viz. Decision Tree (DT), Support Vector Machine (SVM) and Neural Network (NN)] was conducted on two models to compare the results adequately.

Phase V This phase includes the evaluation of the classification performed in the previous phase. A set of appropriate metrics was used to pursue this goal.

Matlab 2012a was used in Phases II–V to analyse the data offline.

2.1 Phase I: Experimental Protocol Definition

According to statistics [28], home is the most common place where European citizens stay during the day. In particular, among most common activities, European people (aged 20–74) spend 36% of their time sleeping, and 18% doing domestic work like preparing food or cleaning dishes. 22% of time is spent on activities related to free time, like watching TV (41%), resting on the sofa (4%) and reading books (4%). 10% is spent on activities related to gainful work and study (i.e. working at a PC).

Starting from these results, an experimental protocol has been defined. Eight daily activities were selected considering four main categories. (i) Work at PC desk,

Table 1 Experimental protocol

Code	Time (min)	Activity	Location
SPC	3	Work at PC desk	Desktop PC
STV	3	Sit on sofa, watching TV	Sofa
LSO	3	Rest on sofa	Sofa
LS	3	Sleep in bed (supine)	Double bedroom
LRS	3	Sleep in bed (on right side)	Double bedroom
SK	3	Sit at kitchen table	Kitchen (near the table)
SB	3	Sit on toilet	Bathroom
CD	3	Wash up	Kitchen (near the sink)

sit on sofa watching TV, and rest on sofa activities were chosen as the "free-time" category. (ii) Two different sleeping poses (supine and on the right side of the bed) were chosen for the "sleeping" category. (iii) Sit at the kitchen table and washing up were chosen for the "domestic work"; and (iv) sit on the WC represented the "personal hygiene" category (Table 1).

These selected activities aimed to underline how user location could increase the accuracy of the activity recognition tasks. For instance, four different activities (SPC, STV, SK, and SB) presented equal "body orientation"; in fact, the user performed different activities while he/she sits in different places. Even the LS and LSO activities presented the same body orientation and similar physiological parameters, but were performed in two different rooms (Fig. 1b).

2.1.1   Instrumentation

The proposed system for daily activity recognition is shown in Fig. 2. It includes appropriate sensors to measure body acceleration, vital signs and the user's location.

Hardware

The hardware agents included in this system were: wireless sensor networks to estimate the user's location and two kinds of wearable sensors to estimate, respectively, the vital signs' and the user's movement.

1. **Vital Signs** (ECG) were measured with a BioHarness Zephyr 3 chest strap, connected through Bluetooth to a computer. ECG was acquired at a frequency of 250 Hz.
2. **Body acceleration** was measured by means of two wireless 3-axial accelerometer sensors, one placed on the chest and the other placed on the lower back, as shown in Fig. 1a. The number of accelerometer sensors and their position were chosen according to literature evidence considering the balance between accuracy and the number of sensors. These sensors sent data through ZigBee protocol to a computer at a frequency of 50 Hz.

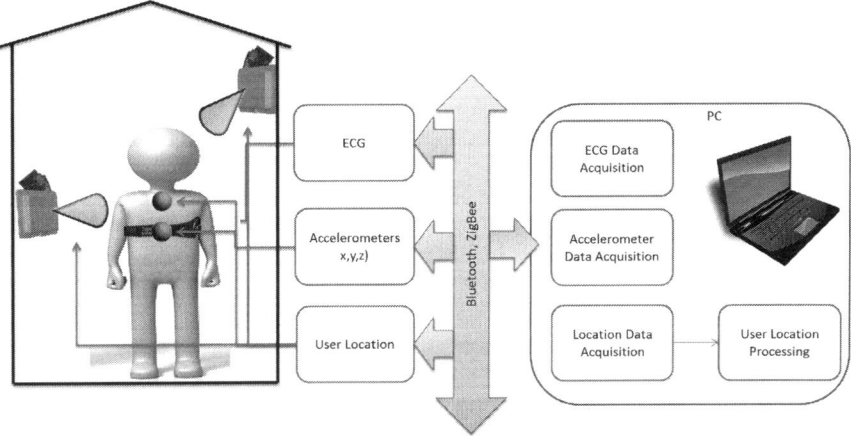

Fig. 2 System architecture. The hardware part is composed of a BioHarness chest band, two accelerometers, one placed on the chest and one in the low back, and the wireless sensor network to estimate the user's location, the MN node is placed on the necklace. A computer collects all the information from these sensors through proper interfaces. Additionally, the user location processing module computes the user's location using the RSS signal

3. The **indoor user location** was estimated through a wireless sensor network, composed of a number of ZigBee wireless radio devices to estimate the user's position with an in-room granularity, developed during the Robot-Era project [23, 29]. This network was designed for the indoor user localisation, observing the Received Signal Strength (RSS) of the messages exchanged between the radios. It was composed of a ZigBee Coordinator (ZC), a Data Logger (DL), a wearable Mobile Node (MN) and a set of ZigBee Anchors (ZAs). The wearable MN periodically sent messages at 1 Hz to all ZAs within one communication hop. Each ZA computed the RSS as the ratio between the received and transmitted electromagnetic power on the received messages, and transmitted this value to the DL. ZAs were instrumented with $60°$ sectorial antennas and installed in a fixed position in the home environment. In particular, they were installed on walls and inside the furniture to monitor the best accessed or interesting areas of the rooms, and to achieve an in-room localisation accuracy. The sectorial antennas were introduced to improve the signal-to-noise ratio of the RSS observations over the selected areas of interest for the user localisation. The MN was instead embedded an omnidirectional antenna for data transmission, to reduce the sensitivity of the localisation system to the user rotations. The DL node was connected to a PC via USB, to upload data for the processing. The entire localisation workspace was 200 m^2, covered by 17 anchors. The overall sensor density was approximately 0.1 device/m^2, but the density was higher in the most accessed areas like the kitchen (~ 0.23 device/m^2), bathroom (~ 0.25 device/m^2) and bedroom (~ 0.20 device/m^2). Additional details on these sensor networks are given in [29].

Software

The software involved in this system includes four different modules developed with Visual Studio (Fig. 2). The ECG data acquisition was able to collect data from BioHarness, implemented using the SDK Zephyr developer kit. The second module was used to collect data from the accelerometers. The final two modules were implemented to collect RSS data from the DL and to compute the user's location with in-room granularity.

The user location processing module [30] was based on a sensor fusion approach implemented by means of a Kalman Filter (KF). The KF inputs were from traditional range-free [31] and range-based [32] localisation methods, according to [20]. The system accounted for a metre-level localisation accuracy (mean localisation error = 0.98 m) [29].

2.2   Phase II: Experimental Setting and Data Acquisition

The experimental protocol was realistically tested in the DomoCasa Lab (Peccioli, Italy), which reproduces a fully furnished apartment of 200 m^2 with a living room, a kitchen, a bathroom, a double bedroom and a single bedroom. The apartment was instrumented with user localisation network as described in [20, 30]. The user location ZigBee anchors were distributed as described in [29].

As a proof of concept, in this study, the experimental session was conducted with three users: one male and two female, whose ages ranged from 27–30 (28.33 ± 1.53).

The user was asked to wear the sensors, the mobile node for user position (as described in Fig. 1a), and to perform each specific activity in the specified room (Table 1) for a total of 3 min. A PC is used to collect the data from the wearable sensors and to compute the user's position using information from the user localisation network.

2.3   Phase III: Feature Extraction

The aim of this phase was to prepare data for the analysis. The accelerometer data consisted of the following attributes: timestamp and acceleration value along the x, y and z directions. The physiological data consisted of the ECG value and timestamp, and the user position data report the user's location estimated with the relative timestamp.

In the first part of the analysis, the data were cut, pre-processed and conveniently filtered to reduce noise. As concern the accelerometer data, a fourth-order low-pass digital Butterworth filter was applied with a 5 Hz cut-off frequency. As for the ECG data, a fourth-order band-pass digital Butterworth filter was applied with 0.05 and 60 Hz cut-off frequencies in order to reject the disturbance properly.

Then, the data were synchronised by means of the timestamp. These time-series were divided with time-window length of 7 s; furthermore, in order to handle transitions more accurately, an overlapping window-time of 50% was chosen.

The next step consisted of the feature extraction. As regard the accelerometer signals, only the time-domain features were considered and included in the analysis [4]. These features were: the mean value (M), the root mean square (RMS), the mean absolute deviation (MAD), the standard deviation (SD) and the variance (VAR). All these features were computed for each axis of the two sensors, for a total of 30 accelerometer features.

Starting from the ECG signal, the inter-beats (RR) interval was computed as the time interval between consecutive heart beats, and was practically measured in the electrocardiogram from the beginning of a QRS complex to the beginning of the next QRS complex. From the RR signal, three different features were extracted: the mean RR value (RRM), the standard deviation (RRSD) and the number of heartbeats per minute (BPM). The final feature of this dataset was represented by the user location, which indicates the micro-area where the activity was performed.

Within this phase, all these 34 features were computed for all the activities listed in the experimental protocol. Consequently, at the end of this phase, a dataset composed of 35 columns (the final column was the label of the activity) was obtained and manually labelled for each user. Table 2 reports all the features involved in the analysis.

2.4 Phase IV: Feature Classification

In this phase, the three users' datasets were merged into a unique dataset in order to reduce the users' physiological variability. Then, this dataset was randomly split

Table 2 Features list

	Features		Number
Accelerometer	M	Mean value	5 × 3 (axis) × 2 (sensors) = 30
	RMS	Root mean square	
	MAD	Mean absolute deviation	
	SD	Standard deviation	
	VAR	Variance	
Vital sign	RRM	Mean RR value	3
	RRSD	Standard deviation	
	BPM	Heartbeat per minute	
User location	User location inside the house, indicated with microarea granularity		1
	Total		34

into two parts (60% training set and 40% test set). The training set was used to build the models, whereas the test set was used for the evaluation phase, as will be described in Sect. 2.5.

Many supervised classification algorithms have already been employed in activity recognition tasks: Decision Tree (C4.5) [26], Fuzzy Logic [33], Support Vector Machine [34] and Hidden Markov Model [35], amongst others. Here, three different algorithms (DT, SVM and NN) were used to perform the recognition tasks. The models were built using (i) Classification Tree with 10 k-fold; (ii) Multiclass Support Vector Machine, adapted from [36], with a linear kernel; and (iii) a Feed-forward neural network. All these models were computed using the machine learning toolbox of Matlab 2012.

In order to evaluate whether user localisation could improve the accuracy, two different classification models were built on the training dataset: one including information on the user's position; the other, not.

2.5 Phase V: Evaluation

Within this phase, the two models were evaluated considering the test set (40% of the original dataset). The results were reported into a confusion matrix. Then, the precision, accuracy, recall, specificity and F-Measure metrics were used to estimate the effectiveness of the models [4] and to compare the performance of the three algorithms used.

Recall is defined as the ratio between the number of correctly classified instances of a class and the number of instances belonging to that class predicted as belonging to other classes. Overall recall is computed as the mean value.

Precision is defined as the ratio of correctly classified in each class to the total number of instances predicted as belonging to that class [33]. Overall precision value is computed as the mean value.

Specificity, also called the true negative rate, is the ratio between the total number of negative instances that were classified as negative, and the total number of negative instances classified in that class. The overall specificity value is computed as the mean value.

F-Measure combines the overall precision value and the overall recall value as follows:

$$F - Measure = \frac{2 \cdot Precision \cdot Recall}{(Precision + Recall)} \tag{1}$$

Overall Accuracy is defined as the ratio between the number of correctly classified instances of a certain class and the total number of instances. It estimates the overall accuracy of the system.

These evaluation metrics were used to compare the activity recognition results gained by applying the DT, SVM and NN over the two models. The difference percentage (Eq. 2) was used to estimate the improvements quantitatively:

$$\text{Difference Percentage} = \frac{P_N - P_Y}{P_N} \cdot 100 \qquad (2)$$

where P_N is the parameter of the model without the user's location and P_Y is the parameter of the other model.

3 Results and Discussion

In this section, the overall evaluation of the results obtained from phase V is reported and discussed. The analysis was conducted considering a total of 482 samples (60%), whereas a total of 193 samples (40%) were included in the evaluation phase.

As shown in Fig. 3, the results obtained in this proof of concept suggest that the inclusion of information on user location could increase the performance of activity recognition (see Table 3). The NN approach presented the highest difference percentage between the two models (Recall +127%, Precision +104%, F-Measure +116%, Specificity +19%, Overall Accuracy +147%) from visual inspection of Fig. 3. The SVM model presented a higher increase in the performance rather than DT (Recall +5%, Precision +5%, F-Measure +5%, Specificity +1%, Overall Accuracy +7%). Finally, the DT comparison values were: Recall +3%, Precision +3%, F-Measure +3%, Specificity +0.4%, Overall Accuracy +2.67%.

In particular, as regards the DT analysis, the overall accuracy was equal to 96.38% for the system without the information on the user's position; this result was comparable to other work that followed a similar approach [37]. On the other hand, the accuracy was equal to 99.24% for the model that included the user's location. Similar results were also obtained for the overall precision, which

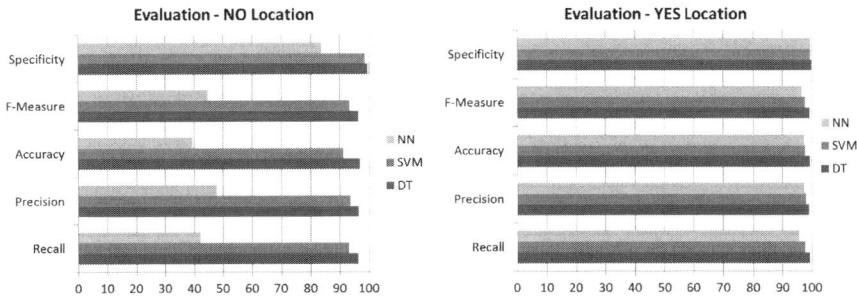

Fig. 3 Performance of the three classification algorithms (NN, SVM, ST)

Table 3 Overall evaluation metrics for the three classification algorithms

		Recall	Precision	Accuracy	F-measure	Specificity
DT	N	96.34	96.43	96.89	96.38	99.57
	Y	99.26	99.22	99.48	99.24	99.93
SVM	N	93.22	93.62	91.19	93.42	98.68
	Y	97.74	98.03	97.93	97.88	99.70
NN	N	42.21	47.62	39.38	44.75	83.52
	Y	95.83	97.40	97.41	96.61	99.64

(Overall precision, overall recall, overall accuracy, f-measure and overall specificity) for the two models (*N* no user location, *Y* user location). The values are expressed as percentages

Table 4 Phase V: DT—evaluation results for each activity. The values are expressed as percentages

DT	No location			Yes location		
	Recall	Precision	Specificity	Precision	Recall	Specificity
STV	100	96	99	100	100	100
SPC	100	100	100	100	100	100
SK	100	75	97	100	94	99
SB	79	100	100	100	100	100
LSO	94	100	100	94	100	100
LS	100	100	100	100	100	100
LRS	100	100	100	100	100	100
CD	98	100	100	100	100	100

increased from 96.43% of the first case to 99.22% of the second case. Comparable trends could be observed also for Recall and F-measure. Specificity was higher than 99% for both cases, meaning that both models were able to classify the negative instances as negative correctly.

For the SVM results, for the model without the user's location, we obtained comparable results to the state-of-the-art [4]. Considering the second model, the overall accuracy was increased from 91.19 to 97.93%, while the precision was increased from 93.62 to 98.03%. Similar results were also obtained for recall and F-Measure. Both models showed similar specificity results; indeed it is the lowest difference percentage obtained in this analysis. NN recognition analysis had the worst recognition results without the user's location (Recall 42.21%, Precision 47.62%, Accuracy 39.38%, F-Measure 44.75%, Specificity 83.52%). However, these results are considerably improved in the model with the user's location. In fact, in this case, the overall accuracy was equal to 96.61%; similar improvements were also obtained for the other metrics. DT and SVM seem to be the best activity recognition approaches (Fig. 3).

Concerning the analysis conducted considering the single activity with the DT algorithm, SB was the worst-recognised activity without user localisation (recall 79%), whereas SK was the activity with the lowest precision value (75%) (Table 4).

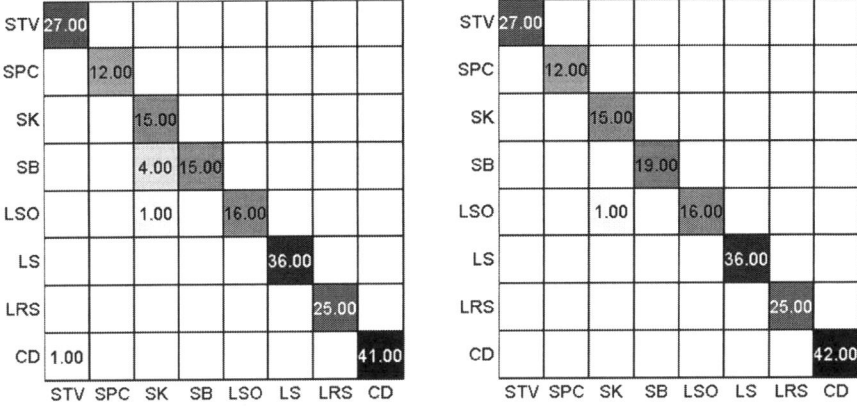

Fig. 4 Phase V—DT confusion matrix of the test set. *Left* results of the dataset without the user localisation. *Right* confusion matrix obtained with the user localisation

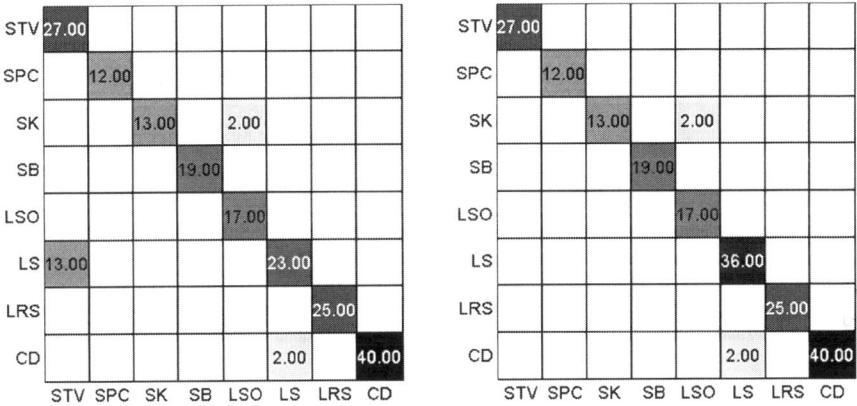

Fig. 5 Phase V—SVM confusion matrix of the test set. *Left* results of the dataset without the user localisation. *Right* confusion matrix obtained with the user localisation

In particular, analysing the two confusion matrices reported in Fig. 4, it is evident how "similar" activities like SB and SK could be easily confused because of the similar body posture and orientation, as shown in the confusion matrix. Consequently, information on the location can provide missing information for activity recognition. In fact, in the second model, the same activities were corrected classified.

For the SVM analysis (Fig. 5), LS were the activities with the lowest recall value (64%), while the activity with the lowest precision and specificity value was STV (68 and 92% respectively). The complete results for SVM models are reported in Table 5.

Table 5 Phase V: SVM—evaluation results for each activity. The values are expressed as percentages

SVM	No location			Yes location		
	Recall	Precision	Specificity	Recall	Precision	Specificity
STV	100	68	92	100	100	100
SPC	100	100	100	100	100	100
SK	87	100	100	87	100	100
SB	100	100	100	100	100	100
LSO	100	89	99	100	89	99
LS	64	92	99	100	95	99
LRS	100	100	100	100	100	100
CD	95	100	100	95	100	100

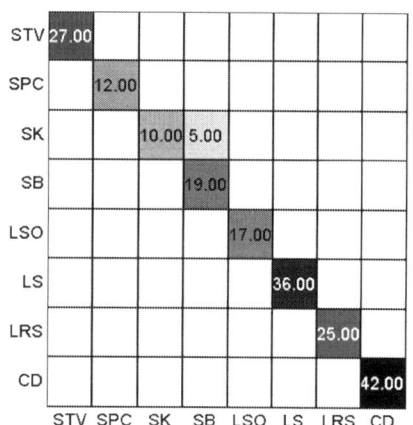

Fig. 6 Phase V—NN confusion matrix of the test set. *Left* results of the dataset without the user localisation. *Right* confusion matrix obtained with the user localisation

On the contrary, as regards the NN results, it is evident how STV, SK, SB and SPC and LRS and LS are mutually confused (confusion matrix: Fig. 6). Their recall values were 26, 0, 74, 58, 52 and 17% respectively. The LSO and LRS activities had the lowest specificity values (69 and 70% respectively). In the second model, the identification of STV, SK, SB, LS, LRS, and CD were improved significantly (Table 6).

Analysing the state-of-the-art, it was evident how aggregate data (vital signs and accelerometer data) could improve activity recognition performance [14]. These preliminary results also suggest that the user's location can improve the accuracy and precision of an activity recognition model.

IoT and connected devices are becoming more common in our daily life. This means that there is much available information that could potentially be included in the analysis. In this proof of concept, user localisation was used as an example;

Table 6 Phase V: NN—evaluation results for each activity. The values are expressed as percentages

NN	No location			Yes location		
	Recall	Precision	Specificity	Recall	Precision	Specificity
STV	26	100	100	100	100	100
SPC	58	58	93	100	100	100
SK	0	0	85	67	100	100
SB	74	37	72	100	79	97
LSO	71	29	69	100	100	100
LS	17	24	79	100	100	100
LRS	52	33	70	100	100	100
CD	40	100	100	100	100	100

other activity and service models can also be generated, including other types of information that comes from the pervasive use of connected devices and smartphones [38].

4   Conclusions

This work has presented a proof of concept where information on user indoor location has been used to reduce the number of wearable devices, therefore increasing the overall accuracy of the system. Indeed, the overall accuracy values were satisfactorily increased (+2.67% DT, +7.39% SVM, +147.37% NN) in the model with information about the user's location.

The presented system was tested in a realistic environment with three users in order to assess the feasibility of the concept design. These results encouraged the use of this approach in activity recognition applications. Thinking to apply and to exploit this method to real-time cases in a cloud computing design, other considerations concerning the processing efficiency, should be made. As stated by Yuan and Hcbcrt [39], DT is the optimal choice to be performed on the cloud in terms of efficiency. However, they found an accuracy of about 95% for DT (and SVM). The method presented in this proof of concept increases the overall accuracy without also increasing the number of sensors placed on the user's body.

Future tests will be performed in order to increase the number of participants in the experimental settings. Future improvement of the systems should also include "movement" activities (i.e. walking, descending/ascending stairs) in order to evaluate whether the user's location can increase the accuracy of these kinds of activities.

Acknowledgements This work was supported in part by the European Community's 7th Framework Program (FP7/2007–2013) under Grant agreement No. 288899 (Robot-Era Project) and Grant agreement No. 601116 (Echord++ project).

References

1. Moschetti A, Fiorini L, Aquilano M, Cavallo F, Dario P (2014) Preliminary findings of the AALIANCE2 ambient assisted living roadmap. In: Ambient assisted living. Springer International Publishing, Switzerland, pp 335–342
2. Aquilano M, Cavallo F, Bonaccorsi M, Esposito R, Rovini E, Filippi M, Dario P, Carrozza MC (2012) Ambient assisted living and ageing: preliminary results of RITA project. In: 2012 annual international conference of the IEEE engineering in medicine and biology society, pp 5823–5826
3. Cook DJ, Schmitter-Edgecombe M, Dawadi P (2015) Analyzing activity behaviour and movement in a naturalistic environment using smart home techniques. IEEE J Biomed Health Inf 19(6):1882–1892
4. Lara OD, Labrador MA (2013) A survey on human activity recognition using wearable sensors. IEEE Commun Surv Tutorials 15(3):1192–1209
5. Yin J, Yang Q, Pan JJ (2008) Sensor-based abnormal human-activity detection. IEEE Trans Knowl Data Eng 20(8):1082–1090
6. Cook DJ, Krishnan NC (2015) Activity learning: discovering, recognizing, and predicting human behavior from sensor data. John Wiley & Sons
7. Foerster F, Smeja M, Fahrenberg J (1999) Detection of posture and motion by accelerometry: a validation study in ambulatory monitoring. Comput Hum Behav 15(5):571–583
8. Kim E, Helal S, Cook D (2010) Human activity recognition and pattern discovery. IEEE Pervasive Comput 9(1):48–53
9. Cook DJ, Crandall AS, Thomas BL, Krishnan NC (2013) CASAS: a smart home in a box. Published in final edited form as: Computer (Long Beach California). 2013 July 46(7): doi:10.1109/MC.2012.328. Published online 2012 Sept 26. doi:10.1109/MC.2012.328
10. Kadam R, Mahamuni P, Parikh Y (2015) Smart home system. Int J Innovative Res Adv Eng 2(1):81–86
11. Continuum Bridge, Internet of thing solution: http://www.continuumbridge.com/. Last accessed June 2016
12. Vera, Smarter Home Control. http://getvera.com/. Last accessed June 2016
13. Gil NM, Hine NA, Arnott JL, Hanson J, Curry RG, Amaral T, Osipovic D (2007) Data visualisation and data mining technology for supporting care for older people. In: Proceedings of the 9th international ACM SIGACCESS conference on computers and accessibility. ACM, pp 139–146
14. Fiorini L, Caleb-Solly P, Tsanaka A, Cavallo F, Dario P, Melhuish C (2015) The efficacy of "Busyness" as a measure for behaviour pattern analysis using unlabelled sensor data: a case study. In: Proceeding of IET international conference on technologies for active and assisted living (TechAAL), London
15. Cook DJ, Krishnan NC, Rashidi P (2013) Activity discovery and activity recognition: a new partnership. IEEE Trans Cybern 43(3):820–828
16. Arning K, Ziefle M (2015) Get that camera out of my house!. Conjoint measurement of preferences for video-based healthcare monitoring systems in private and public places. In: Inclusive Smart Cities and e-Health. Springer International Publishing, Switzerland, pp 152–164
17. Braun A, Dutz T, Alekseew M, Schillinger P, Marinc A (2013) Marker-free indoor localization and tracking of multiple users in smart environments using a camera-based approach. In: Distributed, ambient, and pervasive interactions. Springer, Berlin, pp 349–357
18. Volkhardt M, Mueller S, Schroeter C, Gross HM (2011) Playing hide and seek with a mobile companion robot. In: 2011 11th IEEE-RAS international conference on humanoid robots (humanoids), pp 40–46
19. Zhu C, Sheng W (2012) Realtime recognition of complex human daily activities using human motion and location data. IEEE Trans Biomed Eng 59(9):2422–2430

20. Cavallo F, Limosani R, Manzi A, Bonaccorsi M, Esposito R, Di Rocco M, Dario P et al. (2014) Development of a socially believable multi-robot solution from town to home. Cogn Comput 6(4):954–967
21. Parate A, Chiu MC, Chadowitz C, Ganesan D, Kalogerakis E (2014) Risq: recognizing smoking gestures with inertial sensors on a wristband. In: Proceedings of the 12th annual international conference on mobile systems, applications, and services. ACM, pp 149–161
22. Li Q, Stankovic JA, Hanson MA, Barth AT, Lach J, Zhou G (2009) Accurate, fast fall detection using gyroscopes and accelerometer-derived posture information. In: Sixth international workshop on wearable and implantable body sensor networks, BSN 2009, pp 138–143
23. Weiss GM, Timko JL, Gallagher CM, Yoneda K, Schreiber AJ (2016) Smartwatch-based activity recognition: a machine learning approach. In: 2016 IEEE-EMBS international conference on biomedical and health informatics (BHI), pp 426–429
24. Sharma N, Gedeon T (2012) Objective measures, sensors and computational techniques for stress recognition and classification: a survey. Comput Methods Prog Biomed 108(3):1287–1301
25. Nocua R, Noury N, Gehin C, Dittmar A, McAdams E (2009) Evaluation of the autonomic nervous system for fall detection. In: Annual international conference of the IEEE engineering in medicine and biology society, EMBC 2009, pp 3225–3228
26. Pärkkä J, Ermes M, Korpipää P, Mäntyjärvi J, Peltola J, Korhonen I (2006) Activity classification using realistic data from wearable sensors. IEEE Trans Inf Technol Biomed 10(1):119–128
27. Lara ÓD, Pérez AJ, Labrador MA, Posada JD (2012) Centinela: a human activity recognition system based on acceleration and vital sign data. Pervasive Mobile Comput 8(5):717–729
28. European Commission (2004) Eurostat, "How European Spends their time"? Available at http://www.unece.org/fileadmin/DAM/stats/gender/publications/Multi-Country/EUROSTAT/HowEuropeansSpendTheirTime.pdf. Last accessed Oct 2016
29. Bonaccorsi M, Fiorini L, Cavallo F, Saffiotti A, Dario P (2016) A cloud robotics solution to improve social assistive robots for active and healthy aging. Int J Social Robot 8:393. doi:10.1007/s12369-016-0351-1
30. Bonaccorsi M, Fiorini L, Sathyakeerthy S, Saffiotti A, Cavallo F, Dario P (2015) Design of cloud robotic services for senior citizens to improve independent living in multiple environments. Intelligenza Artificiale 9(1):63–72
31. Wang Y, Jin Q, Ma J (2013) Integration of range-based and range-free localization algorithms in wireless sensor networks for mobile clouds. In: Green computing and communications (GreenCom), IEEE and Internet of Things (iTh-ings/CPSCom), IEEE International Conference on and IEEE Cyber, Physical and Social Computing, pp 957–961
32. Arias J, Zuloaga A, Lázaro J, Andreu J, Astarloa A (2004) Malguki: an RSSI based ad hoc location algorithm. Microprocess Microsyst 28(8):403–409
33. Medjahed H, Istrate D, Boudy J, Dorizzi B (2009) Human activities of daily living recognition using fuzzy logic for elderly home monitoring. In: IEEE international conference on fuzzy systems, 2009. FUZZ-IEEE 2009, pp 2001–2006
34. Anguita D, Ghio A, Oneto L, Parra X, Reyes-Ortiz JL (2012) Human activity recognition on smartphones using a multiclass hardware-friendly support vector machine. In: Ambient assisted living and home care. Springer, Berlin, pp 216–223
35. Lee YS, Cho SB (2011) Activity recognition using hierarchical hidden markov models on a smartphone with 3D accelerometer. In: Hybrid artificial intelligent systems. Springer, Berlin, pp 460–467
36. Mishra A (2016) Multiclass—SVM Matlab toolbox. Available at http://www.mathworks.com/matlabcentral/fileexchange/39352-multi-class-svm. Last accessed Oct 2016
37. Lara ÓD, Labrador MA (2012) A mobile platform for real-time human activity recognition. In: Consumer communications and networking conference (CCNC), 2012 IEEE, pp 667–671

38. Turchetti G, Micera S, Cavallo F, Odetti L, Dario P (2011) Technology and innovative services. IEEE Pulse 2(2):27–35
39. Yuan B, Herbert J (2014) A cloud-based mobile data analytics framework: case study of activity recognition using smartphone. In: 2nd IEEE international conference on mobile cloud computing, services, and engineering (MobileCloud), pp 220–227

An Innovative Speech-Based Interface to Control AAL and IoT Solutions to Help People with Speech and Motor Disability

Massimiliano Malavasi, Enrico Turri, Maria Rosaria Motolese,
Ricard Marxer, Jochen Farwer, Heidi Christensen, Lorenzo Desideri,
Fabio Tamburini and Phil Green

Abstract The main aim of the project described in this paper is to develop an experimental low cost system for environmental control through simplified user interfaces and voice control, to better respond to the needs of users with motor speech impairments (dysarthria). The project is actually being conducted by Area Ausili, a department of Polo Tecnologico Regionale Corte Roncati in Italy, in collaboration with AIAS AT Team and the CloudCAST project. The prototype, that has been implemented in an experimental smart home in Italy, integrates a completely hands free commands recognition function based on the cloud-based voice recognition system developed within the CloudCAST project. The target of the project is to create a tool that is able to overcome the limits of some actual assistive technologies, and to take advantage from the evolution of home automation and internet of things technologies. Future developments of the projects and expected results are discussed.

Keywords Voice recognition · Smarthome · Disability · Internet of things (IoT) · Environmental control · Speech disability

Massimiliano Malavasi: **Area of Interest**—Disability and rehabilitation.

M. Malavasi (✉) · L. Desideri
CRA Centro Regionale Ausili, Area Ausili di Corte Roncati,
Via Sant'Isaia 90, 40123 Bologna, Italy
e-mail: mmalavasi@ausilioteca.org

L. Desideri
e-mail: ldesideri@ausilioteca.org

E. Turri
Università di Bologna, Facoltà di Ingegneria, Bologna, Italy
e-mail: enrico.torre91@yahoo.it

M.R. Motolese
CAAD Bologna, Bologna, Italy
e-mail: mmotolese@ausilioteca.org

R. Marxer · J. Farwer · H. Christensen · P. Green
University of Sheffield, Sheffield, UK
e-mail: r.marxer@sheffield.ac.uk

© Springer International Publishing AG 2017
F. Cavallo et al. (eds.), *Ambient Assisted Living*, Lecture Notes
in Electrical Engineering 426, DOI 10.1007/978-3-319-54283-6_20

1   Introduction

The expansion of the functional control capabilities of home automation systems and Internet of Things (IoT) devices for the needs of users with disability is the subject of a research project currently being conducted by Area Ausili (Assistive Technology Area), a department of Polo Tecnologico Regionale Corte Roncati of the public health system authority of Bologna (Italy). The main aim of this project is to develop experimental low cost systems for environmental control through simplified user interfaces and voice control. Some of the activities have been set within the CloudCAST [1–3] project. Here we report on the first technical achievements of the project and discuss future possible applications within CloudCAST.

1.1   The CloudCAST Project and Environmental Control

The Department of Computer Science at the University of Sheffield (UK), in collaboration with the universities of Toronto (Canada) and West Indies (Jamaica) and AIAS Bologna Onlus, is funded by the Leverhulme Trust to develop a computing resource based in the cloud, for clinical and educational applications related to technologies for speech recognition (CloudCAST: clinical applications of speech technology). The project aims to provide a way for automatic learning and speech recognition technology developments to be put in the hands of professionals who deal with speech problems, such as therapists, pathologists, and teachers, creating a self-sufficient community that continues to grow the resource after the three-year funding period (from January 2015 until December 2017). The project aims to achieve this by creating an internet-based, free resource, which will provide a set of software tools for personalized speech recognition and speech therapy. Moreover, it provides a personalized interactive dialogue; the voice recognition system of CloudCAST is able to adapt to dysarthric speech, or to more general problems of language by adaptation processes which require only a few minutes of training data. This opens up the possibility of providing users with an efficient voice control system, for example in the case where they are unable to use other interfaces like traditional mouse or keyboards.

J. Farwer
e-mail: j.farwer@sheffield.ac.uk

H. Christensen
e-mail: heidi.christensen@sheffield.ac.uk

P. Green
e-mail: p.green@sheffield.ac.uk

F. Tamburini
FICLIT, University of Bologna, Bologna, Italy
e-mail: fabio.tamburini@unibo.it

Home automation systems, often used in combination with other assistive technologies can greatly increase the autonomy and safety of persons with disabilities [4]. This sector can be considered an evolving reality, but can it be advanced by the increasing availability and dispersal of new low cost mobile ICT solutions? Another significant element is the growth, in recent years, of the availability of IoT solutions. It is important to understand how these two factors may change the home automation sector for people with disability. Currently, many home automation systems require substantial changes of the domestic electronics to be integrated with user control interfaces from the assistive technology (AT) field. This type of interfaces is often quite expensive and with a poor choice of smart functions, if compared with those present in smartphones or tablets. In the present contribution, we describe the development of the CloudCAST platform to efficiently control both traditional home automation systems and IoT solutions, using mobile ICT devices.

2 Materials and Methods

2.1 A Single Multi-standard Access Point

The first problem to solve was to create a single multi-standard access point to handle home automation systems and IoT devices which could also be connected to different types of human machine interfaces (HMI). The technical goal was to create a web-server system, possibly based on an open source architecture. Different solutions have been evaluated (see Table 1) to define the architecture underlying the system.

Table 1 Web-server systems for home automation and IoT

Name	Open source	Technologies supported	HMIs available
OpenHAB	Yes	121	iOS and Android Apps Web interface (Classic UI) Web-app (GreenT) XML-based (Comet Visu)
Open remote	Yes	46	iOS and Android Apps Web interface
IKON	No	29	App iOS e Android Web interface
Calaos	Yes	14	iOS and Android Apps Web application Touchscreen user interface
DomotiGa	Yes	92	iOS and Android Apps Web interface
Thinknx	No	44	App Android Web interface
Jeedom	Yes	101	iOS and Android Apps Web interface

The choice fell on OpenHAB (Home Automation Bus) framework [5, 6] which is specifically aimed at creating integrated control systems, not bound to a specific hardware device and capable of using a single communication protocol. The main reasons for this choice was the huge number of different technologies and standards supported, the full open source architecture and the active community of developers and users that is actually supporting the project.

OpenHAB is fully based on OSGI (Open Service Gateway Initiative). It makes it possible to build modular application components (bindings). Any technology, device, social network or integrated cloud platform is supported by a specific binding. These packages are optional and can be added or removed to expand or limit the functionalities of a specific installation. OpenHAB is designed to run independently and brings together different types of field-bus systems, hardware devices and interface protocols for dedicated applications. These allow an application to send and receive commands and status updates, enabling the design of personalized user interfaces with a unique appearance and keeping open the possibility of operating with multiple devices and services. These allow an application to send and receive commands and status updates on the bus enabling the design of personalized user interfaces with a unique appearance while keeping open the possibility of operating with multiple devices and services. It also allows the development of automation logics between the different sections of the system.

2.1.1 Basic Automation Functions Available in the Prototype

As the prototype is based on OpenHAB technology, the basic automation functions are the ones available in a standard OpenHAB server. The principal functions and data types with related commands are described in Table 2.

Table 2 Basic automation functions available in the prototype

Data type	Description	Commands
Color	RGB data	On, Off, Increase, Decrease, Percent, HSB
Contact	State of binary sensors	Open, Closed
DateTime	Date and time data	
Dimmer	Light dimmers data	On, Off, Increase, Decrease, Percent
Group	Useful for creating groups of basic functions	
Location	Location data	
Number	Numeric data in different formats	
Rollershutter	Used for motors, blinds, shutters	Up, Down, Stop, Move, Percent
String	Text data	String
Switch	Used for any kind of switching functions	On, Off

2.2 Implementing the Prototype

The prototype has been developed and implemented in a context of real application (Fig. 1): the two Experimental Domotic Apartments (ADS) of the Polo Tecnologico Regionale Corte Roncati of the public health system authority of Bologna (Italy) [7]. They are used as an exhibition site for assistive and AAL solutions, where end users and professional users can test them. They are also used for temporary residential experiences of independent living within the project "Weekends of Autonomy" dedicated to young people with disability. The goal of this project is to give the opportunity to users with disability to live a few days in a smart home, to test the benefits they would get by installing similar systems in their homes [8]. The two ADS are equipped with a full automation system based on KNX standard. One of the main activities of the project was to integrate this system with the prototype.

Specifically, many function have been integrated such as lighting controls, automation of doors, windows, blinds and shutters, heating/air conditioning systems and environmental sensors (such as temperature, presence, flooding, light and smoke sensors).

2.3 Integrating IoT Devices and Low Cost ICT Solution

In a logic of creating a low cost control system, the webserver has been implemented and tested on a Rasperry Pi 1 system [9]. In the same logic, several IoT devices were integrated in the system and tested, but a full functional integration was possible only with three systems:

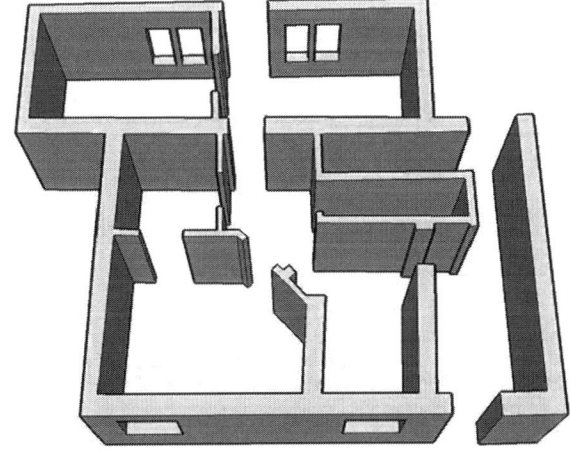

Fig. 1 The ADS 1 Smart Home, Corte Roncati, Bologna

1. RGB Philips Hue bulbs (a lighting system)
2. Netamo Weather Station
3. Logitech Harmony HUB (an infrared universal remote control system).

   The third device is really important for daily use as it can allow target users to control many audio/video home devices.

3   Results and Discussion

3.1   A Completely Hands-Free Home Control Interface

Some smart functions, particularly useful for the needs of target users, were developed and tested:

1. Non-invasive monitoring based on environmental sensors
2. Functions for deaf and blind users
3. Cloud based and remotely controlled functions.

   At present, the voice control of the devices of the two ADS is made through the use of a universal remote control that allows the management of infrared (IR) codes. The device has the capability to learn IR codes directly from other remote controls and the voice recognition module requires a brief user training session. This kind of product belongs to the AT commercial sector. A key feature of the project was therefore to integrate voice control also in the low cost prototype based on mobile devices. The official app of the OpenHAB community allows users to operate the mobile device's microphone and send the recognized text to a specific module of the web server. A specific script was developed to parse the command phrases and decode the single commands to activate the functions available in the ADS apartments. In order to make this service accessible to people with upper limbs disability, it has been developed and integrated with another software unit to provide a complete hands-free voice activation. In the present phase, it uses Google voice recognition services. The major limitation of this system for voice control is the need for an internet connection. Other research projects have involved the use of a computer with voice recognition systems that run locally. On the other hand, the designed solution has an important economic advantage: it only requires a device with Android OS which can be purchased for a few hundred euros.

3.2   The CloudCAST Based Solution

To extend the performance and the functions available, a second prototype, based on CloudCAST technology, was developed. Clinical applications of speech technology face two challenges. The first is the lack of data: there are few corpora available to support the techniques that rely on machine learning and since it is difficult to collect large speech corpus, the only way to address this problem is to collect material which is produced by systems already in use. The second is customization: this field requires individual solutions, and a technology that adapts to its user rather than demanding that the user adapts to it. CloudCAST addresses these two problems making the adaptive technology available at a distance to professionals who work with language. The CloudCAST resources also facilitate the collection of voice data needed to improve the machine learning techniques that are the basis of this technology: it will be able to automatically collect data from systems that are already in use, in addition to providing a system for the collection of databases. From the beginning, it was planned to use a technology based on open-source services, like Kaldi for automatic speech recognition and OpenHAB for home automation control.

Compared to CloudCAST goals, existing solutions for the target user groups are inferior in terms of the choice of recognizer output, the flexibility of the recognition process, the personalization of the speech models and modes of interaction. CloudCAST services include the possibility to provide interactive voice recognition where the user is able to change the grammar, the acoustic models, and other essential parameters. The recognizer may also provide feedback on its own performance, for examples partial decodings and confidence measures. Subsequently, the interaction of different users with CloudCAST should provide data resources to improve the recognition process and the training of future models.

The general architecture of CloudCAST (Fig. 2) can be divided into two sections: the application and the CloudCAST server. The server processes the audio data according to the models and provides the speech recognition results using a Kaldi library. The server also has the task of applying the changes to the parameters of the models concerned for the recognition process; both application and server have access to a common storage database for models, recordings and authentication data. The CloudCAST site will be visible to users who can manage recordings, developers who wish to obtain API keys, professionals who want to create models, and so on.

In the initial stages, in order to facilitate the creation of services that use CloudCAST, a speech recognition client was developed in JavaScript on the basis of dictate.js existing library. The final client is planned to extend CloudCast dictate.js allowing for more types of interaction with the server, such as swapping grammars, models and other parameters, so as to interpret the results provided by different servers.

In the CloudCAST based environmental control prototype (Fig. 3), it was possible to view the same initial interface of OpenHAB in a different format with the possibility to provide feedback of the actions performed by the program in a dialog box. Compared to the initial prototype, in this version, the items and commands to execute were single words rather than sentences. In this other interface, the user navigates the command tree using single commands because the microphone is always active and a word is recognized as soon as it matches with one of those displayed. The system then either proceeds to a submenu or executing the

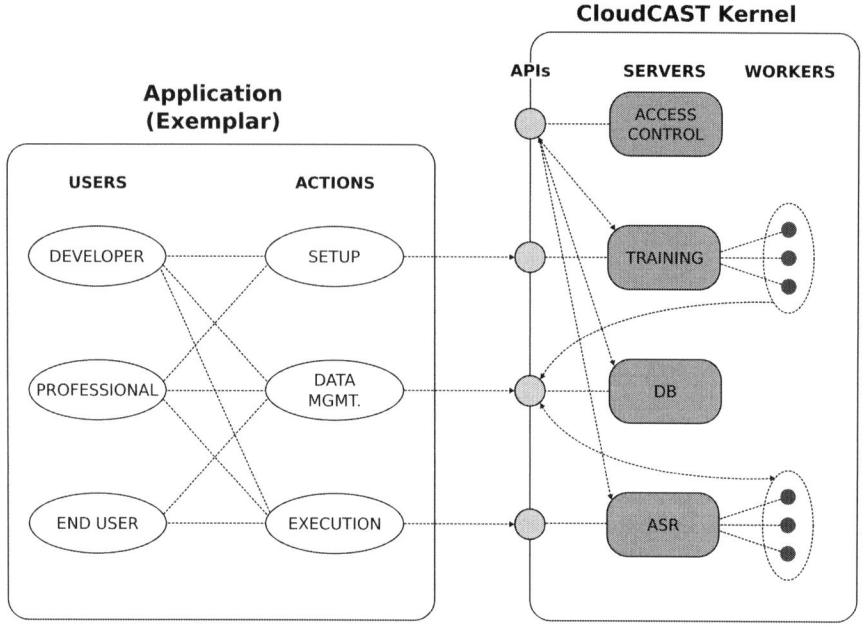

Fig. 2 The CloudCAST architecture

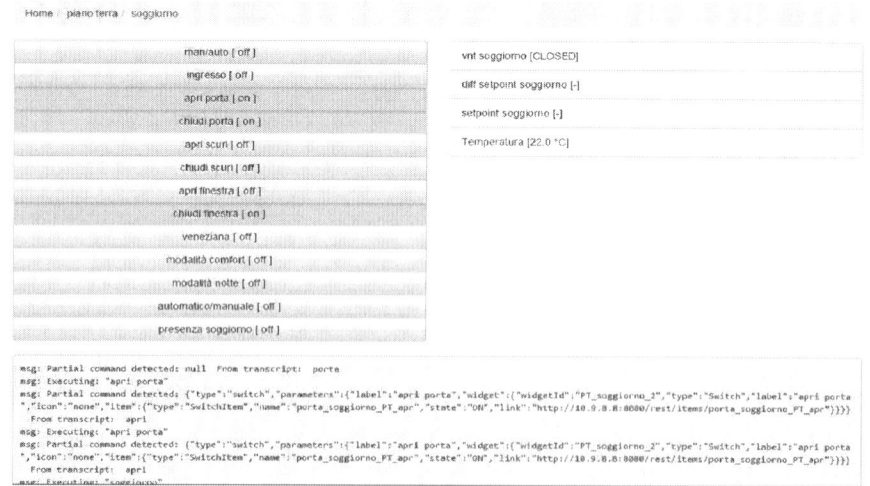

Fig. 3 An early prototype of the CloudCast voice recognition interface for environmental control

command. For example, to open the door of the kitchen, the user will have to pronounce the words in sequence to access the relevant page for the room and finally the object concerned: "ground floor", "kitchen", "open door".

This procedure can appear unnatural, but it's often required for users with severe dysarthric problems, who usually have difficulties in articulating a whole sentence instead of a word at a time. This also helps the CloudCAST voice recognition system since for every access to an interface page, it only needs to consider the possible words by the processing server. The interface is configured to accept the most similar words, before sending a signal declaring its readiness to receive the command. Keeping the grammar simple, with only a few commend options (low perplexity) at every stage of the control sequence, makes the system less prone to error detection.

An improvement has been made to include the function of directly and automatically use the OpenHAB interface in JSON format, without the need to download it. Future developments include the possibility of activating the recognition after the delivery of a specific word and saving an adaptation session in order to make specific recognitions constant and regular for a certain user. The CloudCAST cloud server will be available within the next year, so the tests have been performed using a demo Kaldi version with a standard language model. When the service will be on-line, selecting few options it will be possible to specify a configuration based on a model to be used by dysarthric users.

4 Conclusion

The initial goal of the project was to create a low cost and highly accessible home automation control system, to be tested in two already existent smart homes, and which could be operated from an off the shelf mobile ICT device. The prototype has fully achieved the functional objectives, while the integration with a completely hands free voice recognition function and the connection with the CloudCAST system have created significant added value in relation to the target user needs.

The versatility of the system developed has allowed the creation of a tool that is able to replace specific products belonging to the assistive technology sector for home automation control, which currently have high costs, functional limits and a certain level of obsolescence due to the evolution of home automation and IoT technologies.

Thus, the solution developed can be considered a starting point for the creation of low cost custom home automation systems, useful for improving the levels of independence and autonomy in daily living activities, and particularly dedicated to people with full or partial inability in the use of the upper limbs, but not limited to this: the integration with the cloud based speech recognition systems, provided in CloudCAST, will also allow, in the future, the possibility of an efficient use by dysarthric users.

Acknowledgements CloudCAST is an International Network (IN-2014-003) funded by the Leverhulme Trust.

References

1. Green P, Mrxer R, Cunningham S, Christensen H, Rudzicz F, Yancheva M, Coy A, Malavasi M, Desideri L (2015) Remote speech technology for speech professionals—the CloudCAST initiative. In: Paper accepted for 6th workshop on speech and language processing for assistive technologies, Dresden, Germany, 11 Sept 2015
2. Green P, Mrxer R, Cunningham S, Christensen H, Rudzicz F, Yancheva M, Coy A, Malavasi M, Desideri L, Tamburini F (2016) CloudCAST—remote speech technology for speech professionals. Interspeech 8–12 Sept 2016, San Francisco, USA
3. http://cloudcast.rcweb.dcs.shef.ac.uk/
4. del Zanna G, Malavasi M, Vaccari G (2009) Manuale illustrato per la domotica a uso sociale-la casa flessibile al servizio dell'uomo. Tecniche Nuove
5. https://community.openhab.org/
6. https://github.com/openhab/openhab/wiki
7. Agusto R, Ioele FM, Malavasi M, Martinuzzi S, Motolese MR, Rimondini M (2014) Living in the living lab! Adapting two model Domotic apartments for experimentation in autonomous living in a context of residential use. In: Longhi S, Siciliano P, Germani M, Monteriù A (eds) Ambient assisted living—Italian forum 2013, pp 325–333
8. Krantz O (2012) Assistive devices utilization in activities of everyday life. A proposed framework of understanding a user perspective. Disabil Rehabil Assistive Technol 7:189–198
9. https://it.wikipedia.org/wiki/Raspberry_Pi

Fall Risk Evaluation by Electromyography Solutions

Gabriele Rescio, Alessandro Leone, Andrea Caroppo
and Pietro Siciliano

Abstract Falls are very dangerous events among elderly people. Several automatic fall detectors have been developed to reduce the time of the medical intervention, but they cannot avoid the injures due to the fall. The purpose of this study has been to identify a computational framework for the real-time and automatic detection of the fall risk, allowing the fast adoption of properly intervention strategies, to reduce injuries and traumas due to falls. A wearable, wireless and minimally invasive surface Electromyography (EMG)-based system has been used to measure four lower-limb muscles activities. Eleven young healthy subjects have simulated several fall events (through a movable platform) and normal Activities of Daily Living (ADLs) and their patterns have been analyzed. Highly discriminative features extracted within the EMG signals for the pre impact fall evaluation have been explored and a threshold-based approach has been adopted, assuring the real-time functioning. The threshold level for each feature has been set to distinguish an instability condition from normal activities. The proposed system seems able to recognize all falls with an average lead-time of 840 ms before the impact, in simulated and controlled fall conditions.

Keywords Wearable · Wireless surface electromyography probes · Healthcare · Risk of fall

G. Rescio (✉) · A. Leone · A. Caroppo · P. Siciliano
National Research Council of Italy, Institute for Microelectronics
and Microsystems, Lecce, Italy
e-mail: gabriele.rescio@le.imm.cnr.it

A. Leone
e-mail: alessandro.leone@le.imm.cnr.it

A. Caroppo
e-mail: andrea.caroppo@le.imm.cnr.it

P. Siciliano
e-mail: pietro.siciliano@le.imm.cnr.it

© Springer International Publishing AG 2017
F. Cavallo et al. (eds.), *Ambient Assisted Living*, Lecture Notes
in Electrical Engineering 426, DOI 10.1007/978-3-319-54283-6_21

1 Introduction

The injuries due to a fall remain one of the main cause of accident and wellness issues among older people, resulting in the loss of their independence [1]. Several automatic, miniaturized, wireless and wearable fall detectors have been developed [2, 3]. Even if this kind of technology is more invasive regarding to the vision or acoustic sensors, it presents some important advantages, such as: the re-design of the environments is not required, outdoor operation and the privacy are preserved. The fall detectors appear very important for minimizing the time of medical intervention, however it is desirable the development of a system able to detect falls before the impact on the floor, which working together with an impact reduction systems, prevents some injuries. Several solutions have been proposed in the prevention of falls and high-quality reviews have been presented [4]. They use inertial sensors and above all threshold based techniques for the classification of the events. Their performance suggest that specificity and sensitivity values are high, but the lead-time before the impact is low (less than 400 ms). For this reason a new EMG-based system to detect the risk of fall in a faster mode has been investigated. To reduce the invasiveness, only four EMG sensors, placed through the gelled electrodes, have been considered and used for the measuring of the lower limb muscles activities. The main purpose of the work, deals with the development of a low-power, wireless, real time, automatic and effective fall risk detection EMG based framework. The lead-time before the impact has been evaluated by simulating imbalance condition and fall events through a moveable platform activated by a pneumatic piston. The obtained results show that the system, in simulated and controlled conditions, is able to detect the falls about 840 ms before the impact on the floor.

2 Materials and Methods

2.1 Hardware Architecture

The EMG data are acquired using the BTS FREEEMG1000 device produced by BTS Bioengineering [5]. It is made up of four wireless, wearable surface EMG probes and an USB receiver (Fig. 1a); their main characteristics are summarized in the Tables 1 and 2. The sensors have been worn through the common pre-gelled Ag/AgCl electrodes by using clips, allowing a fast, simple and resistant to the user's movements mounting. Each probe integrates two low noise active electrodes for the sensing and the RF transmitter to send the data according to the Zigbee protocol. The system allows the transmission in a range of more than 20 m in free space and up to 10 m in presence of a 50 cm thick wall. The data can be sent during a period of about 8 h in streaming mode, through the rechargeable lithium-ion integrated batteries. The logical framework for EMG signals acquisition and

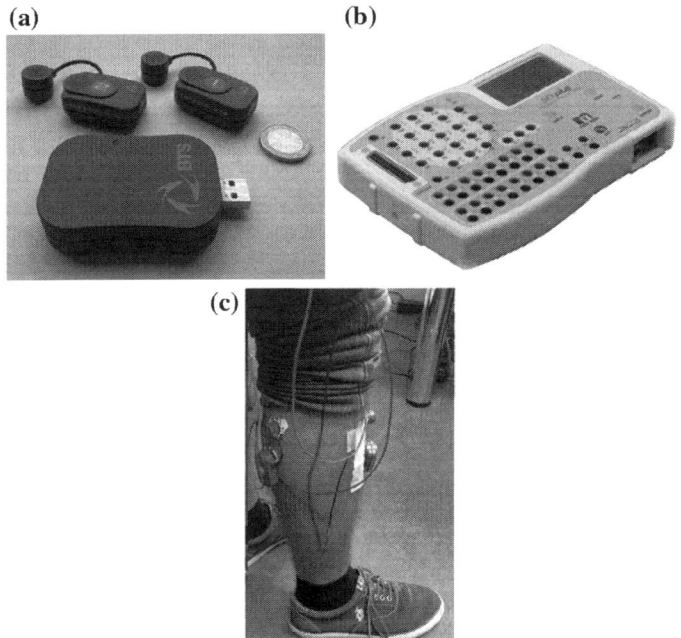

Fig. 1 BTS bioengineering Freeemg 1000 wireless surface EMG probes and USB receiver System (**a**); EEG-EMG MICROMED wired system (**b**); EMG wireless signals validation mounting setup (**c**)

Table 1 Main features of USB receiver

USB receiver	Technical features
EMG channels	Up to 20 probes
Dimensions	82 × 44 × 22.5 mm
Weight	80 g

elaboration is hosted on a Windows PC, composed by a CPU i5@2.20 GHz and 8 GB memory DDR3 RAM. During the first step of the work, the BTS EMG validation signal has been provided through the comparison with the data coming from the certified wired biomedical system EEG-EMG MICROMED (Fig. 1b). In particular five young actors simulated several lower limb muscles contractions, wearing the wired and wireless electrodes on the gastrocnemius and tibialis muscles as shown in Fig. 1c. Based on the results obtained, the signals of BTS and MICROMED systems have shown a high degree of similarity (maximum cross-correlation measured has been more than 0.9 for all simulations).

Table 2 Main features of EMG probe

Wireless probes	Technical features
Resolution	16 bit
Data transmission	Wireless IEEE 802.15.4
Battery	Rechargeable lithium-ion
Autonomy	8 h battery life in streaming mode
Acquisition range	Up to 20 m in free space
Memory	On board solid-state
Certification	Class "IIa"
Weight	10 g
Dimensions	41.5 × 24.8 × 14 mm (mother electrode)
	16 × 12 mm (satellite electrode)

2.2 Software Architecture

To develop and to test the fall risk assessment algorithm a large dataset has been created, conducting a study on 11 young healthy actors with different age (29.5 ± 8.2 years), weight (65.4 ± 11.1 kg), height (1.77 ± 0.2 m) and sex (8 males and 3 females), who have simulated Activities of Daily Living (ADLs) and falls through the movable platform. The research has been focused on the electromyography patterns evaluation of the two lower limbs (tibialis anterior and gastrocnemius lateralis muscles).

The main computational steps of the software architecture have been validated as first on the Mathworks Matlab. They are (a) pre-processing, (b) calibration, (c) feature extraction, (d) classification. During the pre-processing phase, the raw data, coming from each EMG channel, have been band-pass filtered using a 12th order FIR filter, with cut frequencies between 20 and 450 Hz, to reduce the artefacts and to avoid signal aliasing. In Fig. 2 it is reported an example of the EMG signal artifacts, simulated through an external perturbation by tapping the probes, in quiescent condition (a) before and (b) after the filtering.

Then, to compare the EMG-tension relationship the signals have been processed by generating their full wave rectification and their linear envelope, using a 10th order low-pass Butterworth filter, with cut-off frequency of 10 Hz. The calibration procedure has been accomplished after device mounting by recovering the initial condition and the maximum EMG signal amplitude values for muscles of interest. For the feature extraction, the parameters that have shown higher degree of discrimination for the imbalance condition and lower computational cost are: Root Mean Square (RMS), Waveform length (WL), Co-contraction Index (CCI), Zero Crossing (ZC), Integrated EMG (IEMG) and Willison Amplitude (WAMP) [6]. In the end, for the classification of the fall risk event, a single threshold approach has been adopted. This method has been chosen to guarantee a real time operation to detriment of generalization ability.

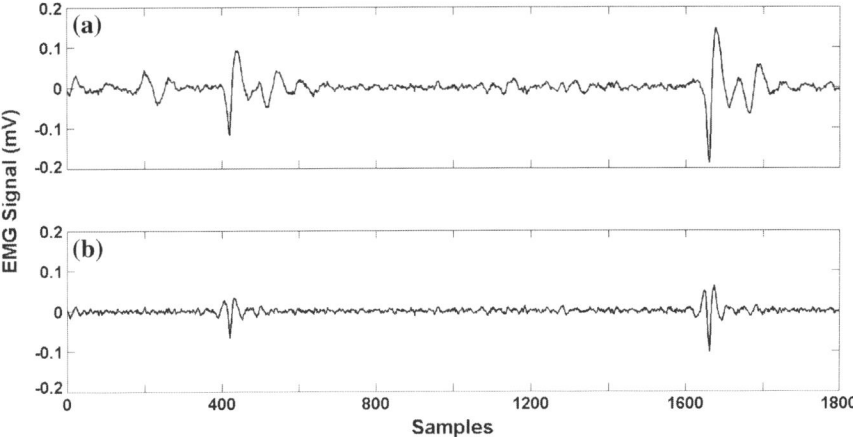

Fig. 2 Example of EMG signals with artifacts in quiescent condition **a** before and **b** after the filtering

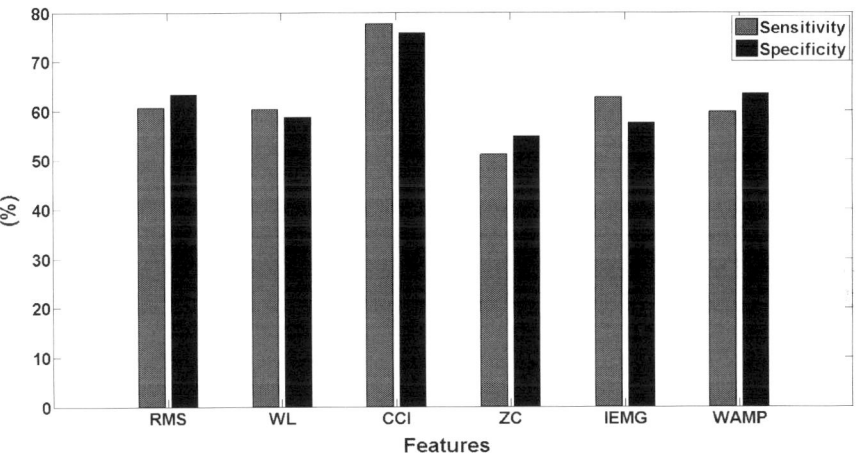

Fig. 3 Sensitivity and Specificity values for the features extracted

3 Results

The performance of the algorithm has been evaluated considering the aforementioned features for more than 250 ADLs and fall events, simulated during the acquisition campaign. In particular, one half of the dataset has been used to calculate the threshold values of features to detect the instability events, while the remaining part has been considered to test the performance in terms of sensitivity and specificity [7]. In Fig. 3 the performance obtained for each feature have been reported. The best results have been achieved with Co-Contraction indices

(77.6% for sensitivity and 75.8% for specificity). To reduce the computational cost, for the feature extraction, only the CCI have been selected.

These results have been obtained considering 1 kHz frequency sampling for the EMG signals. To reduce the computational cost, a performance evaluation on the system according to the down sampling EMG has been conducted. In particular the signals coming from each sensor has been digitally down sampled at 500, 250 and 125 Hz and Co-Contraction Indices have been calculated. Based on the experimental results, the performance remains quite the same from 250 Hz up to 1 kHz sampling frequency; instead significant changes have been measured for 125 Hz. Consequently for the real time application, developed through Microsoft C#, the frequency of 250 Hz has been chosen. For the analysis of the lead-time before the impact and the related gastrocnemius/tibialis muscles behavior, a movable platform to simulate involuntary falls has been considered, according to the work proposed in [8]. It is driven by a pneumatic system that can cause slow and fast involuntary falls. The mat, where the subjects fell, has been sensorized in order to detect the instant of the impact: in this way it has been possible to evaluate the period of time from the onset of the perturbation up to the user impact on the mat. The average of this period was about 1.4 s and the average lead-time before the impact on the mat has been measured in about 840 ms, considering all fall events recognized. From the results obtained, the solution developed appears a good starting point to realize a fast and efficient system for the fall risk assessment. With respect to the inertial fall detection system, the solution proposed could act before the start of falling phase defined in [9], through the monitoring of the electrical activity produced by muscles after an imbalance condition. The performance in terms of sensitivity and specificity could be improved increasing the area of legs monitored (through a larger number of probes). Furthermore, a relevant open issue present in literature regards the wearability of the Ag/AgCl electrodes. In fact they may cause skin irritation and allergies, moreover their signal quality may degrade due to the drying of the gel over time [10, 11]. To address these problems new biocompatible, textile and more comfortable wearable electrodes [10, 11] could be adopted to increase the user acceptability.

4 Conclusion

This work presents a preliminary study on a real-time and minimally invasive pre-fall detection surface Electromyography-based system. Significant performance in terms of lead-time before the impact on the floor has been measured, in simulated conditions, by using only four EMG probes. Future works will be focused to improve the performance and the user acceptability of the system increasing the number of probes and using more biocompatible and comfortable electrodes.

Acknowledgements This work has been carried out within ActiveAging@Home PON Project founded by the Italian Minister of Research, University and Educational. Authors would like to thank the colleague Mr. Flavio Casino for the technical support.

References

1. Chung MC, McKee KJ, Austin C, Barkby H, Brown H, Cash S, Ellingford J, Hanger L, Pais T (2009) Posttraumatic stress disorder in older people after a fall. Int J Geriatr Psychiatry 24(9):955–964
2. Bagalà F, Becker C, Cappello A, Chiari L, Aminian K, Hausdorff JM, Zijlstra W, Klenk J (2012) Evaluation of accelerometer-based fall detection algorithms on real-world falls. PLoS ONE 7:e37062
3. Rescio G, Leone A, Siciliano P (2013) Supervised expert system for wearable MEMS accelerometer-based fall detector. J Sens 2013, Article ID 254629, 11 pages
4. Wu G (2000) Distinguishing fall activities from normal activities by velocity characteristics. J Biomech 33(11):1497–1500
5. http://www.btsbioengineering.com
6. Phinyomark A, Chujit G, Phukpattaranont P, Limsakul C, Huosheng H (2012) A preliminary study assessing time-domain EMG features of classifying exercises in preventing falls in the elderly. In: 9th international conference on electrical engineering/electronics, computer, telecommunications and information technology (ECTI-CON), pp 1, 4, 16–18
7. Noury N, Rumeau P, Bourcke AK, Olaighin G, Lundy JE (2008) A proposal for the classification and evaluation of fall detectors. IRBM 29(6):340–349
8. Rescio G, Leone A, Caroppo A, Casino F, Siciliano P (2015) A minimally invasive electromyography-based system for pre-fall detection. Int J Eng Innov Technol (IJEIT) 5(6)
9. Becker C, Schwickert L, Mellone S, Bagalà F, Chiari L, Helbostad JL, Zijlstra W, Aminian K, Bourke A, Todd C, Bandinelli S, Kerse N, Klenk J (2012) Proposal for a multiphase fall model based on real-world fall recordings with body-fixed sensors. Z Gerontol Geriatr 45(8):707–715
10. Pylatiuk C, Muller-Riederer M, Kargov A, Schulz S, Schill O, Reischl M, Bretthauer G (2009) Comparison of surface EMG monitoring electrodes for long-term use in rehabilitation device control. In: IEEE international conference on rehabilitation robotics (ICORR 2009), pp 300–304
11. Lee SM, Byeon HJ, Lee JH, Baek DH, Lee KH, Hong JS, Lee S-H (2014) Self-adhesive epidermal carbon nanotube electronics for tether-free long-term continuous recording of biosignals. Sci Rep 4:6074

Semantic Knowledge Management and Integration Services for AAL

Gianfranco E. Modoni, Mario Veniero and Marco Sacco

Abstract The integration of a set of heterogeneous data streams coming from different source into a coherent scheme is still one of the key challenges in designing the new generation of AAL system enabling the Smart Home. This paper introduces a service-oriented platform that aims to enhance data integration and synchronization between physical and virtual components of an AAL system. The idea behind this research work goes in the direction to find scalable technological solution in order to answer the continued growth of objects (Things) connected to the network within the domestic environment. Thus, the Smart Objects can operate synergistically on the basis of a shared semantic model, supporting various tailored services that assist elderly users or users with disabilities for a better and healthier life in their preferred living environment. Moreover, a prototype of the platform has been implemented and validated in order to prove the correctness of the approach and conduct a preliminary performance evaluation.

Keywords AAL · Integration services · Internet of things · Semantic web · Knowledge management

G.E. Modoni (✉)
Institute of Industrial Technologies and Automation, National Research
Council, Bari, Italy
e-mail: gianfranco.modoni@itia.cnr.it

M. Veniero
ABMEDICA SPA, Cerro Maggiore, MI, Italy
e-mail: veniero.mario@abmedica.it

M. Sacco
Institute of Industrial Technologies and Automation, National Research
Council, Milan, Italy
e-mail: marco.sacco@itia.cnr.it

© Springer International Publishing AG 2017
F. Cavallo et al. (eds.), *Ambient Assisted Living*, Lecture Notes
in Electrical Engineering 426, DOI 10.1007/978-3-319-54283-6_22

1 Introduction

Today's homes are environments where various devices perform separate and isolated tasks. Instead, future homes can become systems of distributed and interconnected smart objects (SO) working together in a reliable and predictable manner [1]. In fact, on the basis of the increasingly widespread protocol of the Internet of Things (IoT), the SO can acquire, handle and share the knowledge about the home inhabitants in order to meet the goal of achieving their comfort and well-being [2], thus enabling the model of Smart Home (SH) [3].

One of the main application of the SH is in the field of the Ambient Assisted Living (AAL), where the SH can provide tailored services that support users with disabilities for a better, healthier and safer life in their everyday living environment; e.g. such services can be used to drive the behaviors of users through the processing of the context information. However, the implementation of the SH entails a wide range of technological and scientific problems to be tackled. One of the most relevant is represented by the lack of interoperability between the various involved smart objects which often isolates significant data sets and emphasizes the "existing problem of too much data and not enough knowledge" [4]. This issue is mainly due to the adoption of different communication interfaces, since devices often are produced from various vendors, which use different programming languages, operating systems, and hardware. Moreover, even many standards have been defined also in the AAL field, this issue still remains to be faced.

Under these conditions, it is necessary to adopt a new model of collaboration among the various involved sources, regardless the information representation formats. In order to address this problem, various generic models of interoperability have been proposed by researchers. Sacco et al. have proposed the Virtual Home Framework (VHF) [5], that represents a possible pattern based on Sematic Web technologies to be applied to solve such issue of integration. On the basis of this reference model, the research introduced in this paper analyzes and designs a service-oriented platform [6] for ambient assisted living (AAL) systems, in which information coming from different types of SO are enriched with semantic metadata, thus contributing to seamlessly integrate, aggregate and synchronize the various SO. The platform, which is one of the main outcomes of the ongoing Italian research project "Design for All" (D4A) [5], allows to handle and maintain near real-time shared semantic representation of the available knowledge, while enabling new, implicit knowledge inferencing, based on semantic derivation rules and ontology entailments. A relevant role here is played by the *Integration Services* and specifically by a publish/subscribe middleware enabling messages exchange among all the loosely coupled SO and applications included in the AAL system. A prototype has been also implemented and validated in order to prove the correctness of the approach and to perform a preliminary performance evaluation.

The remainder of the paper is structured as follows. Section 2 examines the motivation for this research work, whereas Sect. 3 illustrates the main characteristics on the basis of the service-oriented platform. Section 4 presents the conducted experiments. Finally, Sect. 5 draws the conclusions, summarizing the main outcomes.

2 The Vision

The proposed approach mainly addresses the data integration issue, which is particularly relevant when talking about complex domain models often expressed as huge, intensive, and multisource data [7]. The idea behind this work is to provide AAL applications and tools with a common and high-level interfacing means, the *Integration Services* (Fig. 1), allowing them to access a shared domain knowledge managed by the *Semantic Repository*, contributing to simplify collaboration among applications.

This approach represents a common best-practice when dealing with Enterprise Information Systems [8, 9]. Applications can easily interoperate while the handled data are integrated, aggregated and shared or dispatched through mechanisms that are transparent to their clients. In the context of the D4A project, *Integration Services* foster the semantic integration among several different domestic devices and tools, contributing to enhance their near real-time synchronization capabilities and making them smarter. In fact, the *Integration Services* allow to abstract from implementation details of each given device, hiding the complexity of their different interfaces. In this sense, *Integration Services* enable a proper SO interaction and enhance their capability to exchange information providing a seamless view on high-quality data extracted through a common and generalized interface providing the following main functionalities:

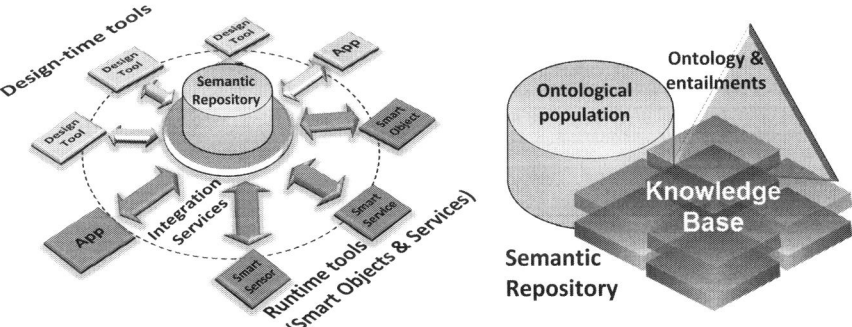

Fig. 1 General vision behind the integration services

1. acquisition of information from any SO;
2. storing, interpreting and properly managing the information received;
3. sharing or proactively dispatching information when a SO asks for them or a needed information becomes available.

Integration Services comprise a specific service (the *Information Dispatching Service*) which makes available the changed information to a whatever application through a multi agent server enabling the near real time semantic signaling. Under these conditions, the *Information Dispatching Service* plays the role of an IoT middleware that supplies the central point which join heterogeneous devices communicating through heterogeneous interfaces. It also implements the major functionalities that Sacco et al. [5] conceived for the Virtual Home Manager, the component of the reference framework that enables the bidirectional connection between the two worlds of the real home and the digital home.

The proposed service-oriented platform has been implemented and tested in the context of D4A project activities to integrate both AAL design tools and runtime smart services and objects included in an AAL system (Fig. 1). In order to test and validate the proposed platform, some demonstration scenarios have been identified, which are thought to represent habits and activities occurring on a regular basis in a domestic environment. A significant one focuses on the user during the grocery shopping; in this situation the idea is to monitor food inventory through a smart interaction between a refrigerator and a smart phone. Performances has been evaluated considering not only the pure execution time but also the feasibility and ergonomics w.r.t. developers and systems integrators.

3   The Integration Services

The *Integration Services* provides the following capabilities:

- *Authoring*, which allow each application to manipulate shareable owned knowledge through the operations of insert, update and delete;
- *Retrieval*, which allow the extraction (retrieval) of both asserted and inferred knowledge from the shared domain;
- *Signaling*, allowing socially connected applications to register themselves and receive alert related to the changing of the state of one or more interesting elements.

Through these capabilities, the *Integration Services* allow each application or smart object distributed in the AAL environment to translate information expressed according to its own applicative ontology into application expressed according to the shared domain ontology and vice versa, thus contributing to create a shared common understanding of the relevant knowledge of the domestic environment.

Figure 2 reports the main steps of this knowledge sharing process in a processing pipeline from authoring to retrieval. Sharable legacy data, whose definition

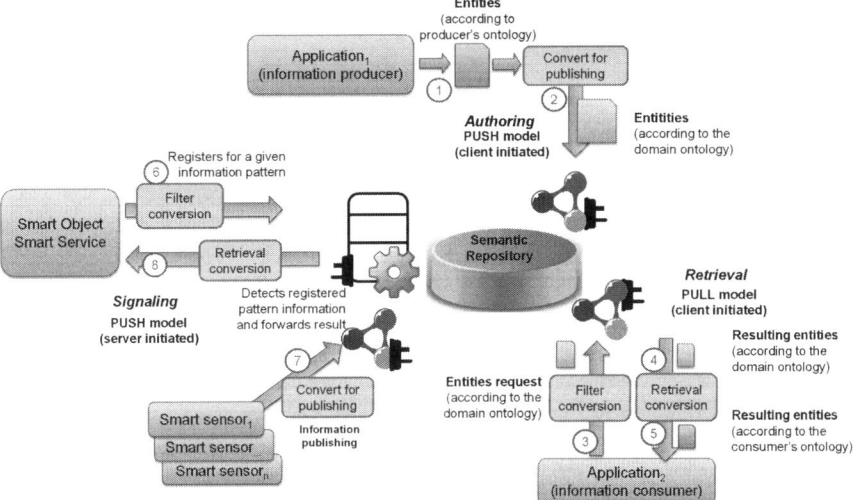

Fig. 2 The processing pipeline concerning the *Integration Services*

is given with respect to the specific application's ontology, will be translated according to the shared D4A domain ontology (Step 1). Once translated, this common representation is forwarded to the SR (Step 2) in order to be stored by means of semantic data manipulation languages and tools. On the other side, by means of search criteria conveniently converted in a SR understandable form (Step 3), domain ontology represented entities are retrieved (Step 4) by semantically querying shared knowledge, and successively converted in the requestor under-standable form (Step 5).

In order to support the aforementioned capabilities, the *Integration Services* comprises the three following components (Fig. 2):

- *Data mash-up services.* It implements the typical data access layer in a multi-tier application architecture, allowing to manage application sharable data. Designed specifically for each application, it is in charge of translating forth and back data entities from the application's specific format to the shared domain ontology representation.
- *Semantic data access service.* In the form of a shared common application library, is in charge of translating received SPARQL requests into corresponding HTTP request, according to SPARQL 1.1 Protocol for RDF, which is the adopted standard way to compose the semantic query. In this way, the translated request will be served through the cloud integration services component.
- *Information dispatching service*, allowing to real-time distribute emerging information to interested subsystems (services, applications and so on).

3.1   Supporting the Signaling Capabilities Through the Information Dispatching Service

The *Integration Services* provide near real-time signaling capabilities to all the networked Smart Objects and Services involved in the AAL environment thanks to the *Information Dispatching Service*, which is a multi agent and semantic based signaling server. In particular, the *Information Dispatching Service* plays the role of an effective IoT middleware, allowing applications to register for interesting information and receive back alerts about the changing state or the emergence of interesting knowledge. Moreover, it abstracts and hides the complexities of the hardware or software components, involved within the system.

Under these conditions, this architecture resembles the one of Enterprise 2.0 Social Software (E2.0) [10–12] since it supports social and networked applications concurrently accessing and modifying a shared knowledge domain. The evaluation of the emersion of the asked information is proactively activated by the agent upon recognizing an update of the knowledge-base. Each agent can act as a publisher to send changed information and as a subscriber to receive all the updates related to subscribed information. Figure 2 reports the processing pipeline concerning the *Information Dispatching Service* (Step 6, Step 7, Step 8). These services has the potential to significantly reduce the bandwidth cost of busy spin semantic queries, as well as the required workload both at the client application and knowledge base sides. Moreover, it enables an effective and performant semantic event-driven model to support design and development in the field of AAL; thus reducing the development cost, while also increasing interoperability, quality and portability.

3.1.1   The Architectural Model

The implementation of the *Information Dispatching Service* leverages the specifications of the Foundation for Intelligent Physical Agents (FIPA) [13], which include a full set of computer software standards for specifying how agents should communicate and interoperate within a system. In particular, it has been take into account the FIPA Subscribe-like interaction protocol (IP) specification [14] that defines messages to be exchanged, as well as their sequencing according to a Request-Reply Enterprise Integration Pattern [15].

The *Information Dispatching Service* is enabled by a messaging system, supporting both the publish/subscribe pattern and message queue models. The first allows the specific receivers (subscribers) to express interest in one or more information and only receive messages that are of interest, while the second enables an asynchronous inter-process communications protocol. In this implementation, the selected messaging system is the Apache ActiveMQ™ [16], an open source messaging platform through which clients can make a subscription specifying the SPARQL query of interest, the content type of the expected response and the authorization credentials for accessing the repository (username and password). The

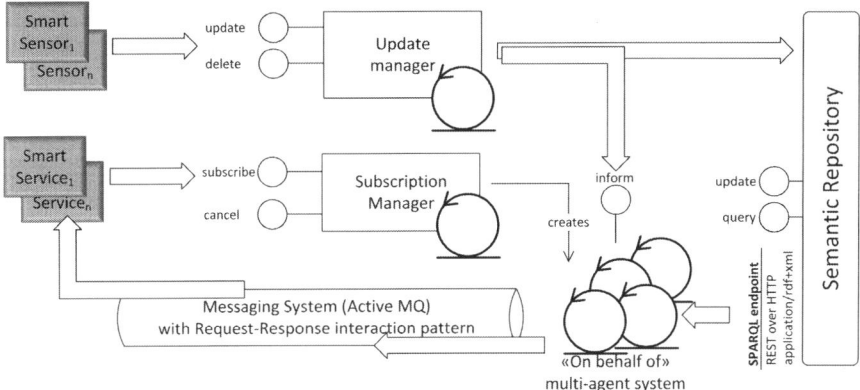

Fig. 3 The architectural model

presented infrastructure is paired with a web server based on the Jersey framework [17] which allows to expose a notification service of the state of the knowledge base changes.

Through the Apache ActiveMQ™, the *Information Dispatching Service* is always listening on the queue that manages the new subscriptions (*SubscriptionManager*) (Fig. 3). Whenever it receives a subscription request from a network client, it activates server-side an agent (the *ClientAgent*) which takes care of the client interests.

The subscription requires that the client sends the following information:

1. the *client-ref*, a unique identifier of the client;
2. the *req-id*, a unique identifier of the query of interest;
3. the SPARQL query of interest, the credentials (username and password) for the authentication, and a boolean flag, *reasoning*, which tells the system whether to activate the reasoning during the query execution (in order to extract implicit knowledge).

After the transmission of the subscription, the client waits for subsequent notifications provided by the *SubscriptionManager* whenever the knowledge base is changed and the corresponding query produces a result different from that previously transmitted. The changes applied to the knowledge base are notified to *SubscriptionManager* through appropriate communication interface (e.g. a REST, etc.). Notifications are automatically (transparently) carried by the operator SPARQL endpoint at each interaction of type SPARQL Update. In summary, the main operations performed server-side by the *Information Dispatching Service* are:

1. the activation of a queue listening on new subscriptions;
2. the activation of a queue listening on new notifications of the knowledge base changes;
3. the execution of the subscribed queries, reports any change to the listening client;

while the main operations performed client-side are:

1. the creation of a temporary queue of messages specific for the client;
2. the preparation of the message for the subscription and listening of notifications;
3. the sending by the client of the request for subscription to one or more of the queries;
4. the cancellation of the registration, by closing the connection.

3.1.2 The Subscription Protocol

The client starts the interaction with the server through a subscription message containing the description of the information of interest (specified in a query) with the minimum refresh rate in milliseconds, together with a unique identifier of the request (*req-id*) and a reference (pointer, address, etc.) of the client (*client-ref.*) to which forward the discovered information.

The query transmitted from the client is expressed through the SPARQL 1.1 syntax and may be a SELECT, ASK or CONSTRUCT that refers to semantic model contained in the repository. The server processes the subscription request and decides whether to accept it. If it is rejected, the repository sends to the client the rejection condition ending the interaction. If it is accepted, at each interval of minimum refresh rate, the server updates the evaluation of the subscribed queries and transmits an information message (*inform-result* to the client) containing the result of the executed query (*query-result*) if the result is not empty (SELECT or CONSTRUCT query type) or positive (ASK query type), according to the chosen response format.

The server continues to broadcast type messages (*inform-result*) as long as one of the following conditions happen:

1. the client deletes the subscription request by the cancellation request (see next section);
2. an error occurs for which the server is no longer able to communicate with the client or to process queries.

All interactions are identified by a unique identifier other than zero (*req-id*) assigned by the initiator of the protocol and valid for it (*client-ref*). This allows stakeholders to manage their communication strategies and activities. Moreover, since it can be important to preserve the sequence of the messages, the transport layer has to preserve the order of the messages (reliable transport layer). Thanks to the oneness of the *req-id*, each client can participate in multiple signaling at the same time. Figure 4 reports the overall workflow of the subscription process.

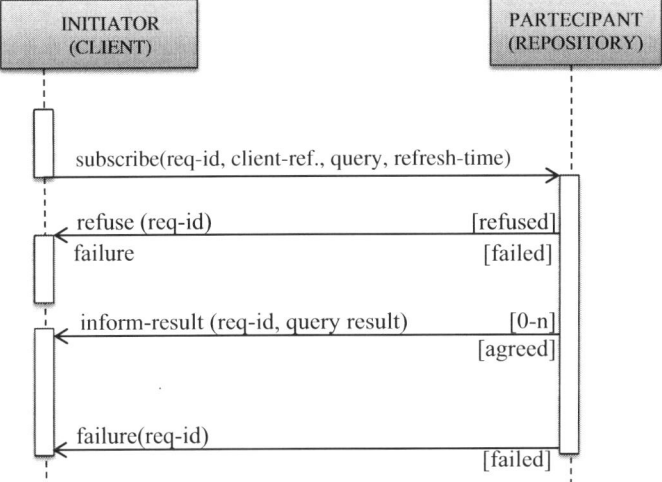

Fig. 4 Subscription and notification workflow

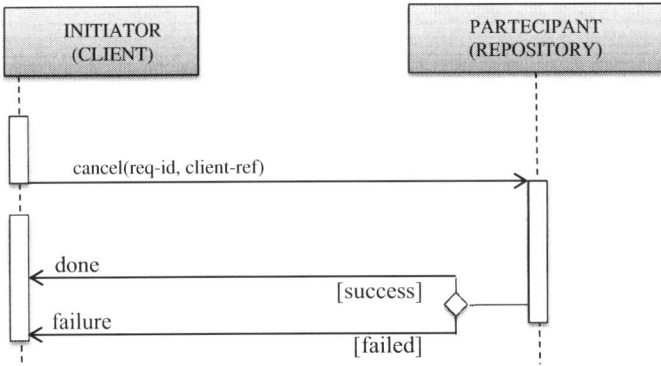

Fig. 5 Workflow of the cancellation of the subscription

3.1.3 Cancelling Subscriptions

At any time, the client may cancel a subscription request by transmitting a cancel request to the server. In such a request, the parameters *req-id-ref* and *client* identify the interaction to be stopped (Fig. 5). The server inform then the client if the interruption succeeded (done) or that it was not possible to break the interaction due to an error (failure).

3.2 The Data Persistence Through the Semantic Repository

A significant study during this research has regarded the identification of a valid Semantic Repository (SR) capable to handle large amount of Semantic data, also in the form of Big Data [18]. Managed data comprise:

- the domain ontology, as representation of the knowledge about home environment;
- the ontological population, compliant to the domain ontology;
- the derivation rules needed to properly entail the implicit knowledge.

This component must also provide reasoning capability in order to automatically infer new knowledge about the concepts and their relationships, starting from the explicitly asserted facts [19].

A study of the state of the art of a set of existing semantic repositories has been carried out, considering the reasoning capability as main criteria of evaluation, since it represents an essential requirement for the platform currently under development. The result of the survey is that majority of reasoners are still far away from conformance to the full specification of the OWL (Ontology Web Language) [20], the standard language used to represent semantic data. One of the causes is the great expressivity allowed by OWL that results in difficult (if not impossible) reasoner implementations. OWL, in its full specification, is undecidable. (i.e. query answering for an OWL ontology needing reasoning could require infinite time). Since decidability is an important property in real world scenarios, a decidable syntactic subset of OWL has been defined. This leads to an enormous amount of possible implementations, and appears to disrupt the standardization effort made by product developers. In the context of this project, we have evaluated and finally adopted Stardog [21], since it supports the largest subset of OWL compared to other solutions, thus, allowing an higher level of expressivity to represent the derivation rules.

Moreover, the here presented platform attempts to deal with the horizontal scalability. This can be also addressed through the enabling technologies of the cloud computing [22]. The Infrastructure as a Service (IaaS) paradigm, characterized in that the providers offer computers (physical or virtual machines) and also other resources, has been used for the tests of the platform, since it is the only offering valid solution compliant with the Semantic Web technologies.

4 The Conducted Experiments

One out of the defined experimental settings is a context aware *Situation Identification System (SIS)* designed and prototyped by ab medica, one of the D4A project partners. The SIS is aimed at identifying ongoing situations that are relevant from a cognitive point of view in the reference scenario and selecting services to be activated based on the contextual and situational profile.

The main features of this system are:

- Gathering, analyzing and semantically annotating brain signals, as well as several other bioelectrical and medical information. All these information are to be merged with contextual information acquired by ubiquitous home-automation sensors;
- Extraction of all those features useful to identify situations that are relevant from a cognitive perspective, in the reference scenario;
- Contextual profiling of the observed user and identification of status and behavioral patterns;
- Activation of needed services, identified according to the current contextual and situational user profile.

As can be seen in Fig. 6, the general architecture of *SIS* recalls the Endsley model for Situation Awareness [23] and is based on an specific knowledge base feeding and sustaining situational models for identification and elicitation. These model and their underlying knowledge are, in their turn, modeled according to an application ontology focused on modeling and reasoning on medical and behavioral features of a observer subject. SIS exploits D4A Integration Services by getting contextual information coming from smart sensors and objects deployed in the environment such aa internal and external temperature, light levels, devices activation, receipt execution, etc. At the same time *SIS* is able to feed back the repository with information related to the current state of the user and his current health profile.

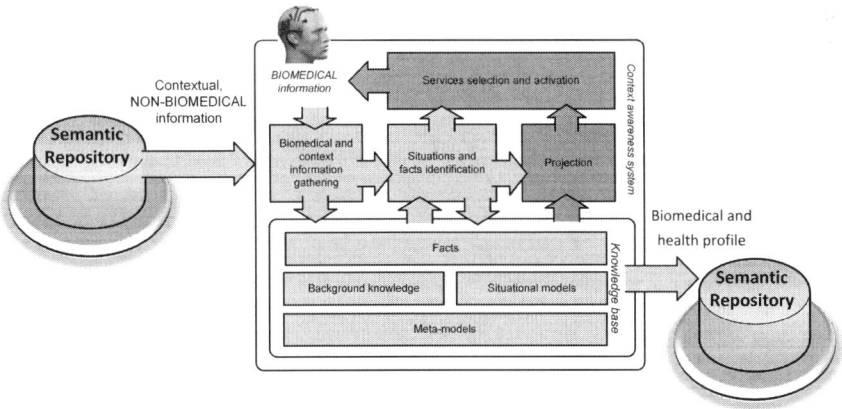

Fig. 6 Situation identification system's architecture and its interaction in the AAL platform

5   Conclusion

This paper has introduced a service-oriented platform for ambient assisted living which contributes to enable a smarter interaction of the various devices distributed within the domestic environment. Devices can cooperate through the integration of the knowledge about home environment, thanks to a strategy leveraging the central role of the Semantic Web Technologies. The proposed platform is particularly relevant in the context of AAL, in the perspective of moving away from more traditional assistive technologies towards an approach that takes into account the full range of human diversity. Nevertheless some issues continues to limit the potential usage of the platform, especially when dealing with legacy systems whose knowledge models are huge or too complex to make the integration process simply economically unaffordable [24]. This problem represents the most relevant technological gap to be addressed in the future developments of the platform [25]. Future work also concerns a quantitative analysis of performance, also exploiting new benchmarks that are currently under study.

Acknowledgements This work has been co-funded by the Ministry of University and Research of Italy within the cluster "Tecnologie per gli ambienti di vita—Technologies for Ambient Assisted Living" initiatives, with the overall objective of increasing the quality of life in the domestic environments through the use of the modern technologies.

References

1. Perumal T, Ramli AR, Leong CY, Mansor S, Samsudin K (2008) Interoperability for smart home environment using web services. IJSH 2:1–16
2. Koskela T, Vaananen-Vaino-Mattila K (2004) Evolution towards smart home environments: empirical evaluation of three user interfaces. Pers Ubiquit Comput 8(3–4):234–240
3. Harper R (2003) Inside the smart home. Springer Science & Business Media
4. Sheth AP, Sahoo SS (2008) Semantic sensor web. IEEE Internet Comput 12(4):78–83
5. Sacco M, Caldarola EG, Modoni G, Terkaj W (2014) Supporting the design of AAL through a SW integration framework: the D4All project. In: Universal access in human-computer interaction. Design and development methods for universal access. Springer, pp 75–84
6. Jammes F, Smit H, Martinez Lastra JL, Delamer IM (2005) Service-oriented paradigms in industrial automation. IEEE Trans Ind Inf 1(1):62–70
7. Modoni GE, Sacco M, Terkaj W (2016) A telemetry-driven approach to simulate data-intensive manufacturing processes. 49th procedia CIRP-CMS 2016
8. Hinchcliffe D (2007) The state of enterprise 2.0. ZDNET.com, London
9. Cook N (2008) Enterprise 2.0: how social software will change the future of work. Gower Publishing Ltd.
10. Bellifemine F, Caire G, Greenwood D (2007) Developing multi-agent systems with JADE. Wiley. ISBN 978-0-470-05747-6
11. McAfee AP (2006) Enterprise 2.0: the dawn of emergent collaboration. MIT Sloan Manage Rev 47(3):21
12. McAfee A (2009) Enterprise 2.0: new collaborative tools for your organization's toughest challenges. Harvard Business Press

13. FIPA Communicative Act Library Specification. Foundation for intelligent physical agents, 2000. http://www.fipa.org/specs/fipa00037/
14. IEEE Computer Society, IEEE foundation for intelligent physical agents (FIPA) standards committee [Online]. Available http://www.fipa.org/. Retrieved Oct 2016
15. Hohpe G, Woolf B (2003) Enterprise integration patterns. Addison-Wesley, 650 pages. ISBN 0321200683
16. Apache ActiveMQ™ [Online]. Available http://activemq.apache.org. Retrieved Oct 2016
17. Project Jersey [Online]. https://jersey.java.net/. Retrieved Oct 2016
18. Modoni G, Sacco M, Terkaj W (2014) A survey of RDF store solutions. In: Proceedings of the 20th international conference on engineering, technology and innovation, Bergamo
19. Modoni GE, Sacco M, Terkaj W (2014) A semantic framework for graph-based enterprise search. Appl Comput Sci 10(4):66–74
20. [Online]. Available from http://www.w3.org/TR/2012/REC-owl2-primer-20121211/. Retrieved Oct 2016
21. Stardog [Online]. Available http://stardog.com/. Retrieved Oct 2016
22. Sriram I, Khajeh-Hosseini A (2010) Research agenda in cloud technologies. arXiv preprint arXiv:1001.3259
23. Endsley MR (2000) Theoretical underpinnings of situation awareness: a critical review. In: Endsley MR, Garland DJ (eds) Situation awareness analysis and measurement. LEA, Mahwah, NJ
24. Canfora G, Fasolino AR, Frattolillo G, Tramontana P (2006) Migrating interactive legacy systems to web services. In: Conference on software maintenance and reengineering (CSMR'06). IEEE, 10 pp
25. Modoni GE, Doukas M, Terkaj W, Sacco M, Mourtzis D (2016) Enhancing factory data integration through the development of an ontology: from the reference models reuse to the semantic conversion of the legacy models. Int J Comput Integr Manuf 1–17

Part III
Experiments, Evaluation and Lessons Learnt

ASTRO: Autism Support Therapy by RObot Interaction

Massimo Pistoia, Marco Pistoia and Paolo Casacci

Abstract "Autism" is a syndrome that, according to the latest surveys, affects 1 child out of 100 and is the most characteristic group of pervasive developmental disorders. This work describes the experience gained through the "ASTRO" Project to develop a product able to support, by the means of new technologies, pre-school and school-aged children affected by Autism Spectrum Disorders and that can serve as a proper tool to be used during educational and rehabilitation activities. The goal was pursued by an ICT platform, endowed with a robotic platform, aimed at facilitating treatment of autistic children by ABA (Applied Behavior Analysis) methodology.

Keywords Living labs · Autism · Dyslexia · Robot · Learning · LMS

1 Introduction

Even though children affected by autism present different functional deficits, however, they are often able to use surprisingly different technologies such as PCs, MP3 player, TV, video games: tools used daily at home and sometimes at school. Teaching can find then a "rich soil" for what concerns the use of new technologies in order to foster learning by children suffering from autism and by taking into consideration that achieving new competences can go through those already learned, using technological devices as operational tools [1].

M. Pistoia (✉) · M. Pistoia · P. Casacci
eResult s.r.l., Piazzale Luigi Rava n.46, 47522 Cesena (FC), Italy
e-mail: massimo.pistoia@eresult.it

M. Pistoia
e-mail: info@eresult.it

P. Casacci
e-mail: Paolo.Casacci@eresult.it

© Springer International Publishing AG 2017
F. Cavallo et al. (eds.), *Ambient Assisted Living*, Lecture Notes
in Electrical Engineering 426, DOI 10.1007/978-3-319-54283-6_23

The ASTRO project, co-financed by the Apulia Region in Italy by means of the Apulian ICT Living Labs programme, meant to create a multimedia robotic system integrated with the OMNIACARE software platform, developed by eResult, which enables to cope with diverse disability-related conditions. This was achieved by extending the features of the so-called OMNIACARE software platform for the delivery of didactical and cognitive exercises, in order to enable an interaction mediated by a robot to act as an intermediary in the process of socialization, reducing stress introduced by the absence of emotional inferences [2]. The realized system is suitable for domestic use as well, allowing the teacher to intervene in telepresence assisted by a parent. The development of human-machine interaction integrating IT tools with robotic devices provides a solution that contains flexible and customizable activities to suit different needs and characteristics. Such characteristics can be summarized as shift of the focus from learning to "doing", in an educational design, organized and articulated, careful about timing and method of use, along with spurring self-use of the tool in order to enhance technical skills as well, increase self-esteem and gratification [3, 4].

2 Materials and Methods

The main goal of the ASTRO project was to develop a product able to support, by the means of new technologies, pre-school and school-aged children affected by Autism Spectrum Disorders and that can serve as a proper tool to be used during educational and rehabilitation activities. The goals of the project were pursued using a kit consisting of an anthropomorphic robot, NAO™, developed by the French company Aldebaran Robotics, and an LMS (Learning Management System) platform, developed on the OMNIACARE system, devised and produced by eResult [5, 6].

The ASTRO system, along with the services it provides have been shaped around the UCD methodology. It is a design philosophy and a process, which focuses the attention on the user's need, expectations and limits in respect to the final product. The user is placed at the center of each step of the development process in order to maximize the usability and acceptance of the product, optimizing it around the needs of the users. The UCD methodology is characterized by a multi-level co-design and problem solving process. It requires designers to not only analyze and foresee how the user will utilize the final product, but to test and validate their assumptions at the same time by taking into consideration the end user's behavior during the usability and accessibility tests (test of user-experience) into the real world. The UCD methodology leads to the creation of the final product through an iterative and interactive process that provides the development of a first prototype and a following test and assessment stage based on which to proceed with the development of the next prototype. Each cycle therefore leads to the creation of a product that is closest to the real and practical needs of the user. The aim of the UCD is to move from a high-fidelity prototype with a focus on users' identified needs to an innovation. This means to include both business model aspects as well as designing a fully functioning innovation. The main objective is to re-design the innovation according to feedback gained in earlier phases.

The activities spent in the design and testing phases were conducted side-by-side with therapists who apply the ABA (Applied Behavior Analysis) methodology and with a parent association of autistic children. ABA is a program that is based on the principles of behavior modification, and which aims to intervene in children of preschool age with the mediation of parents and the support of operators. The ABA intervention has proven to be particularly effective in intellectual functioning, in the understanding of language and learning of social skills in adaptive behavior, in understanding and linguistic expression.

All the work was scientifically supervised by an independent third party represented by the University of Foggia (Italy). The project team designed and implemented a set of exercises for the autistic children, which aimed to improve parent-child relation by initially stimulating attention with actions initiated by the robot, later substituted by the parent to continue the interaction. All in all, the robot acted as a facilitator for the parents to gain attention from their children.

3   Technology

The ASTRO project was realized using two main ICT technologies, one hardware and one software. The hardware platform was a NAO™ robot, while the software application was OMNIACARE.

NAO™ is a hi-tech robotic device characterized by 25 degrees of freedom, which allow it to perform even the most complex motions and it is suitable for structured and unstructured environments. It is equipped with:

- Ultrasonic proximity sensors pointing towards different directions, that allow to detect and evaluate the physical distance;
- Pressure sensors located under the lower limbs;
- Advanced multimedia system with 4 microphones and 2 speakers;
- 2 CMOS cameras designed for speech synthesis, space location, face and object recognition;
- Interaction sensors such as 3 touch areas above the head of the robot;
- 2 infrared led and 2 contact sensors on the front of the lower limbs.

The OMNIACARE platform is a multi-functional hardware and software system, specifically developed by eResult for the remote monitoring and assistance of frail users. By providing tools to patients and caregivers, the system improves quality of life of those people who need particular assistance in daily living and to those who take care of them. OMNIACARE's software architecture is modular: each element realizes some specific functions, as to be able to dynamically adapt to a variety of situations and environments. The system allows exploitation of more or less functionalities in a seamless way, by using specific elements, while the overall system keeps running. The system architecture is open to any potential development by just adding new modules.

To cover the aspect of support to children affected with learning or developmental disorders, the platform implements a Learning Management System that administers provision of multimedia exercises, aided by Information and Communication Technology tools, to make the learning or therapy process more playful, usable and effective. The system also records the pupils' answers and feedbacks to ease teachers and therapists in their effort to properly assess children's capacity evolution and growth.

OMNIACARE comprises the following elements:

- Central Server;
- Home Server;
- External hardware systems (robot, sensors, interaction and parameter collecting devices);
- Webcam;
- Smartphone and tablet (Android-based).

The webcam is connected to the Internet through a Wi-Fi router. Operators and therapists can use it to monitor the local environment and to support patients and caregivers by working on the system themselves, through the Central and Home Servers. This is an optional feature that can be disabled by the end user for privacy reasons.

The Central Server (CS) is the main element of the system. User profiles, device configurations and all system data reside on the CS. The CS also provides the web interface that operators and therapists use to interact with the system, in order to customize exercises and therapy for pupils. Configurations can be done on the CS by the tutors only, to avoid unauthorized modifications by the users or caregivers. The Home Server and the hand-held device periodically synchronize data and download configurations from and to the CS. The CS has been built on the eResult's OMNIAPLACE software development platform, and it inherits its inner characteristics (Fig. 1):

- Hierarchical data structure.
- Web-based user interface.
- Advanced data navigation, display and search.
- Extensive data export functionalities.
- Granular user privilege management.
- Structured system event management.
- Information traceability.

The Home Server (HS) acts as a gateway that interfaces with detection sensors and external devices managing all of the diverse communication protocols. The HS collects data from the devices and provides configuration data exchange to proper manage them. The HS also consolidates and conditions data and sends them to the

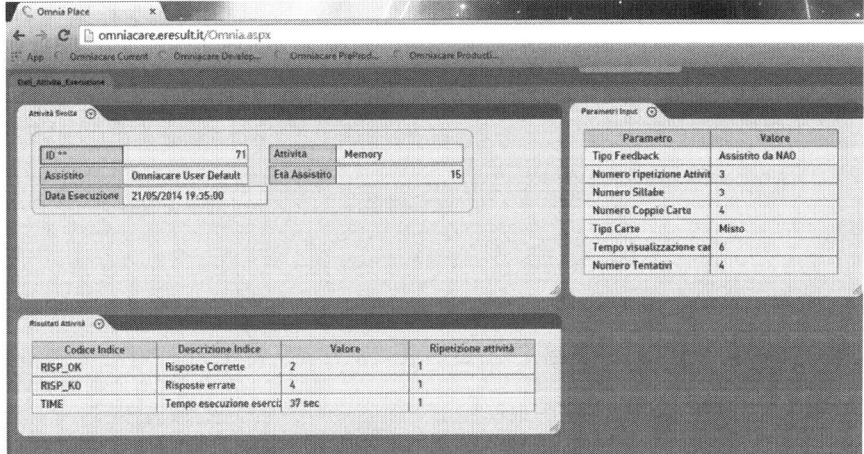

Fig. 1 OMNIACARE central server (CS)

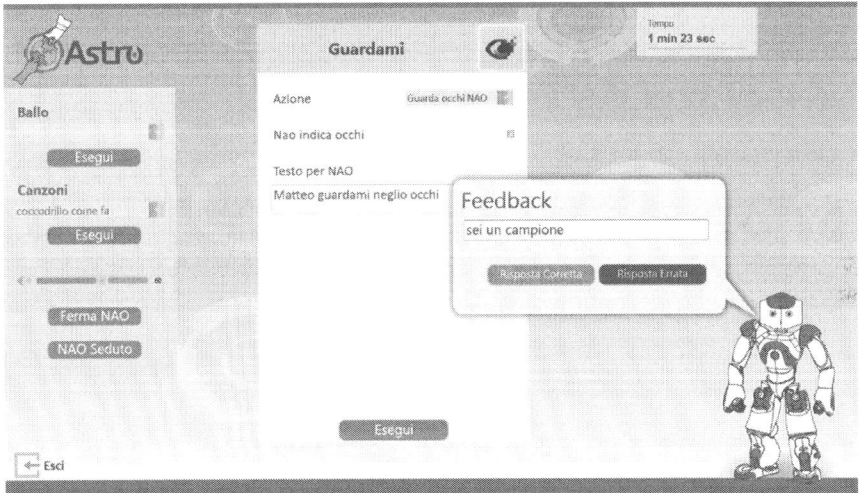

Fig. 2 OMNIACARE home server LMS screen

CS, according to the established rules and timing, while at the same time providing warning or alerts in case of a detected anomaly.

As concerns the LMS system, the HS also contains the software engine used for exercise administration and the user interface module to display such exercises to the pupil, along with the interaction control dashboard for the therapist/teacher to manage behaviors of the NAO™ robot (Fig. 2).

Different access to information and functions can be granted on the HS-based LMS platform to different users, according to their needs and competences, by a web interface present on the CS configuration page [7].

4 Results

The ASTRO Project result assessment revealed that 63% of involved children positively reacted to the robot's presence, showing curiosity, happiness, interest; 18.5% showed negative reactions; 18.5% of children showed an alternate behavior, sometimes afraid or indifferent, sometimes curious. In some cases, negative expressions depended on technical problems interfering with, or blocking, the experimentation session. 48.1% of children satisfactorily responded also to direct interaction with the robot. It was important for the experimentation to note how easily children would physically approach the robot, spontaneously approached and touched in most cases.

As to families, parents were actively involved in the ASTRO co-design and experimentation phases. 81.5% of families declared themselves satisfied by the experimentation, in some cases expressing amazement for "the progress obtained [by their children]". Even those who were doubtful in the beginning of the project, progressively gained confidence during the course of experimentation, due to the gradual successful improvement in their children's interaction. In 90 sessions, parents participated in exercise execution, using the system and stimulating children to establish a direct contact with the robot, by singing and dancing with it and giving expressions of encouragement. This allowed the robot to play a role of functional game and raising interest and curiosity in autistic children, unlike the stereotyped games they typically use in a solitary manner. Thus, the robot facilitated the relation between child and parents. Parents, on their side, discovered a new way of living a joyful and playful moment with their children, at the same time useful to stimulate their cognitive and behavioral abilities [8].

In a limited number of cases, intensive intervention and help by the therapist was necessary, because the parent was not able to properly use the PC and thus easily discouraged; or, for the fact that the parent, while desiring to cooperate, was not able to oversee the child and use the system at the same time. Some families decided to leave the project because the exercises from the system were too simple for the chronological age of the children. This criticality emerged as a side effect of the need to experiment the possibilities offered by the system as a mediator in the parent/child relation. In fact, the proposed exercises were rather simple, in order to ensure the active involvement of parents allowing them to carry out the session autonomously, with the simple supervision of the therapist. This prevented the system to adapt to the need of the single patient. From the experimentation, it nonetheless emerged how the preparation and behavior of therapists are critical to the success of the session. It is important that they invest time in preparing the setting before the session itself, eliminating any distractors and arranging preliminary plans along with required procedures.

The ASTRO project led to the conclusion that the realized intervention, designed to make parents protagonists in their children's treatment, makes a step in the right direction towards the awareness of the possibilities they have to make a difference with their own kids [9]. Parents were all available to further experiment and gave suggestions for improvements.

Acknowledgments The authors thank Prof. Stefania Pinnelli from University of Salento and Dr. Giovanna Avellis from Innovapuglia SpA for the essential contribution to this paper. This work has been funded by Apulia Region, under Regional Operational Programme ERDF 2007–2013 Action 1.4.2 supporting the growth and the development of SMEs specialized in the delivery of digital contents and services.

References

1. Dillon G, Underwood J (2012) Computer mediated imaginative storytelling in children with autism. Int J Hum Comput Stud 70:169–178
2. Goodrich MA, Colton M, Brinton B, Fujiki M, Atherton JA, Robinson L, Ricks D, Maxfield MH, Acerson A (2012) Incorporating a robot into an autism therapy team. IEEE Intell Syst 27:52–59
3. Lee J, Takahashi H, Nagai C, Obinata G, Stefanov D (2012) Which robot features can stimulate better responses from children with autism in robot-assisted therapy? Int J Adv Robot Syst 2012:9. doi:10.5772/51128
4. Nuria Aresti Bartolome N, Garcia Zapirain B (2014) Technologies as support tools for persons with autistic spectrum disorder: a systematic review. Int J Environ Res Public Health 2014 (11):7767–7802
5. Petric F (2014) Robotic autism spectrum disorder diagnostic protocol: basis for cognitive and interactive robotic system. Available at http://www.fer.unizg.hr/en/search?sq=%22robotic+autism%22&sm%5B%5D=16&s_count=25&sortby=2&s_skip=0
6. Tapus A, Peca A, Aly A, Pop C, Jisa L, Pintea S, Rusu AS, David DO (2012) Children with autism social engagement in interaction with Nao, an imitative robot—a series of single case experiments. Interact Stud 13:315–347
7. Pinnelli S (2014) Reading difficulties and technologies: design and development of an educational ICT training. Conference/proceedings/book: international conference on education and new developments 2014 (END 2014), Madrid 27/29 June 2014
8. Turkle S, Taggart W, Kidd CD, Dasté O (2006) Relational artifacts with children and elders: the complexities of cybercompanionship. Connection Sci 18(4):347–361
9. Lester JC, Converse SA (2006) The persona effect: affective impact of animated pedagogical agents. Proceedings of the ACM SIGCHI conference on human factors in computing systems, pp. 359–366

MARIO Project: A Multicenter Survey About Companion Robot Acceptability in Caregivers of Patients with Dementia

Daniele Sancarlo, Grazia D'Onofrio, James Oscar,
Francesco Ricciardi, Dympna Casey, Keith Murphy,
Francesco Giuliani and Antonio Greco

Abstract In the frame of the European Community funded MARIO, caregivers of 139 dementia patients were recruited in National University of Ireland (NUIG), in Geriatrics Unit of IRCCS "Casa Sollievo della Sofferenza"-Italy (IRCCS) and in Alzheimer Association Bari-Italy (AAB) for a multicenter survey on to determine the needs and preferences of caregivers for improving the assistance of dementia patients, and guiding technological development of MARIO. A six minute video on technological devices and functions of MARIO was showed, and all caregivers fulfilled a 43-item questionnaire that explored four areas: (A) Acceptability, (B) Functionality, (C) Support devices, and (D) Impact. Caregivers declared that to

---

Grazia D'Onofrio—Macroarea of interest: Disability and rehabilitation.

D. Sancarlo · G. D'Onofrio (✉) · A. Greco
Geriatrics Unit & Laboratory of Gerontology and Geriatrics, Department of Medical
Sciences, IRCCS "Casa Sollievo Della Sofferenza", San Giovanni Rotondo, Foggia, Italy
e-mail: graziadonofrio@libero.it; g.donofrio@operapadrepio.it

D. Sancarlo
e-mail: sancarlodaniele@yahoo.it

A. Greco
e-mail: a.greco@operapadrepio.it

J. Oscar · D. Casey · K. Murphy
National University of Ireland, Galway, Ireland
e-mail: oscar.ben.james@gmail.com

D. Casey
e-mail: dympna.casey@nuigalway.ie

K. Murphy
e-mail: Kathy.murphy@nuigalway.ie

F. Ricciardi · F. Giuliani
ICT, Innovation and Research Unit, IRCCS "Casa Sollievo Della Sofferenza",
San Giovanni Rotondo, Foggia, Italy
e-mail: f.ricciardi@operapadrepio.it

F. Giuliani
e-mail: f.giuliani@operapadrepio.it

© Springer International Publishing AG 2017
F. Cavallo et al. (eds.), *Ambient Assisted Living*, Lecture Notes
in Electrical Engineering 426, DOI 10.1007/978-3-319-54283-6_24

311

facilitate acceptance (over 17.5%) and to improve functionality of MARIO (over 29%) should be important/likely/useful. Over 20.3% of caregivers reported that following support devices in MARIO could be useful for their patients: (1) for monitoring bed-rest and movements, (2) for monitoring the medication use, (3) for monitoring the ambient environmental conditions, (4) for regulating heating, humidity, lighting and TV channel, (5) for undertaking comprehensive geriatric assessment, (6) for link to care planning, (7) for monitoring physiological deterioration, and (8) for monitoring cognitive deterioration. Over 21.8% of caregivers declared that MARIO should be useful to improve quality of life, quality of care, safety, emergency communications, home-based physical and/or cognitive rehabilitation programs, and to detect isolation and health status changes of their patients. MARIO is a novel approach employing robot companions, and its effect will be: (1) to facilitate and support persons with dementia and their caregivers, and (2) reduce social exclusion and isolation.

Keywords Building resilience for loneliness and dementia · Comprehensive geriatric assessment · Caring service robots · Acceptability · Quality of life · Quality of care · Safety

1 Introduction

Europe has the highest prevalence of dementia in the world; seven million people are currently affected and this is projected to increase to 13.4 million by 2050 [1]. Across EU countries, participation of people with dementia in family and civic life is diminished by cultures of exclusion and stigmatisation [2]. Less severe and even more widespread, loneliness, isolation and depression are becoming increasingly important within Social Care. The increased mortality risk associated with the effects of these conditions is 200% greater than that of clinical obesity and comparable to the effects of smoking 15 cigarettes a day [3]. These effects include impaired immune functions, increased blood pressure, inflammation, anxiety, increased risk for heart disease, stroke and others [4]. Dementia is characterised by impaired mental functioning, language and thinking [5]. These impairments are often accompanied by personality, functional and behavioural changes.

To fight loneliness and the effects suffered by person with dementia, effective techniques include those that target change of a person's perception of loneliness and those that increase a person's resilience. Resilience is an adaptive capacity that refers to one's ability to 'bounce back' and cope in the face of adversity.

ICT solutions can be used to increase psychological skills like resilience [6], and to manage active and healthy aging with the use of caring service robots as will be explored with the EU funded MARIO project [7].

In this project specific technological tools are adopted that try to create real feelings and affections making it easier for the patient to accept assistance from a robot when—in certain situations—in return the human can also support the machine.

The approach targeted in MARIO is the Comprehensive Geriatric Assessment (CGA) on which the Multidimensional Prognosis Index (MPI) [8] is based. Used effectively, the MPI can improve dramatically diagnostic accuracy, optimize medical treatment and health outcomes, improve function and quality of life, reduce use of unnecessary formal services, and institute or improve long-term care management.

In MARIO, the service robot will provide information to MPI survey and evaluation process based on its observation of the instrumental activities of daily living and detection of changes regarding them.

The aim and ambition of the project are:

- to address and make progress on the challenging problems of loneliness, isolation and dementia in older persons through multi-faceted interventions delivered by service robots
- to conduct near project length interaction with end users and assisted living environments to enable iterative development and preparation for post project uptake
- to assist caregivers and physicians in the CGA of subjects at risk to loneliness, isolation or dementia through the use of service robots
- the use of near state of the art robotic platforms that are flexible, modular friendly, low cost and close to market ready in order to realize field contributions in the immediate future
- to make Mario capable to support and receive "robot applications" similar to the developer and app community for smartphones. This will empower development and creativity, enable the robot to perform new functionalities over time, and support discovery and improve usefulness for end users while lowering costs
- through novel advances in machine learning techniques and semantic analysis methods to make Mario more personable, useful, and accepted by end users (e.g. gain perception of non-loneliness).

To bring MARIO service robot concepts out of the lab and into industry by addressing licensing aspects via Apache, the integration of telecommunication aspects and application hosting environment.

In the first stage of the project, a series of mini-workshops locally at the pilot sites with partner organizations to introduce MARIO to both end users and stakeholders were done. After an interview about determining the needs and preferences of patients were performed.

The caregivers play a pivotal role in the management of the health and care of dementia patients, but although caregiving may be rewarding, providing care to a family member is stressful [9]. These negative consequences can affect the quality of life of patients and informal caregivers, and finally the quality of care of the patients and increase the likelihood of institutionalization [10].

The informal caregivers of dementia patients are early overwhelmed by care responsibilities and others showing stability or even decreases in the burden over time [11].

It was shown that the amount of time of informal care is the frequent reporting of up to 24 h per day, leading to very high cost estimates that may overlook aspects of joint production (i.e. caregivers performing multiple tasks simultaneously) [12]. Several studies were shown that the caregiver burden leads to higher levels of depression and anxiety [13, 14], use of psychotropic medication more frequently [15], engagement in fewer protective health behaviours, and increased risk of medical illness [16, 17] and mortality [18].

In this perspective, the ICT may provide promising new tools to improve the functional and cognitive assessment of patients with dementia and related disorders [19]. Development and implementation of novel computer-based ICT applications in the field of cognitive impairment mitigation and rehabilitation [20], emerging ICT applications based on virtual reality environments, including Augmented Reality technology, are become important game changers [19]. The ICT concept and approach can support the range of activities of daily living [21], monitor the circadian rhythm [22] for dementia patients.

The goal of this paper was to determine the needs and preferences of formal and informal caregivers for improving the assistance of dementia patients, and guiding the technological development of the MARIO though a questionnaire.

2 Materials and Methods

This study fulfilled the Declaration of Helsinki, the guidelines for Good Clinical Practice, and the Strengthening the Reporting of Observational Studies in Epidemiology guidelines. The approval of the study for experiments using human subjects was obtained from the local ethics committees on human experimentation. Written informed consent for research was obtained from each patient or from relatives or a legal representative in the case of severe demented patients. Caregivers of dementia patients consecutively recruited from May 2015 to February 2016 in the National University of Ireland (NUIG, Galway, Ireland), in the Geriatrics Unit of the Casa Sollievo della Sofferenza Hospital (IRCCS, San Giovanni Rotondo, Italy), and in the Alzheimer Association Bari (AAB, Bari, Italy) were screened for eligibility.

Inclusion criteria were: (1) caregiver of patients with diagnosis of dementia according to the criteria of the National Institute on Aging-Alzheimer's Association (NIAAA) [23]; and (2) the ability to provide an informed consent or availability of a proxy for informed consent. Exclusion criteria were: caregivers of patients with serious comorbidity, tumors and other diseases that could be causally related to cognitive impairment (ascertained blood infections, vitamin B12 deficiency, anaemia, disorders of the thyroid, kidneys or liver), history of alcohol or drug abuse, head trauma, psychoactive substance use and other causes of memory impairment.

The following parameters were collected by a systematic interview about the caregivers: gender, age, educational level (in years), and caregiving type [Informal caregiver (unpaid), Informal caregiver (paid), Formal caregiver (Geriatrician), Formal caregiver (Psychologist) and Forma caregiver (Nurse)].

To all caregivers were shown a video on the technological devices and the functions that should been implemented in MARIO (video weblink: https://www.youtube.com/watch?v=v1s2Hbad1l0).

Shortly after watching the video, a questionnaire was administered to all caregivers (MARIO Questionnaire) designed to find out their perceptions about robot companions, especially what they would like such a robot to do for them, and how robots could be designed to build their resilience.

The MARIO Questionnaire (Appendix 1) included 43 items that explored four areas: (A) Acceptability; (B) Functionality; (C) Support devices; and (D) Impact.

It was a quantitative questionnaire based on a Likert scale of "Extremely important/likely/useful" and "YES, very useful" to "Not at all important/likely/useful" and "Not useful at all".

All the analyses were made with the SPSS Version 20 software package (SPSS Inc., Chicago, IL). For dichotomous variables, differences between the groups were tested using the Fisher exact test. This analysis was made using the 2-Way Contingency Table Analysis available at the Interactive Statistical Calculation Pages (http://statpages.org/). For continuous variables, normal distribution was verified by the Shapiro–Wilk normality test and the 1-sample Kolmogorov–Smirnov test. For normally distributed variables, differences among the groups were tested by the Welch 2-sample t test or analysis of variance under general linear model. For non normally distributed variables, differences among the groups were tested by the Wilcoxon rank sum test with continuity correction or the Kruskal–Wallis rank sum test. Test results in which the p value was smaller than the type 1 error rate of 0.05 were declared significant.

3 Results

During the enrolment period, 130 caregivers were recruited: 39 caregivers were from NUIG (M = 4, F = 35), 70 caregivers from IRCCS (M = 28, F = 42), and 21 caregivers from AAB (M = 8, F = 13). Table 1 shows that the demographic and clinical characteristics of the three groups of caregivers according to their residence country. The three groups of caregivers did not differ in following parameters: gender distribution (p = 0.876) and mean age (p = 0.473). Significant differences were observed in educational level (NUIG = 18.88 vs. IRCCS = 14.90 vs. AAB = 15.61 years, p = 0.006). NUIG and IRCCS showed an higher presence of nurses (NUIG = 56.1% and IRCCS = 38.6%), and IRCCS showed an high presence of Informal caregivers unpaid (IRCCS = 72.7%), Informal caregivers paid (IRCCS = 85.7%) and Formal caregivers (Geriatrician) (IRCCS = 94.7%) with a significance of p < 0.0001 compared to other caregivers types.

Table 1 Characteristics of dementia caregivers

	ALL	NUIG	IRCCS	AAB	*P* value
	N = 130	N = 39	N = 70	N = 21	
Gender (M/F)	36/55	4/35	28/42	8/13	0.004
Age (years)[a] Range	48.12 ± 15.81 23–88	–	48.74 ± 14.90 23–88	45.72 ± 19.25 24–82	0.473
Educational level (years)[a] Range	16.09 ± 6.00 0–24	18.88 ± 1.22 18–23	14.90 ± 7.06 0–23	15.61 ± 5.30 5–24	0.006
Caregiving types					
Informal caregiver (unpaid) N(%)	33 (25.3)	0 (0)	24 (72.7)	9 (27.3)	<0.0001
Informal caregiver (paid) N(%)	7 (5.4)	0 (0)	6 (85.7)	1 (14.3)	
Formal caregiver (Geriatrician) N(%)	19 (14.6)	0 (0)	18 (94.7)	1 (5.3)	
Formal caregiver (Psychologist) N(%)	7 (5.4)	0 (0)	0 (0)	7 (100.0)	
Formal caregiver (Nurse) N(%)	57 (43.9)	32 (56.1)	22 (38.6)	3 (5.3)	
Not indicated (N%)	7 (5.4)	7 (100.0)	0 (0)	0 (0)	

[a]Values are presented as mean ± standard deviation

3.1 Acceptability and Functionality of Caring Service Robot

As shown in Table 2 within 60.4% of caregivers of dementia patients declared that the Section A Items should be very important/likely/useful or extremely important/likely/useful to facilitate acceptance of caring service robot.

Within 52.8% of caregivers of dementia patients declared that the Section B Items should be very important/likely/useful or extremely important/likely/useful to improve the functionality of caring service robot.

3.2 Support Devices and Impact of Caring Service Robot

As shown in Table 3 within 65.9% of caregivers reported that following support devices in MARIO could be very useful or moderately useful for their patients:

Table 2 Percentage of responses by caregivers of dementia patients to the MARIO questionnaire (Section A: Acceptability, and Section B: Functionality)

Items	Extremely important/likely/useful N(%)	Very important/likely/useful N(%)	Moderately important/likely/useful N(%)	Slightly important/likely/useful N(%)	Not at all important/likely/useful N(%)
Section A: Acceptability					
1	69 (53.5%)	33 (25.6%)	22 (17.1%)	0 (0%)	5 (3.9%)
2	72 (55.8%)	39 (30.2%)	15 (11.6%)	1 (0.8%)	2 (1.6%)
3	72 (56.2%)	30 (23.4%)	17 (13.3%)	4 (3.1%)	5 (3.9%)
4	45 (49.5%)	29 (31.9%)	14 (15.4%)	0 (0%)	3 (3.3%)
5	55 (43.0%)	38 (29.7%)	26 (20.3%)	5 (3.9%)	4 (3.1%)
6	61 (48.0%)	41 (32.3%)	18 (14.2%)	2 (1.6%)	5 (3.9%)
7	61 (47.7%)	40 (31.6%)	22 (17.2%)	0 (0%)	5 (3.9%)
8	50 (40.0%)	31 (24.8%)	25 (20.0%)	14 (11.2%)	5 (4.0%)
9	47 (36.7%)	25 (19.5%)	33 (25.8%)	16 (12.5%)	7 (5.5%)
10	52 (40.9%)	35 (27.6%)	28 (22.0%)	8 (6.3%)	4 (3.1%)
11	48 (37.5%)	38 (29.7%)	23 (18.0%)	14 (10.9%)	5 (3.9%)
12	53 (42.1%)	50 (39.7%)	20 (15.9%)	0 (0%)	3 (2.4%)
13	60 (46.9%)	46 (35.9%)	15 (11.7%)	3 (2.3%)	4 (3.1%)
14	52 (40.6%)	40 (31.2%)	23 (18.0%)	8 (6.2%)	5 (3.9%)
15a*	35 (60.3%)	11 (19.0%)	8 (13.3%)	4 (6.9%)	0 (0%)
15b*	31 (54.4%)	17 (29.8%)	5 (8.8%)	2 (3.5%)	2 (3.5%)
15c*	24 (42.1%)	10 (17.5%)	18 (31.6%)	4 (7.0%)	1 (1.8%)
15d*	27 (46.6%)	13 (22.4%)	4 (6.9%)	7 (12.1%)	7 (12.1%)
15e*	13 (22.4%)	18 (31.0%)	9 (15.5%)	11 (19.0%)	7 (12.1%)
15f*	16 (27.6%)	16 (27.6%)	10 (17.2%)	10 (17.2%)	6 (10.3%)
15g*	19 (32.8%)	13 (22.4%)	10 (17.2%)	12 (20.7%)	4 (6.9%)

(continued)

Table 2 (continued)

Items	Extremely important/likely/useful N(%)	Very important/likely/useful N(%)	Moderately important/likely/useful N(%)	Slightly important/likely/useful N(%)	Not at all important/likely/useful N(%)
Section B: Functionality					
1	58 (45.7%)	49 (38.6%)	13 (10.2%)	4 (3.1%)	3 (2.4%)
2	63 (49.6%)	46 (36.2%)	14 (11.0%)	1 (0.8%)	3 (2.4%)
3	59 (46.5%)	43 (33.1%)	22 (17.3%)	1 (0.8%)	3 (2.4%)
4	63 (49.6%)	43 (33.9%)	18 (14.2%)	0 (0%)	3 (2.4%)
5	56 (44.4%)	43 (34.1%)	17 (13.5%)	7 (5.6%)	3 (2.4%)
6	59 (46.8%)	45 (35.7%)	17 (13.5%)	2 (1.6%)	3 (2.4%)
7	59 (46.8%)	45 (35.7%)	19 (15.1%)	0 (0%)	3 (2.4%)
8	57 (45.2%)	46 (36.5%)	20 (15.9%)	0 (0%)	3 (2.4%)
9	62 (48.8%)	45 (35.4%)	17 (13.4%)	0 (0%)	3 (2.4%)
10	60 (48.4%)	45 (36.3%)	15 (12.1%)	1 (0.8%)	3 (2.4%)
11	50 (40.0%)	42 (33.6%)	25 (20.0%)	1 (0.8%)	7 (5.6%)
12	67 (52.8%)	37 (29.1%)	19 (15.0%)	1 (0.8%)	3 (2.4%)
13	45 (48.4%)	32 (34.4%)	12 (12.9%)	1 (1.1%)	3 (3.2%)

*Extremely important/likely/useful = 6–7 ranks; Very important/likely/useful = 4–5 ranks; Moderately important/likely/useful = 3 rank; Slightly important/likely/useful = 2 rank: Not at all important/likely/useful = 1 rank

Table 3 Percentage of responses by caregivers of dementia patients to the MARIO Questionnaire (Section C: Support Devices, and Section D: Impact)

Items	YES, very useful	YES, moderately useful	YES, low level of usefulness	Not useful at all
Section C: Support devices				
1	80 (65.0%)	28 (22.8%)	13 (10.6%)	2 (1.6%)
2	81 (65.9%)	25 (20.3%)	14 (11.4%)	3 (2.4%)
3	80 (65.0%)	29 (23.6%)	12 (9.8%)	2 (1.6%)
4	66 (53.7%)	37 (30.1%)	16 (13.0%)	4 (3.3%)
5	60 (48.8%)	37 (30.1%)	20 (16.3%)	6 (4.9%)
6	65 (52.8%)	36 (29.3%)	16 (13.0%)	6 (4.9%)
7	70 (57.4%)	35 (28.7%)	13 (10.7%)	4 (3.3%)
8	70 (56.9%)	35 (28.5%)	15 (12.2%)	3 (2.4%)
Section D: Impact				
1	65 (52.4%)	38 (30.6%)	18 (14.5%)	3 (2.4%)
2	65 (52.4%)	40 (32.3%)	16 (12.9%)	3 (2.4%)
3	67 (54.0%)	36 (29.0%)	16 (12.9%)	5 (4.0%)
4	80 (64.5%)	27 (21.8%)	14 (11.3%)	3 (2.4%)
5	71 (57.3%)	36 (29.0%)	13 (10.5%)	4 (3.2%)
6	71 (57.3%)	35 (28.2%)	14 (11.3%)	4 (3.2%)
7	70 (57.4%)	34 (27.9%)	15 (12.3%)	3 (2.5%)

(1) Devices for monitoring bed-rest and movements, (2) Devices for monitoring the medication use, (3) Devices for monitoring the ambient environmental conditions, (4) Devices for regulating heating, humidity, lighting and TV channel, (5) Devices for undertaking comprehensive geriatric assessment, (6) Devices that link to care planning, (7) Devices for monitoring physiological deterioration, and (8) Devices for monitoring cognitive deterioration.

Within 64.5% of caregivers of dementia patients declared that MARIO should be very useful or moderately useful to improve quality of life, quality of care, safety, emergency communications, home-based physical and/or cognitive rehabilitation programs, and to detect isolation and health status changes of their patients.

3.3 Effects of Sex and Age of the Caregivers

As shown in Table 4 the caring service robot were deemed more useful in supporting the female than male in following items: Section A Item 1 ($p = 0.008$), Item 2 ($p < 0.0001$), Item 4 ($p = 0.004$), Item 6 ($p = 0.047$), Item 12 ($p = 0.020$), and Item 13 ($p = 0.010$); Section B Item 1 ($p = 0.003$), Item 4 ($p = 0.024$), Item 7 ($p = 0.011$), Item 10 ($p = 0.009$), Item 11 ($p = 0.018$), Item 12 ($p = 0.018$), and Item 13 ($p = 0.001$); Section C Item 1 ($p = 0.015$), Item 3 ($p = 0.037$), Item 4 ($p = 0.019$), Item 6 ($p = 0.015$), Item 7 ($p < 0.0001$) and Item 8 ($p = 0.005$);

Table 4 Effects of sex and age of the caregivers of dementia patients on the "Extremely important/likely/useful" and "Very important/likely/useful responses" to the MARIO Questionnaire (Section A: Acceptability, and Section B: Functionality, Section C: Support Devices, and Section D: Impact)

Items	SEX			AGE			
	M	F	P value	20–34 years	35–49 years	≥ 50 years	P value
Section A: Acceptability							
1	26 (65.0%)	76 (85.4%)	0.008	11 (68.8%)	29 (85.3%)	32 (84.2%)	**0.323**
2	28 (70.0%)	83 (93.3%)	<0.0001	13 (81.2%)	30 (88.2%)	31 (81.6%)	**0.700**
3	32 (82.1%)	70 (78.7%)	**0.660**	13 (81.2%)	31 (91.2%)	34 (89.5%)	**0.574**
4	24 (66.7%)	50 (90.9%)	0.004	11 (68.8%)	30 (88.2%)	32 (84.2%)	**0.224**
5	26 (65.0%)	67 (76.1%)	**0.190**	9 (56.2%)	27 (79.4%)	29 (76.3%)	**0.199**
6	28 (70.0%)	74 (85.1%)	0.047	11 (68.8%)	27 (79.4%)	32 (84.2%)	**0.437**
7	29 (72.5%)	72 (81.8%)	**0.231**	12 (75.0%)	28 (82.4%)	32 (84.2%)	**0.722**
8	24 (60.0%)	57 (67.1%)	**0.441**	8 (50.0%)	26 (76.5%)	31 (81.6%)	**0.050**
9	24 (60.0%)	48 (54.5%)	**0.564**	7 (43.8%)	27 (79.4%)	30 (78.9%)	0.016
10	26 (65.0%)	61 (70.1%)	**0.564**	8 (50.0%)	28 (82.4%)	30 (78.9%)	0.036
11	25 (62.5%)	61 (69.3%)	**0.446**	9 (56.2%)	31 (91.2%)	28 (73.7%)	0.018
12	28 (70.0%)	75 (87.2%)	0.020	10 (62.5%)	31 (91.2%)	29 (76.3%)	**0.052**
13	28 (70.0%)	78 (88.6%)	0.010	11 (68.8%)	31 (91.2%)	30 (78.9%)	**0.132**
14	26 (65.0%)	66 (75.0%)	**0.243**	8 (50.0%)	31 (91.2%)	29 (76.3%)	0.005
Section B: Functionality							
1	28 (70.0%)	79 (90.8%)	0.003	12 (75.0%)	27 (79.4%)	31 (81.6%)	**0.861**
2	31 (77.5%)	78 (89.7%)	**0.068**	13 (81.2%)	28 (82.4%)	32 (84.2%)	**0.959**
3	29 (72.5%)	72 (82.8%)	**0.183**	13 (81.2%)	28 (82.4%)	32 (84.2%)	**0.959**
4	29 (72.5%)	77 (88.5%)	0.024	13 (81.2%)	29 (85.3%)	33 (86.8%)	**0.869**
5	28 (70.0%)	71 (82.6%)	**0.110**	12 (75.0%)	27 (79.4%)	33 (86.8%)	**0.528**
6	30 (75.0%)	74 (86.0%)	**0.128**	12 (75.0%)	29 (85.3%)	33 (86.8%)	**0.538**
7	28 (70.0%)	76 (88.4%)	0.011	10 (62.5%)	27 (79.4%)	33 (86.8%)	**0.129**

(continued)

Table 4 (continued)

Items	SEX			AGE			
	M	F	P value	20–34 years	35–49 years	≥ 50 years	P value
8	29 (72.5%)	74 (86.0%)	**0.067**	11 (68.8%)	28 (82.4%)	33 (86.8%)	**0.288**
9	30 (75.0%)	77 (88.5%)	**0.052**	11 (68.8%)	29 (85.3%)	31 (81.6%)	**0.378**
10	29 (72.5%)	76 (90.5%)	0.009	12 (75.0%)	29 (85.3%)	32 (84.2%)	**0.641**
11	24 (60.0%)	68 (80.0%)	0.018	12 (75.0%)	28 (82.4%)	30 (78.9%)	**0.829**
12	28 (70.0%)	76 (87.4%)	0.018	13 (81.2%)	28 (82.4%)	31 (81.6%)	**0.994**
13	24 (66.7%)	53 (93.0%)	0.001	12 (75.0%)	30 (88.2%)	31 (81.6%)	**0.487**
Section C: Support devices							
1	31 (77.5%)	77 (92.8%)	0.015	13 (81.2%)	32 (94.1%)	32 (84.2%)	**0.315**
2	33 (82.5%)	73 (88.0%)	**0.412**	13 (81.2%)	32 (94.1%)	35 (92.1%)	**0.317**
3	32 (80.0%)	77 (92.8%)	0.037	13 (81.2%)	32 (94.1%)	33 (86.8%)	**0.367**
4	29 (72.5%)	74 (89.2%)	0.019	12 (75.0%)	32 (94.1%)	32 (84.2%)	**0.162**
5	28 (70.0%)	69 (83.1%)	**0.095**	11 (68.8%)	32 (94.1%)	31 (81.6%)	**0.062**
6	28 (70.0%)	73 (88.0%)	0.015	10 (62.5%)	32 (94.1%)	31 (81.6%)	0.020
7	27 (69.2%)	78 (94.0%)	<0.0001	12 (75.0%)	32 (94.1%)	32 (84.2%)	**0.162**
8	29 (72.5%)	76 (91.6%)	0.005	13 (81.2%)	32 (94.1%)	32 (84.2%)	**0.315**
Section D: Impact							
1	28 (70.0%)	75 (89.3%)	0.007	10 (62.5%)	31 (91.2%)	32 (84.2%)	0.041
2	30 (75.0%)	75 (89.3%)	0.039	12 (75.0%)	32 (94.1%)	32 (84.2%)	**0.162**
3	30 (75.0%)	73 (86.9%)	**0.098**	10 (62.5%)	32 (94.1%)	33 (86.8%)	0.012
4	30 (75.0%)	77 (91.7%)	0.012	13 (81.2%)	32 (94.1%)	33 (86.8%)	**0.367**
5	31 (77.5%)	76 (90.5%)	**0.050**	12 (75.0%)	31 (91.2%)	35 (92.1%)	**0.163**
6	31 (77.5%)	75 (89.3%)	**0.082**	11 (68.8%)	31 (91.2%)	34 (89.5%)	**0.074**
7	29 (72.5%)	75 (91.5%)	0.006	11 (68.8%)	31 (91.2%)	33 (86.8%)	**0.106**

The significative *p*-values (<0.050) should be in bold

Table 5 Effects of educational level of the caregivers of dementia patients on the "Extremely important/likely/useful" and "Very important/likely/useful responses" to the MARIO Questionnaire (Section A: Acceptability, and Section B: Functionality, Section C: Support Devices, and Section D: Impact)

Items	Low education	High school diploma	Degree	P value
Section A: Acceptability				
1	23 (88.5%)	5 (55.6%)	66 (77.6%)	**0.114**
2	22 (84.6%)	5 (55.6%)	77 (90.6%)	0.012
3	24 (92.3%)	7 (77.8%)	65 (77.4%)	**0.236**
4	22 (84.6%)	6 (66.7%)	45 (84.9%)	**0.390**
5	23 (88.5%)	5 (55.6%)	59 (69.4%)	**0.081**
6	23 (88.5%)	7 (77.8%)	64 (76.2%)	**0.404**
7	24 (92.3%)	6 (66.7%)	64 (75.3%)	**0.124**
8	24 (92.3%)	6 (66.7%)	48 (58.5%)	0.006
9	23 (88.5%)	5 (55.6%)	40 (47.1%)	0.001
10	23 (88.5%)	7 (77.8%)	54 (63.5%)	0.046
11	22 (84.6%)	4 (44.4%)	57 (67.1%)	**0.059**
12	23 (88.5%)	4 (44.4%)	71 (84.5%)	0.007
13	22 (84.6%)	6 (66.7%)	72 (84.7%)	**0.378**
14	22 (84.6%)	5 (55.6%)	61 (71.8%)	**0.197**
Section B: Functionality				
1	23 (88.5%)	6 (66.7%)	71 (83.5%)	**0.317**
2	24 (92.3%)	6 (66.7%)	72 (84.7%)	**0.177**
3	23 (88.5%)	8 (88.9%)	66 (77.6%)	**0.385**
4	24 (92.3%)	8 (88.9%)	68 (80.0%)	**0.303**
5	24 (92.3%)	8 (88.9%)	62 (73.8%)	**0.097**
6	24 (92.3%)	8 (88.9%)	67 (79.8%)	**0.292**
7	24 (92.3%)	8 (88.9%)	66 (78.6%)	**0.239**
8	24 (92.3%)	8 (88.9%)	65 (74.3%)	**0.193**
9	23 (88.5%)	7 (77.8%)	71 (83.5%)	**0.718**
10	23 (88.5%)	8 (88.9%)	67 (81.7%)	**0.654**
11	22 (84.6%)	6 (66.7%)	59 (71.1%)	**0.346**
12	23 (88.5%)	7 (77.8%)	70 (82.4%)	**0.687**
13	22 (84.6%)	6 (66.7%)	47 (85.5%)	**0.366**
Section C: Support devices				
1	24 (92.3%)	7 (77.8%)	76 (89.4%)	**0.586**
2	23 (88.5%)	9 (100.0%)	71 (83.5%)	**0.244**
3	23 (88.5%)	8 (88.9%)	76 (89.4%)	**0.990**
4	23 (88.5%)	7 (77.8%)	72 (84.7%)	**0.734**
5	23 (88.5%)	7 (77.8%)	66 (77.6%)	**0.476**
6	23 (88.5%)	7 (77.8%)	70 (82.4%)	**0.687**
7	23 (88.5%)	7 (77.8%)	73 (86.9%)	**0.710**
8	23 (88.5%)	7 (77.8%)	73 (85.9%)	**0.730**

(continued)

Table 5 (continued)

Items	Low education	High school diploma	Degree	P value
Section D: Impact				
1	23 (88.5%)	8 (88.9%)	70 (81.4%)	**0.628**
2	23 (88.5%)	8 (88.9%)	72 (83.7%)	**0.793**
3	23 (88.5%)	8 (88.9%)	69 (80.2%)	**0.547**
4	23 (88.5%)	8 (88.9%)	73 (84.9%)	**0.869**
5	24 (92.3%)	9 (100.0%)	71 (82.6%)	**0.206**
6	24 (92.3%)	9 (100.0%)	70 (81.4%)	**0.167**
7	23 (88.5%)	8 (88.9%)	70 (83.3%)	**0.768**

The significative p-values (<0.050) should be in bold

Section D Item 1 (p = 0.007), Item 2 (p = 0.039), Item 4 (p = 0.012), and Item 7 (p = 0.006).

The caring service robot were deemed more useful in supporting the caregivers who had an age ≥ 35 years than younger in following items: Section A Item 9 (p = 0.016), Item 10 (p = 0.036), Item 11 (p = 0.018), and Item 14 (p = 0.005); Section C Item 6 (p = 0.020); Section D Item 1 (p = 0.041) and Item 3 (p = 0.012).

3.4 Effects of Educational Level and Caregiving Types of the Caregivers

As shown in Table 5 the caring service robot were deemed more useful in supporting the caregivers who had a low educational level in following items: Section A Item 2 (p = 0.012), Item 8 (p = 0.006), Item 9 (p = 0.001), Item 10 (p = 0.046) and Item 12 (p = 0.007).

As shown in Table 6, the caring service robot were deemed more useful in supporting the informal caregivers (unpaid or paid) than formal caregivers in following items: Section A Item 5 (p = 0.048), Item 8 (p = 0.013) and Item 9 (p = 0.001); Section D Item 1 (p = 0.002) and Item 6 (p = 0.010).

4 Discussion

The MARIO robot were deemed very useful in supporting the informal caregivers (unpaid and paid) who were female and had an age ≥ 35 and with low educational level. Indeed, the informal caregivers had more difficulty to manage the dementia patients at home; moreover, who were female, younger and with a lower educational level clearly found even more complexity in management of dementia patients, requiring even more help from the companion robot.

Table 6 Effects of caregiving types of the caregivers of dementia patients on the "Extremely important/likely/useful" and "Very important/likely/useful responses," to the MARIO Questionnaire (Section A: Acceptability, and Section B: Functionality, Section C: Support Devices, and Section D: Impact)

Items	Informal caregiver (unpaid)	Informal caregiver (paid)	Formal caregiver (Geriatr.)	Formal caregiver (Nurse)	Formal caregiver (Psychol.)	P value
Section A: Acceptability						
1	25 (75.8%)	7 (100.0%)	16 (84.2%)	41 (73.2%)	6 (85.7%)	**0.482**
2	24 (72.7%)	7 (100.0%)	16 (84.2%)	51 (91.1%)	7 (100.0%)	**0.078**
3	29 (87.9%)	7 (100.0%)	16 (84.2%)	40 (72.7%)	7 (100.0%)	**0.133**
4	24 (72.7%)	7 (100.0%)	16 (84.2%)	21 (84.0%)	6 (85.7%)	**0.474**
5	25 (75.8%)	7 (100.0%)	14 (73.7%)	40 (71.4%)	2 (28.6%)	0.048
6	28 (84.8%)	7 (100.0%)	14 (73.7%)	42 (76.4%)	5 (71.4%)	**0.498**
7	27 (81.8%)	7 (100.0%)	14 (73.7%)	40 (71.4%)	7 (100.0%)	**0.213**
8	26 (78.8%)	6 (85.7%)	13 (68.4%)	32 (60.4%)	1 (14.3%)	0.013
9	25 (75.8%)	6 (85.7%)	14 (73.7%)	22 (39.3%)	2 (28.6%)	0.001
10	27 (81.8%)	6 (85.7%)	13 (68.4%)	37 (66.1%)	2 (28.6%)	**0.058**
11	23 (69.7%)	6 (85.7%)	16 (84.2%)	36 (64.3%)	3 (42.9%)	**0.216**
12	24 (72.7%)	6 (85.7%)	16 (84.2%)	46 (83.6%)	6 (85.7%)	**0.728**
13	25 (75.8%)	6 (85.7%)	16 (84.2%)	48 (85.7%)	5 (71.4%)	**0.727**
14	24 (72.7%)	6 (85.7%)	16 (84.2%)	38 (67.9%)	4 (57.1%)	**0.506**
Section B: Functionality						
1	27 (81.8%)	7 (100.0%)	14 (73.7%)	48 (85.7%)	6 (85.7%)	**0.555**
2	28 (84.8%)	7 (100.0%)	14 (73.7%)	48 (85.7%)	7 (100.0%)	**0.348**
3	28 (84.8%)	7 (100.0%)	14 (73.7%)	44 (78.6%)	6 (85.7%)	**0.566**
4	29 (87.9%)	7 (100.0%)	14 (73.7%)	44 (78.6%)	7 (100.0%)	**0.257**
5	29 (87.9%)	7 (100.0%)	13 (68.4%)	40 (72.7%)	6 (85.7%)	**0.193**
6	30 (90.9%)	7 (100.0%)	14 (73.7%)	43 (78.2%)	7 (100.0%)	**0.163**
7	30 (90.9%)	7 (100.0%)	13 (68.4%)	45 (81.8%)	5 (71.4%)	**0.174**

(continued)

Table 6 (continued)

Items	Informal caregiver (unpaid)	Informal caregiver (paid)	Formal caregiver (Geriatr.)	Formal caregiver (Nurse)	Formal caregiver (Psychol.)	P value
8	30 (90.9%)	7 (100.0%)	13 (68.4%)	43 (78.2%)	6 (85.7%)	**0.182**
9	28 (84.8%)	7 (100.0%)	14 (73.7%)	48 (85.7%)	6 (85.7%)	**0.551**
10	29 (87.9%)	7 (100.0%)	14 (73.7%)	43 (81.1%)	7 (100.0%)	**0.301**
11	26 (78.8%)	7 (100.0%)	14 (73.7%)	36 (66.7%)	7 (100.0%)	**0.139**
12	27 (81.8%)	7 (100.0%)	14 (73.7%)	48 (85.7%)	6 (85.7%)	**0.555**
13	25 (75.8%)	7 (100.0%)	16 (84.2%)	24 (88.9%)	5 (71.4%)	**0.410**
Section C: Support devices						
1	27 (81.8%)	7 (100.0%)	16 (84.2%)	50 (89.3%)	7 (100.0%)	**0.498**
2	30 (90.9%)	7 (100.0%)	16 (84.2%)	45 (80.4%)	7 (100.0%)	**0.344**
3	28 (84.8%)	7 (100.0%)	16 (84.2%)	50 (89.3%)	7 (100.0%)	**0.621**
4	26 (78.8%)	7 (100.0%)	16 (84.2%)	46 (82.1%)	7 (100.0%)	**0.494**
5	26 (78.8%)	7 (100.0%)	16 (84.2%)	43 (76.8%)	7 (100.0%)	**0.367**
6	26 (78.8%)	7 (100.0%)	16 (84.2%)	47 (83.9%)	4 (57.1%)	**0.298**
7	27 (81.8%)	7 (100.0%)	16 (84.2%)	47 (85.5%)	7 (100.0%)	**0.589**
8	27 (81.8%)	7 (100.0%)	16 (84.2%)	47 (83.9%)	7 (100.0%)	**0.588**
Section D: Impact						
1	28 (84.8%)	7 (100.0%)	16 (84.2%)	49 (86.0%)	2 (28.6%)	0.002
2	28 (84.8%)	7 (100.0%)	16 (84.2%)	48 (84.2%)	5 (71.4%)	**0.697**
3	29 (87.9%)	7 (100.0%)	16 (84.2%)	46 (80.7%)	4 (57.1%)	**0.238**
4	29 (87.9%)	7 (100.0%)	16 (84.2%)	47 (82.5%)	7 (100.0%)	**0.549**
5	31 (93.9%)	7 (100.0%)	16 (84.2%)	47 (82.5%)	5 (71.4%)	**0.309**
6	31 (93.9%)	7 (100.0%)	16 (84.2%)	48 (84.2%)	3 (42.9%)	0.010
7	29 (87.9%)	7 (100.0%)	16 (84.2%)	47 (85.5%)	4 (57.1%)	**0.217**

The significative p-values (<0.050) should be in bold

Limitations of the present study should also be considered in interpreting our findings. In particular, the differences in educational levels of the caregivers across the three sites of the MARIO Project reflected the caregiving type of each sites: NUIG is a nursing home where the nurses are more numerous and present, IRCCS is an hospital where formal and informal caregivers are present almost in equal measure, and AAB is an association where psychologists and informal caregiver are more present.

Questionnaires similar to the that developed for the MARIO Project were the HOPE Questionnaire developed for the HOPE Project [24] and the AL.TR.U.I.S.M. Questionnaire developed for the AL.TR.U.I.S.M. Project [25]. Regarding the HOPE Project, the caregivers considered that the ICT system could be useful to improve the management of patients with Alzheimer's disease (AD), especially if they are aged 75–84 years and with moderate dementia. Older and low educated caregivers had higher expectations on the potential role of ICT systems in improving the management of AD patients. Regarding the AL.TR.U.I.S.M. Project, the caregivers considered that a Virtual Personal Trainer (VPT) can improve the functional, nutritional, cognitive, affective, neuropsychiatric state, and quality of life of the patients with AD. The caregiver of masculine sex had higher expectations on the potential role of a VPT in improving the management of AD patients.

So the HOPE and AL.TR.U.I.S.M. Questionnaire results seem otherwise than those obtained in our study.

A previous report from the Keeping In Touch Everyday (KITE) Project demonstrated how a user-centered design process involving people with dementia and their relatives/caregivers could lead to the development of devices which are more acceptable and relevant to their needs [26]. Other projects [27–29] did not report data of questionnaires used to evaluate the preferences of caregivers and their dementia patients.

Our analysis represented a point of crucial importance not only in developing and improving the system by taking into considerations the end-users' (both patients and caregivers) expectations and needs, but also in leading to the development of a first prototype and to the experimentation stage as well.

5   Conclusion

The testing stages are still ongoing in order to improve the working patterns of the system and to better integrate all of its elements with particular and always renewed regard to the end-users and their needs, limits and requirements.

This first stage of experimentation activity aimed mainly at drawing clear conclusions on the interaction between the user and the MARIO and in general on the acceptability level of this service robot by the patient.

These data, however, are of great importance since they not only give useful indications to assess what has been accomplished up to now, but also they provide important guidelines in order to improve the system while specific clinical experimentation stages are expected to be carried out over the next months.

The work achieved through a fruitful and continuous interaction among the different subjects involved in the process of development of the system and stakeholders enabled the implementation of a platform which can be further and easily integrated and improved.

Finally, the collected and abovementioned data show a satisfactory integration between the patient and the system along with a great level of acceptability of MARIO by the end-user, both the patients themselves and the caregivers or medical providers, those who, day by day, take care and assist their patients.

Acknowledgements The research leading to the results described in this article has received funding from the European Union Horizons 2020—the Framework Programme for Research and Innovation (2014–2020) under grant agreement 643808 Project MARIO 'Managing active and healthy aging with use of caring service robots'.

Appendix 1: Mario Questionnaire on the Use of Companion Robotics

Section A: Acceptability

1. How Important is that MARIO has a human like appearance?

Not at all important	Slightly important	Moderately important	Very important	Extremely important

2. How important is it that MARIO has a human sounding voice?

Not at all important	Slightly important	Moderately important	Very important	Extremely important

3. How important is it that MARIO has a familiar voice?

Not at all important	Slightly important	Moderately important	Very important	Extremely important

4. How important is it that MARIO has an exterior or covering that people like to touch?

Not at all important	Slightly important	Moderately important	Very important	Extremely important

5. How Important is that MARIO height is adjustable?

Not at all important	Slightly important	Moderately important	Very important	Extremely important

6. How important is it that MARIO can communicate non verbally e.g. smiling or raising eyebrows?

Not at all important	Slightly important	Moderately important	Very important	Extremely important

7. How important is it that MARIO displays emotional expression?

Not at all important	Slightly important	Moderately important	Very important	Extremely important

8. To what extent do you think it likely that your patients would agree to having MARIO for daily assistance in the home to remind them to take medicines, eat and drink, buy food, a tracking mechanism to find easily Important personal objects (keys, teeth, purse or glasses), etc.:

Not at all likely	Slightly likely	Moderately likely	Very likely	Extremely likely

9. To what extent do you think that your patients would agree to having MARIO monitor and track their movements in the house, or outside the house?

Not at all likely	Slightly likely	Moderately likely	Very likely	Extremely likely

10. To what extent do you think that your patients would agree to having MARIO provide entertainment, mind games (e.g. showing pictures of family members), a reminder for favourite TV programmes etc.

Not at all likely	Slightly likely	Moderately likely	Very likely	Extremely likely

11. To what extent do you think that your patients would accept MARIO as to stay connected to and communicate with family, friends and professional caregivers, (e.g. an easy to use touch screen with pictures and names of the family members)?

Not at all likely	Slightly likely	Moderately likely	Very likely	Extremely likely

12. How important is it that the robot can be quiet?

Not at all important	Slightly important	Moderately important	Very important	Extremely important

13. How important is it that the robot takes up no more room than a person while moving about?

Not at all important	Slightly important	Moderately important	Very important	Extremely important

14. How important is it that the robot require internet connection (house without broadband coverage)?

Not at all important	Slightly important	Moderately important	Very important	Extremely important

15. Please rank in order of importance from 1–7 (with 1 being the most Important and 7 being the least important) the features of appearance listed below:

Appearance features	Ranking 1–7
a. Human like appearance	
b. Human sounding voice	
c. Familiar voice	
d. Has an exterior or covering that people like to touch	
e. Adjustable height	

(continued)

(continued)

Appearance features	Ranking 1–7
f. Displays emotional expression	
g. Communicates non verbally	

Section B: Functionality

1. How important is it that MARIO has face recognition?

Not at all important	Slightly important	Moderately important	Very important	Extremely important

2. How important is it that MARIO has voice recognition?

Not at all important	Slightly important	Moderately important	Very important	Extremely important

3. How important is it that MARIO can distinguish individuals within a group?

Not at all important	Slightly important	Moderately important	Very important	Extremely important

4. How important is it that MARIO has the capacity for natural dialogue?

Not at all important	Slightly important	Moderately important	Very important	Extremely important

5. How important is it that MARIO has a detachable device that can be used outside the house (e.g. GPS function for shopping)?

Not at all important	Slightly important	Moderately important	Very important	Extremely important

6. How Important is it that MARIO can provide prompts for appointments/social events/date and time?

Not at all important	Slightly important	Moderately important	Very important	Extremely important

7. How important is it that MARIO can store and utilise information from a person's life history?

Not at all important	Slightly important	Moderately important	Very important	Extremely important

8. How important is it that MARIO can utilise multimedia to communicate (e.g. read a book, Skype, play music)?

Not at all important	Slightly important	Moderately important	Very important	Extremely important

9. How important is it that MARIO has voice activation?

Not at all important	Slightly important	Moderately important	Very important	Extremely important

10. How important is it that MARIO has gesture recognition?

Not at all important	Slightly important	Moderately important	Very important	Extremely important

11. How important is it that MARIO could help subjects with walking or stand-up?

Not at all important	Slightly important	Moderately important	Very important	Extremely important

12. How important is it that MARIO can understand dialects?

Not at all important	Slightly important	Moderately important	Very important	Extremely important

13. How useful would a detachable device be that allowed MARIO to provide advice and support when you are ou of the house? Eg (GPS function for finding the way to the shops and back home again)

Not at all useful	Slightly useful	Moderately useful	Very useful	Extremely useful

Section C: Support Devices

To what extent do you think that the following support devices in MARIO could be useful for your patients:

1. Devices for monitoring bed-rest and movements of your patient, such as integrated video/sound systems and imbalance sensors, inside of his/her home to reduce the risk of falls	☐ Not useful at all ☐ YES, low level of usefulness ☐ YES, moderately useful ☐ YES, very useful
2. Devices for monitoring the medication use, such as pill dispenser and/or time schedule reminder system, to avoid errors in drug use by your patients	☐ Not useful at all ☐ YES, low level of usefulness ☐ YES, moderately useful ☐ YES, very useful
3. Devices for monitoring the ambient environmental conditions, (i.e. security systems to control temperature, gas-smoke, lights, humidity, entrance-exits of main doors etc.) to improve the safety and wellness of your patients	☐ Not useful at all ☐ YES, low level of usefulness ☐ YES, moderately useful ☐ YES, very useful
4. Devices for regulating heating, humidity, lighting, TV channel	☐ Not useful at all ☐ YES, low level of usefulness ☐ YES, moderately useful ☐ YES, very useful
5. Devices for undertaking comprehensive geriatric assessment	☐ Not useful at all ☐ YES, low level of usefulness ☐ YES, moderately useful ☐ YES, very useful
6. Devices that link to care planning	☐ Not useful at all ☐ YES, low level of usefulness ☐ YES, moderately useful ☐ YES, very useful
7. Devices for monitoring physiological deterioration	☐ Not useful at all ☐ YES, low level of usefulness ☐ YES, moderately useful ☐ YES, very useful
8. Devices for monitoring cognitive deterioration	☐ Not useful at all ☐ YES, low level of usefulness ☐ YES, moderately useful ☐ YES, very useful

Section D: Impact of Mario

To what extent do you think MARIO could be useful in order to:	
1. Improve the quality of life of your patients	☐ Not useful at all ☐ YES, low level of usefulness ☐ YES, moderately useful ☐ YES, very useful
2. Improve the quality of care that you provide to your patients	☐ Not useful at all ☐ YES, low level of usefulness ☐ YES, moderately useful ☐ YES, very useful
3. Improve the safety in the daily living activities of your patients	☐ Not useful at all ☐ YES, low level of usefulness ☐ YES, moderately useful ☐ YES, very useful
4. Carry out emergency communication/alert messages	☐ Not useful at all ☐ YES, low level of usefulness ☐ YES, moderately useful ☐ YES, very useful
5. Improve the care provided; home-based physical and/or cognitive rehabilitation programs of your patients	☐ Not useful at all ☐ YES, low level of usefulness ☐ YES, moderately useful ☐ YES, very useful
6. Detect when a person is becoming more lonely and isolated	☐ Not useful at all ☐ YES, low level of usefulness ☐ YES, moderately useful ☐ YES, very useful
7. Detect health status changes	☐ Not useful at all ☐ YES, low level of usefulness ☐ YES, moderately useful ☐ YES, very useful

8. What other functions do you think MARIO should have to increase independent living for your patients?

_____

_____

_____

_____

DEMOGRAPHICS

Please tick (√) the appropriate box as indicated

Gender:

Male   ☒

Female   ☒

Current Occupation: _____

Please indicate the highest level of education attained:

No Formal education	☒	Primary Education	☒
Secondary	☒	Post leaving Cert	☒
Third Level- Non Degree	☒		
Technical/Vocational Qualification	☒	Please Specify_____	
Third Level- Degree or above	☒	Please Specify_____	
Professional Qualification	☒	Please Specify_____	
Other	☒	Please Specify_____	

References

1. Prince M, Jackson J (2009) Alzheimer's disease international. World Alzheimer report. http://www.alz.co.uk/research/worldreport/ (Advance access published May 2016)
2. Murphy K, Casey D (2015) http://www.alzheimer-europe.org/Conferences/Previous-conferences/2015-Ljubljana/Detailed-programme-abstracts-and-presentations/PO1-Dementia-Friendly-Society (Advance Access published May 2016)
3. Holt-Lunstad J, Smith TB, Layton JB (2010) Social relationships and mortality risk: a meta-analytic review. PLoS Med 7(7):e1000316
4. Steptoe A, Shankar A, Demakakos P, Wardle J (2013) Social isolation, loneliness and all-cause mortality in older men and women. In: Proceedings of the national academy of sciences of the USA (PNAS), 10.1073/pnas.1219686110. 25 Mar 2013
5. O'Shea E (2007) Implementing policy for dementia care in Ireland. The time for action is now. In Irish Centre for Social Gerontology, National University of Ireland, Galway
6. Norris FH, Stevens SP, Pfefferbaum B, Wyche KF, Pfefferbaum RL (2008) Community resilience as a metaphor, theory, set of capacities, and strategy for disaster readiness. Am J Community Psychol 41:127–150
7. http://www.mario-project.eu/portal/
8. Pilotto A, Ferrucci L, Franceschi M, D'Ambrosio LP, Scarcelli C, Cascavilla L, Paris F, Placentino G, Seripa D, Dallapiccola B, Leandro G (2008) Development and validation of a multidimensional prognostic index for 1-year mortality from the comprehensive geriatric assessment in hospitalized older patients. Rejuvenation Res 11:151–161
9. Schulz R, Martire L (2004) Family caregiving of persons with dementia: prevalence, health effects and support strategies. Am J Geriatr Psychiatry 12:240–249
10. Gaugler JE, Kane RA, Langlois J (2000) Assessment of family caregivers of older adults. In: Kane RL, Kane RA (eds) Assessing older persons: measures, meaning and practical applications. Oxford University Press, New York, pp 320–359
11. Gaugler JE, Davey A, Pearlin LI, Zarit SH (2000) Modeling caregiver adaptation over time: the longitudinal impact of behavior problems. Psychol Aging 15:437–450
12. Jönsson L, Wimo A (2009) The cost of dementia in Europe: a review of the evidence and methodological considerations. Pharmacoeconomics 27(5):391–403
13. Schulz R, O'Brien AT, Bookwala J, Fleissner K (1995) Psychiatric and physical morbidity effects of dementia caregiving: prevalence, correlates, and causes. Gerontologist 35:771–791
14. Mahoney R, Regan C, Katona C, Livingston G (2005) Anxiety and depression in family caregivers of people with Alzheimer disease: the LASER-AD study. Am J Geriatr Psychiatry 13:795–801
15. Clipp EC, George LK (1990) Psychotropic drug use among caregivers of patients with dementia. J Am Geriatr Soc 38:227–235
16. Vitaliano PP, Zhang J, Scanlan JM (2003) Is caregiving hazardous to one's physical health? A meta-analysis. Psychol Bull 129:946–972
17. Son J, Erno A, Shea DG, Femia EE, Zarit SH, Stephens MA (2007) The caregiver stress process and health outcomes. J Aging Health 19:871–887
18. Schulz R, Beach SR (1999) Caregiving as a risk factor for mortality: the Caregiver health effects study. JAMA 282:2215–2219
19. König A, Aalten P, Verhey F, Bensadoun G, Petit PD, Robert P et al (2014) A review of current information and communication technologies: can they be used to assess apathy? Int J Geriatr Psychiatry 29:345–358
20. D'Onofrio G, Sancarlo D, Ricciardi F, Ruan Q, Yu Z, Giuliani F, Greco A (2016) Cognitive stimulation and information-communication technologies (ICT) in Alzheimer's disease: a systematic review. In: Garza P (ed) Cognitive control: development, assessment and performance. https://www.novapublishers.com/catalog/product_info.php?products_id=58756. Nova Science

21. McKenzie B, Bowen ME, Keys K, Bulat T (2013) Safe home program: a suite of technologies to support extended home care of persons with dementia. Am J Alzheimers Dis Other Demen 28(4):348–354

22. Espie CA, Kyle SD, Williams C, Ong JC, Douglas NJ, Hames P et al (2012) A randomized, placebo-controlled trial of online cognitive behavioral therapy for chronic insomnia disorder delivered via an automated media-rich web application. Sleep 35(6):769–781

23. McKhann GM, Knopman DS, Chertkow H, Hyman BT, Jack CR Jr, Kawas CH et al (2011) The diagnosis of dementia due to Alzheimer's disease: recommendations from the National Institute on Aging-Alzheimer's Association workgroups on diagnostic guidelines for Alzheimer's disease. Alzheimers Dement 7:263–269

24. Pilotto A, D'Onofrio G, Benelli E, Zanesco A, Cabello A, Margelí MC, Wanche-Politis S, Seferis K, Sancarlo D, Kilias D (2011) Information and communication technology systems to improve quality of life and safety of Alzheimer's disease patients: a multicenter international survey. J Alzheimers Dis 23(1):131–141

25. Caroppo A, Leone A, Siciliano P, Sancarlo D, D'Onofrio G, Giuliani F et al (2014) Cognitive home rehabilitation in Alzheimer's disease patients by a virtual personal trainer. Ambient assisted living, pp 147–155

26. Robinson L, Brittain K, Lindsay S, Jackson D, Olivier P (2009) Keeping In Touch Everyday (KITE) project: developing assistive technologies with people with dementia and their carers to promote independence. Int Psychogeriatr 21:494–502

27. Duff P, Dolphin C (2007) Cost-benefit analysis of assistive technology to support independence for people with dementia—Part 1: development of a methodological approach to the ENABLE cost-benefit analysis. Technol Disabil 19:73–78

28. Duff P, Dolphin C (2009) Cost-benefit analysis of assistive technology to support independence for people with dementia—Part 2: results from employing the ENABLE cost-benefit model in practice. Technol Disabil 19:79–90

29. Virone G, Sixsmith A (2008) Monitoring activity patterns and trends of older adults. Conf Proc IEEE Eng Med Biol Soc 2008:2071–2074

Enhancing the Interactive Services of a Telepresence Robot for AAL: Developments and a Psycho-physiological Assessment

Gabriella Cortellessa, Francesca Fracasso, Alessandra Sorrentino, Andrea Orlandini, Giulio Bernardi, Luca Coraci, Riccardo De Benedictis and Amedeo Cesta

Abstract This paper describes the work done on a telepresence robot named GIRAFF and part of a telecare AAL system derived from the GIRAFFPLUS project for supporting and monitoring elderly people at home. Specifically, from the long term trials in real houses, a number of user requirements have emerged that inspired changes and improvements on the robotic platform. The implementation of both multimodal communication capabilities and enhanced information services introduced new interesting questions related to human-robot interaction and specifically to *usability*, *valence* of interaction, and *cognitive load* required to interact with and through the robot. An experimental session based on a combination of physiological and psychological methods showed that the enhanced platform is usable, the interaction pleasant and the required *workload* limited. The analysis of

G. Cortellessa (✉) · F. Fracasso · A. Sorrentino · A. Orlandini ·
G. Bernardi · L. Coraci · R. De Benedictis · A. Cesta
CNR—Italian National Research Council, ISTC, Rome, Italy
e-mail: gabriella.cortellessa@istc.cnr.it

F. Fracasso
e-mail: francesca.fracasso@istc.cnr.it

A. Sorrentino
e-mail: alessandra.sorrentino@istc.cnr.it

A. Orlandini
e-mail: andrea.orlandini@istc.cnr.it

G. Bernardi
e-mail: giulio.bernardi@istc.cnr.it

L. Coraci
e-mail: luca.coraci@istc.cnr.it

R. De Benedictis
e-mail: riccardo.debenedictis@istc.cnr.it

A. Cesta
e-mail: amedeo.cesta@istc.cnr.it

© Springer International Publishing AG 2017
F. Cavallo et al. (eds.), *Ambient Assisted Living*, Lecture Notes
in Electrical Engineering 426, DOI 10.1007/978-3-319-54283-6_25

psychophysiological correlates supported the findings from self-report measures and provides further information. It has been possible to discriminate physiological responses between multimodal interaction and the use of new services. Specifically, while usability can be specifically related to the usage of multichannel commands, positive emotions elicited by the interaction with GIRAFF seems to be mostly ascribable to the usage of services provided for the communication with another person.

Keywords Human-robot interaction · Personalization · Ambient assisted living · Active aging · Technology for health monitoring

1 Motivation and Context

The increasing attention for the topic of "prolonging independent living" has generated several initiatives all over the world on the needs of the aging population and triggered funding programs like the Ambient Assisted Living (AAL), promoted by the European Commission in the FP7 and H2020 research programs. The general aim is the one of promoting a healthier society constituting a main social and economic challenge. In fact, most elderly people aim at remaining in their homes as long as possible as this is in general conducive of a richer social life and paramount to maintaining established habits. Most of these efforts in the AAL projects share the idea of having on one side "disappearing technology" that does not impact on the house of the assisted persons, on the other, the idea of having a "central component" that very often is a robotic platform that act as the mediator between the "hidden technology" and the user, or alternatively the mediator between the older user's world and the external world.

This paper describes the improvements of a telepresence robot that is integrated in a telecare system named GIRAFFPLUS. Specifically, starting from real experimentation of the telecare system in real houses, a set of requirement for improvement emerged that suggested the enhancement of the robotic telepresence platform. The challenge of the work has been to increase the functionalities of the system while maintaining the simplicity of use given that the robotic platform is devoted to a specific target group of users that is the one of older persons living alone at home. In this respect a combined evaluation session that exploits psychological and physiological assessment has been carried out to assess aspects of usability, mental workload and overall user satisfaction with respect to the improved version of the system. The reminder of the paper is organized as follows: the rest of this section introduces the general idea of the GIRAFFPLUS system and highlights the user requirements emerged from fielded tests; Sect. 2 describes the technical improvements implemented on top of the robotic platform; Sect. 3 describes the experimental session carried out to assess the new platform; Sect. 4 provide a final discussion.

1.1 The GIRAFFPLUS Telecare System

The GIRAFFPLUS project [2012–2014] built and evaluated a complete system able to collect elderly's daily behavior and physiological measures from distributed sensors in living environments as well as to organize the gathered information so as to provide customizable visualization and monitoring services for both primary and secondary users. The GIRAFFPLUS solution (see Fig. 1) integrates a smart sensor environment, several user oriented software services (e.g., one for data analytics, and one for user personalization) and a state of the art telepresence robot, called GIRAFF, that ensure the communication (mostly social contact) among the primary users (older users at home) and the secondary users (their caregivers both formal and informal) outside the house. The basic loop is: data are continuously gathered in the house from sensors; a certain number of potential alarms are also continuously monitored and, when occurring, communicated to secondary users; data are presented to different users according to their different needs in a personalized way; secondary users can communicate with the primary users by means of the GIRAFF telepresence robot. In order to visualize data to users, a Data Visualization, Personalization and Interaction Service (DVPIS) has been realized to manage interaction with the different actors in such AAL scenario. In particular, two different instances of the DVPIS have been provided: one for use "outside the home" (DVPIS@Office), and another dedicated to the primary user (DVPIS@Home) that is the one studied in details in this paper. The benefit pursued by the GIRAFFPLUS system is twofold: primary users can access the information on their own health condition, enabling them to better manage their health and lifestyle; secondary users are supported by a flexible and efficient monitoring tool while taking care of old persons (relatives/patients).

1.2 User Needs from Fielded Deployment

A long-term experimentation of the GIRAFFPLUS technology into real houses emphasized some concrete needs from the end users mainly devoted to the robotic component of the telecare system. In this work we explain the technical implementation derived from this new requirements and present the user evaluation of the improved version with a combination of psychological and physiological assessment. Having a technological artifact in contact with real end users for long time is a unique opportunity to gather concrete observations, and direct real experiences that identify possibilities of extension, new challenges and wishes that can foster additional added value in new proposals. The findings from this long-term experimentation can be summarized in the following requirements for improvements of the robotic platform:

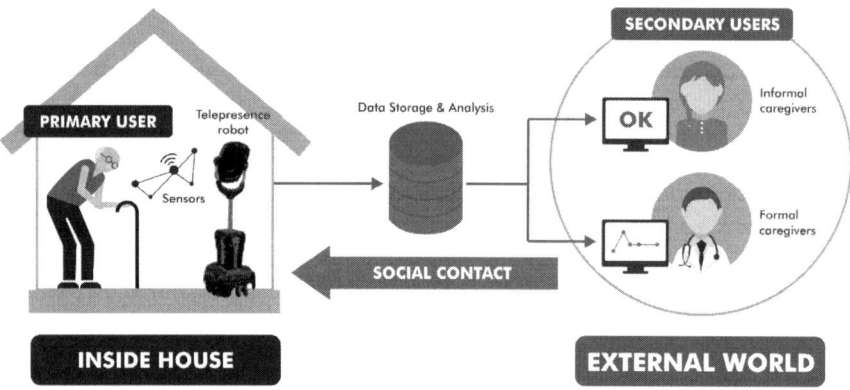

Fig. 1 Sketchy idea of the GIRAFFPLUS system

- **Communication was perceived as too limited**—the video call ensured by the robot was positively judged but still the users were expecting additional communication modality like the possibility to send or receive video and audio messages also in an asynchronous way.
- **The robot's services were judged limited**—connected to the comment above, users expressed the desire to have additional services like the possibility to share material with remote users (e.g., to talk about their health status, to share video and photos) also when not connected through the videoconferencing systems; additionally reminders for taking the medicine were also judged as positive improvements of the system.
- **The users want to be in control**—another important aspect that emerged was related to the fact that the user felt to be too passive and not in control of the robotic platform. In fact they felt passive spectators of interaction, having to wait to be called by someone to be able to see the robot in motion and to interact with it and not having any possibility to command the robot.

These findings suggested us to improve the robotics platform in different directions and specifically motivated the development of additional functionalities that can be summarized in the following components:

- **@Home Services**: an additional services build on top of the robotics platform to ensure further services and communication abilities;
- **Multimodal Communication Module**, that allows maneuvering the robotic platform through gestures and voice commands.

The next section gives details of these two additional services built of top of the robotic platform.

2 Technological Improvements of the Robotic Platform

2.1 @Home Services

The @Home aims at enriching the features already provided by the standard GIRAFF robot exposing additional information services to the primary user. This is done by enlarging the capabilities of the telepresence robot. In fact, we decided to use the telepresence robot as a means to provide services to the primary users and this is also in line with what emerged from the feedback gathered during iterative evaluation sessions. The conceived version of @Home can be seen in Fig. 2. Three main functionalities are available from the @Home:

- *Standard video call (Avatar)*: this functionality preserves the "telepresence" service that the GIRAFF robot provides. The GIRAFF application has been indeed embedded within the @Home so as to maintain the possibility for secondary users to visit the older user's apartment through the telepresence robot.
- *Messages/reminders*: an environment has been designed to allow the primary user to receive messages from secondary users or reminders and suggestions. Messages and reminders maintain both the textual and the spoken form. Besides being able to receive text messages from a secondary user, primary users can receive and send voice messages too: this feature is somewhat similar to a voicemail service. In fact, it is not practical to send text messages from the robot using an on-screen keyboard, particularly for an elder person, while recording a voice message is just a matter of choosing the recipient from the list of secondary users, tapping "record" button and then "send" when finished.
- *Shared Space*: one of the comment from the evaluation session was related to the need to show personal data to the primary user (e.g., physiological measures), and to endow the system with a shared space between the primary user and the secondary users that could foster a discussion on the health status and habits of the old person. The general aim is to improve his/her awareness and also to encourage responsible behaviors for increasing his/her well being. In this light the DVPIS@Home includes an environment that allows such a dialog and that is shown in Fig. 2 (Shared Space). The pursued idea is that a secondary user (e.g., an Health Professional) calls a primary user via the Giraff robot and then uses this environment to discuss about the health related data to both explain them to the assisted person and possibly deepen the understanding of them through questions to the old person. Indeed any type of media materials can be sent through this environment such as photos or videos to be shared between primary and a generic secondary user (not necessarily the caregiver). Some of the services have bee introduced following some user's requests from long term use. For example, a user expressed the desire of being able to make his mother listen to some music of her son's choice. Through the shared space, functionality has been added to play YouTube videos through the robot. The actions are initiated by the secondary user who can define a playlist, play, pause, seek to a certain position, advance to a specific video in the playlist and so on: the

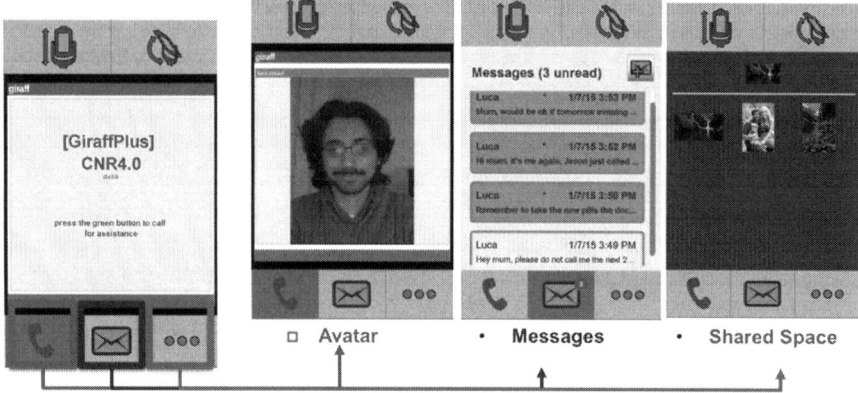

Fig. 2 @Home services

DVPIS@Home acts thus like a remote TV, even if the primary user is not completely passive as they are endowed by some control over the playback process; namely, they can play, pause, seek, advance/go back in the playlist, mute the volume.

2.2 Multimodal Communication Module

The Multimodal Communication module allows the primary user to control the robot through some specific gestures and speech commands. To realize it, the robot as been equipped with a Kinect Sensor. This device is used to implement the following functionalities:

1. the vision part collecting the user's real time body information
2. the audio part capturing sounds come from surrounding area.

The backbone structure is characterized by three different software packages. First, the Kinect Software Developed Kit released by Microsoft has been used to detect and classify image, depth and audio data simultaneously. Second, the robot motion control software, which is responsible for moving the robot towards the target (human) based on the gestures and audio recognized.

Finally, an inter-process communication (IPC) based on the MQTT[1] protocol has been developed. This kind of communication allow to share data across the Kinect and the robot, by just using a publish/subscribe design pattern. It is possible to implement this kind of communication between processes that are working on

---

[1]http://www.mqtt.org/.

the same machine without realizing a network configuration, thus allowing a fast information sharing. The Multimodal Communication module is designed to be user-friendly and safe for human-robot interaction. A visual and audio feedback system has been integrated in order to make the user aware of the command recognized by the robot. The module structure is shown in Fig. 3.

2.2.1 Robot Actions

The robot is now able to: go forward, go backward; turn left, turn right and rotate; stop, be locked and be unlocked; undock from the charging station; turn the screen up and down; adjust its orientation to speaker side; keep doing the previous action; move closer to the user; follow the user. The last two actions are implemented on a distance-based control loop algorithm, while the others are realized combining GIRAFF functionalities. All the robot actions are showed in Fig. 4 and can be evoked by means of both gesture and voice commands.

2.2.2 Gesture e Speech Recognition

The gesture recognition algorithm is able to track the user's arm joint configuration defining specific arm gestures, causing the robot to perform the commanded robot motion according to the corresponding gesture detected. The speech recognition algorithm has been implemented using the Speech Recognition API (SAPI) supplied by Microsoft. This algorithm filters the associated command from the user's speech and classifies it according to the word's sets implemented. Figure 5 shows examples of gestures commands video recorded during the experimental sessions.

Fig. 3 Multimodal communication system structure

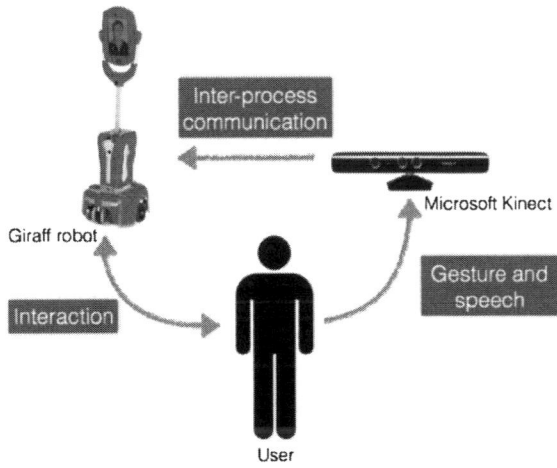

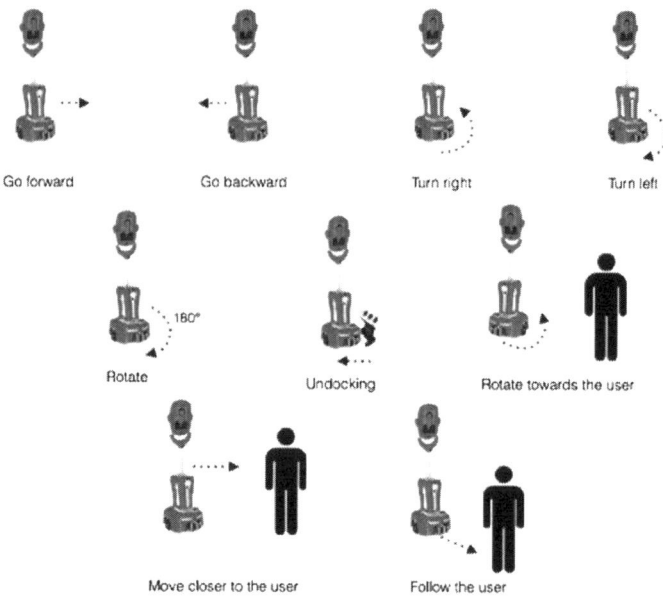

Fig. 4 Robot's actions

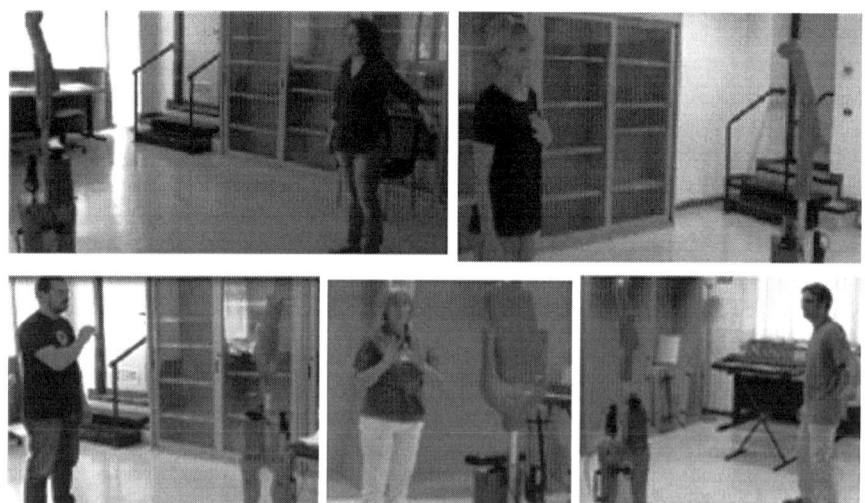

Fig. 5 Gesture examples (from top to bottom, from left to right): *Turn Left; Go Forward; Go Backward; Stop, Turn Left*

3 User Evaluation and HRI Experiments

The improvements on the robotic platform described in the previous section have been subjected to an evaluation based on a combination of psycho-physiological measures. The main aim of this experimentation was to assess the attitude of users toward such improvements. In fact, since we wanted to exclude that a combination of additional functionalities could overburden the user, we wanted to assure that such advancements represent a benefit for users and do not add any obstacles for a satisfactory interaction with the robot. For this reason, the conceived experiment had a twofold aim: (a) to assess the robustness and usability of the technological improvements both for the @Home services and for the Multimodal Communication Module; (b) to investigate Human-Robot Interaction aspects entailed by the introduction of the new functionalities like *cognitive workload*, *affective response* to technology, perceived *usefulness* and *emotional reaction*. As mentioned previously, the chosen approach combined the use of psychological and physiological methods: on one hand we relied on self-report measures, on the other we gathered physiological responses—and specifically cardiovascular activity—to the interaction with the GIRAFF robot. The overall idea is to have an objective indication of the psychological status from a sample of healthy people in terms of emotional valence, workload, and usability experience that can be used to determine the overall reaction of people to the enhanced robotic platform. Our intuition on the use of the GIRAFF robot is that it will not have a negative impact on persons. More specifically, from subjective ratings, we expect a positive response in terms of affective state/emotional experience, and we hypothesize that GIRAFF will be judged to be a pleasant stimulus. Moreover, we speculate that the usage of just learned channels of communication do not negatively affect the interaction with the robot.

Additionally, we want to investigate the impact of the robot by analyzing the physiological responses to the interaction and trying to relate such responses to self-ratings on usability, affective status and workload in order to support findings from questionnaires administration. We would like to focus on autonomous nervous system (ANS) activity. ANS is composed by two complementary systems, the parasympathetic nervous system (PSNS), which is responsible for regulating the body's unconscious actions, those that support the regular body's vital functions. It is wide known that cardiovascular activity reflects the activity of the ANS and in HRI research its activity has been related to emotional status like anxiety [1, 2], to the valence of an interaction experience [3], and an increase has been related to anthropomorphous features of the robot [4]. Moreover, cardiovascular activity can be also informative of cognitive load during a task [5, 6]. Eventually, the evaluation and interpretation of human physiological responses to the physical characteristics and behavior of a robot offer valuable material for understanding the level of application of a robot based on the context of use, the type of task to perform, on the modality of interaction and on needs and preferences of users, and the particular goal within this experimentation is to provide objective evidences from psychophysiology supporting the subjective perception of users.

3.1 Method

3.1.1 Participants

Inclusion criteria for the evaluation were the following: absence of any lifetime history of cardiac complications or any major disease, nor treatment with any medication that could affect the autonomic nervous system activity. The subjects were also asked to refrain from smoking or drinking coffee and alcohol for at least 1 h before the ECG recording. Nineteen participants (9 females, 10 males) have been involved in this evaluation session. Their mean age was 41.52 (SD = 14.6) years old, and they all get a master degree or above (4 of them), except for three users with high school diploma. Participants were also asked about their overall opinion on technology: the major part of them reported a good opinion on technology (n = 14), while four expressed an extremely positive opinion, and only one stated non to have a clear idea upon it.

3.1.2 Materials and Instruments

The questionnaires and instruments explained in Table 1 have been used in order to gather feedback on their experience with the robot and its services.

3.1.3 Experimental Procedure

At their arrival to the laboratory, participants have been asked to sign a consent form and subsequently they have been informed about the tasks of the experiment. The experimental procedure envisaged two main sessions. A first training session devoted to make each participant familiar with the MultiModal Communication interaction (voice and gesture), and a second session which represent the actual experimental session where the participants were asked to perform a set of tasks reproducing a scenario that entails both the use of the Multimodal Communication Module and the @Home services. During the whole experimental session, users have been invited to wear a cardiac holter in order to record their cardiac activity during the interaction with GIRAFF.

- *Training session.* This phase has been dedicated to the participants' familiarization with the two interaction modalities. The training has been, in turn, divided into two sub-sessions, one for gesture interaction learning and one for speech interaction learning. The choice to separate the two modalities has been taken in order to allow the participant to better focus on one modality per time. Participants were allowed to interact with the robot in one single manner until they felt confident enough to move forward. At the end of each sub-section participants were asked to fill in the SUS questionnaire referred to the specific

Table 1 Questionnaires and instruments

Psychological measures	
CSUQ (IBM Computer System Usability Questionnaire; [19])	From this instrument it is possible to get information on the overall satisfaction score (OVERALL), system usefulness (SYSUSE), information quality (INFOQUAL) and interface quality (INTERQUAL)
SUS (System Usability Scale; [20])	The SUS has been administered in order to investigate the two different interaction modalities envisaged by the system (SUS gesture, and SUS speech). Moreover, it has been administered both at the end of the training session and at the end of the experimental session in order to investigate whether a more complex scenario could somehow affect the interaction with the robot
Ad hoc questionnaires on @home services	An ad hoc questionnaire (adapted for each of three services) has been developed in order to investigate the following areas: *Task Ease, System Understanding; User expertise, Expected Behavior, Interaction Pace, System Responsiveness, System Efficiency, System Usefulness, Future Use*. Each item was rated on a five-point Likert scale. The internal consistency for each questionnaire has been assessed through the Cronbach's alpha computation. Good reliability emerged for all the three versions, on message services (a = 0.78), multimedia exchange service (a = 0.92), and video call service (a = 0.91)
NASA-TLX (The NASA Task Load Index; [21])	NASA-TLX is a multidimensional rating procedure that derives an overall workload score based on a weighted average of ratings on six subscales. These subscales include Mental Demands, Physical Demands, Temporal Demands, Own Performance, Effort and Frustration. It can be used to assess workload in various human-machine environments
PANAS (The Positive and Negative Affect Schedule; [22]).	This instrument comprises two mood scales, one that measures positive affect (PA) and the other which measures negative affect (NA)
Physiological measures	
Cardiac holter	A one-channel electrocardiograph (Custo Guard transmitter by Custo Med) was used to record the surface ECG from the subjects. The analogue ECG signals were immediately converted into digital signals by analogue-to-digital converter with a sampling rate of 125 Hz, and data have been sent to the Custo software as RR intervals

interaction modality just learned. The administration order of each sub-section was balanced among participants.

- *Experimental session.* During this session, participants were invited to perform a set of tasks within a fixed scenario reproducing the experience of free interaction with the robot by assuring the testing of the three new services implemented on top of GIRAFF. The scenario started with a message received on the robot parked at the docking station; the participant was invited to command the robot to get closer in order to check the message. As the robot was comfortably close to the person, the service of message exchange started by texting with an experimenter's colleague. Subsequently, a video call started (call service), and some multimedia files were sent and checked by the participants (multimedia services). Right after each service, the participants were asked to fill in the ad hoc questionnaire on the specific service. The experimental session terminated with the participants guiding the GIRAFF back to the docking station through gesture or speech commands. The remaining questionnaires have been administered at the end of the experimental session.

3.1.4 Signal Processing

Off-line signal processing was performed to analyze the acquired ECG signals with Kubios 2.2. RR intervals have been extracted from the recordings and data have been corrected for artifacts by detecting RR intervals bigger/smaller than 0.25 s compared to the local average. Detrending has been performed by applying the smoothness prior method with l = 300. RR series has been interpolated with piecewise cubic spline at 4 Hz interpolation rate. Parameters of the spectral analysis were computed from the sequence of normal RR intervals in order to get information from frequency domain by using Fast Fourier Transform (FFT). Whelch's periodogram used a windows width of 256 s with 50% overlap. Accordingly to the signal processing results, one participant has been excluded from the subsequent data analysis. The parameters mentioned above, have been computed for each one of the three epochs that have been extracted from the recording, accordingly to three different conditions we used for the investigation. Specifically, the baseline (hereafter *Baseline* condition) has been analyzed in order to obtain the individual basal values of autonomic system, and two experimental conditions: the interaction with the services of @Home (@*home* condition) and the interaction with GIRAFF through gestures and speech (*Multimodality* condition). This operation served the computing of the difference between the baseline and each experimental condition (*HB* = @*home*—*baseline*; *MB* = *Multimodality*—*baseline*), and the difference between the @*home* and the *Multimodality* conditions (*HM* = @*home*—*Multimodality*). This choice has been made in order to assess the impact of the interaction with the robot in terms of variation from physiological basal values, and to assess whether this variation could be explained through emotional or cognitive impact, and usability perception on the users by relating these variations to psychological measures.

The following parameters from the frequency domain have been considered for the analysis: LF (Low Frequency; 0.04–0.15 Hz), Normalized Low Frequency (LFn.u.), Relative Low Frequency (LF%), HF (High Frequency; 0.15–0.4 Hz), Normalized High Frequency (HFn.u.), Relative High Frequency (HF%), Total Power (TP), LF/HF Ratio.

3.1.5 Statistical Analysis

Statistical analysis have been performed with SAS 9.2. Preliminary descriptive analysis have been carried out on self-report measures in order to get an overview of user's perception toward the robotic platform, more specifically its usability and its impact on emotional and cognitive status. Ratings of PANAS, CSUQ, and NASA-TLX have been analyzed through Pearson's correlations to investigate possible associations. Usability scores obtained for the interaction modalities with the robot (SUS gesture and SUS speech) have been compared through *t test* statistics in order to find out possible differences between gesture and speech interaction, and pre *versus* post usage of such commands within a complex scenario (SUS administered after the Training session *versus* SUS administered after the Experimental session). Subsequently, in order to investigate whether possible differences in physiological responses among conditions were affected by any psychological factors, separate repeated measures analysis of variance (glm procedure) were applied to each physiological index. Statistical design applied for the analysis envisaged the within-group variable Condition (*Baseline*, *@home*, and *Multimodality*), and a self-report measure as independent continuous variable (PANAS-NA, PANAS-PA, NASA-TLX, CSUQ and sub-scales, SUS). Post hoc analyses have been carried out through contrast analysis. Further investigations have been performed through Pearson's correlation analysis in order to investigate the relationship between individual psychological attitude and the changes of cardiac responses among conditions. Indeed, the computed difference between conditions (*HB, MB, HM*), and self-report measures (CSUQ, SUS, PANAS, and NASA-TLX), have been subjected to correlation analysis in order to investigate possible association between physiological variations and psychological attitude toward GIRAFF and its services.

3.2 Results

3.2.1 Psychological Self-report Measures

The first part of this section is devoted to outline an overview of participants' attitude toward the enhanced robot, assessed through their ratings to the questionnaires. Figure 6 shows how the robot was perceived as usable by participants (M = 5.94, SD = 0.60). It has been considered as useful SYSUSE: (M = 5.91, SD = 0.65), the information provided in order to accomplish the tasks was good (INFOQUAL: M = 5.86, SD = 0.73), and the interface has been judged appropriate (INTERQUAL: M = 6.16, SD = 0.72) for the purpose of the experimental tasks. Moreover, when asking for specific feedback on usability of multimodal interaction, namely on gesture and speech interaction, no significant differences emerged. Additionally, the *@Home* services have been rated positively. As depicted in Fig. 7, all services have been assessed as valuable by participants (Messages

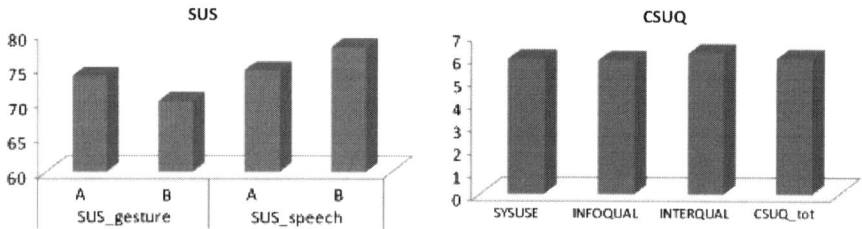

Fig. 6 Results from usability assessment related to the overall experience (CSUQ) and to the multimodal interaction (SUS)

Fig. 7 Results from
questionnaires on @Home

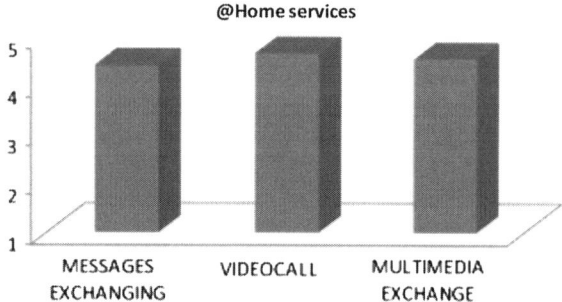

exchange: M = 4.46, SD = 0.41; Videocall: M = 4.68, SD = 0.37; Multimedia exchange: M = 4.59, SD = 0.5). Significant correlation emerged between the Positive Affect of PANAS and some usability dimensions (CSUQ: $r = 0.51$, $p = 0.02$; SYSUSE: $r = 0.52$, $p = 0.02$), suggesting a relationship between perceived usability and positive mood elicited by the interaction with GIRAFF. Moreover, such findings suggest how the usability perception was not affected by an increment of task load due to a more complex scenario and additional tasks to accomplish.

Finally, these results could also be explained considering that users did not experience high degree of workload when participating at the experimental session, and they reported to have felt mostly positive emotions during their participation to the scenario (see Table 2).

3.2.2   Results on Physiological Correlates

This first part aimed to provide an overview of the physiological activation pattern during the experimental sessions. When extracting physiological parameters for different conditions, higher values for LF and lower values for HF emerged respectively for the *Baseline* and for the *@home* condition, and an inverse pattern emerged in the *Multimodality* condition (see Fig. 8). Taken together, these results suggested a prominent activity of the sympathetic system—and a complementary suppression of the parasympathetic activity—when interacting with GIRAFF.

Table 2 Mean score (M) and standard deviation (SD) of PANAS and NASA-TXL

	PANAS-PA	PANAS-NA	NASA-TLX
M	36.27	11.72	50.11
SD	5.50	2.24	11.59

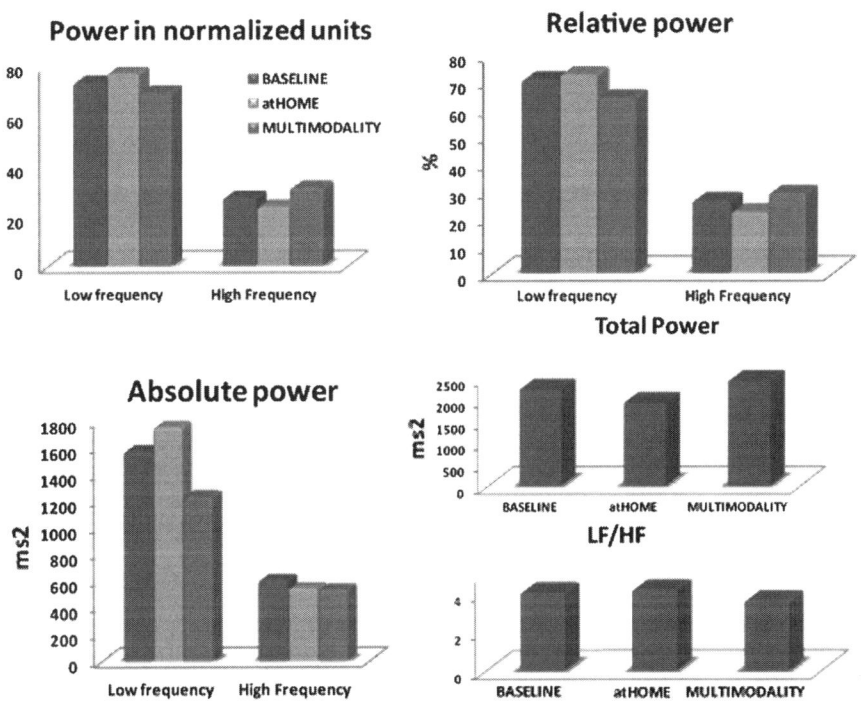

Fig. 8 Results from frequency-domain analysis

Analysis of variance with values from frequency-domain unveiled interesting findings with regard to the interaction of Positive Affect (PA) and usability ratings (CSUQ, SYSUSE subscale, and SUS gesture) when inserting the variables as factors in the GLM procedure. No significant results emerged when including NASA-TLX as independent variable. The two following sections are devoted to the presentation of analysis of variance with the introduction respectively of usability and positive affect as factors.

Psychophysiological correlates of usability

Analysis of variance performed on physiological indexes with the CSUQ variable as between-subject factor produced additional interesting results. First of all, on LF % analysis, a significant interaction CSUQ X Condition emerged ($F_{(4,32)} = 3.79$;

$p = 0.033$), and post hoc contrasts unveiled that the difference between the *Baseline* and the *Multimodality* conditions ($F_{(2,16)} = 9.35$; $p = 0.007$) resulted significant for the overall usability experienced by the users.

Analysis on HF% produced both a main effect of Condition ($F_{(2,32)} = 4.09$; $p = 0.026$), and a significant interaction CSUQ X Condition ($F_{(2,32)} = 4.38$; $p = 0.020$). The same trend emerged for normalized units of LF and HF. With regard to low frequencies, a main effect of Condition ($F_{(2,32)} = 3.94$; $p = 0.029$), and a significant interaction CSUQ X Condition ($F_{(4,32)} = 4.32$; $p = 0.021$) emerged from the analysis. As for low frequencies, high ones reported significant main effect of Condition ($F_{(2,32)} = 3.96$; $p = 0.029$), and a significant interaction CSUQ X Condition ($F_{(4,32)} = 4.34$; $p = 0.021$). The last analysis of variance with the CSUQ as between factor has been made on LF/HF values. It emerged a main effect of Conditions ($F_{(2,32)} = 3.56$; $p = 0.040$), and a significant interaction CSUQ X Condition ($F_{(4,32)} = 3.75$; $p = 0.034$). In every case, post hoc analysis revealed significant differences between the *Baseline* and the *Multimodality* conditions.

When introducing the sub-scale of the CSUQ, System Usefulness (SYSUSE), some interesting results emerged. First of all, a main effect of Conditions in analysis of HF ($F_{(2,32)} = 5.14$; $p = 0.011$) suggested significant differences between the *Baseline* and *Multimodality* conditions ($F_{(1,16)} = 7.63$; $p = 0.013$), and the *Multimodality* and *@home* conditions ($F_{(1,16)} = 8.06$; $p = 0.011$). Analysis of variance on HF% reported significant main effect of Condition ($F_{(2,32)} = 3.38$; $p = 0.046$), and a significant interaction SYSUSE X Condition ($F_{(4,32)} = 3.65$; $p = 0.037$). For normalized values of LF, significant effects for the interaction SYSUSE X Condition ($F_{(4,32)} = 3.48$; $p = 0.043$) emerged from the analysis. The same trend emerged for normalized values of HF, with significant effects for the interaction SYSUSE X Condition ($F_{(4,32)} = 3.50$; $p = 0.042$). Again, post hoc analysis suggested significant differences between the *Baseline* and *the Multimodality* condition.

Generally speaking, it is interesting to notice that usability ratings only influence the interaction with GIRAFF when the user is supposed to provide commands to the robotic platform.

The correlation analysis depicted in Table 3 help in better understanding the interaction of usability perception and the physiological impact of robot usage. Significant associations emerged just when correlating the self-report measures to the variation of autonomic activation from baseline values to the activation elicited by the interaction through gestures and speech. It emerged how usability perception of the robotic platform can be related to the capability to interact with it, specifically to the capability to provide commands and to get those command accomplished by GIRAFF. An increase on usability ratings emerged to be associated with lower difference between basal values and values measured during the interaction with GIRAFF. The lower difference could be due to an increase on sympathetic activity —and decreased parasympathetic—considering that our sample showed to be slightly less aroused during multimodal interaction with respect to the baseline. It can be argued that an increment on sympathetic activity related to higher usability

Table 3 Correlation analysis on physiological correlates of autonomic variability among conditions differences and CSUQ and SYSUSE (only significant results are reported)

		LF%[MB]	HF%[MB]	LFn.u.[MB]	HFn.u.[MB]	LFHF[MB]
CSUQ	r	−0.06	0.65	−0.63	0.63	−0.53
	p	0.00	0.00	0.00	0.00	0.02
SYSUSE	r	−0.52	0.60	−0.58	0.58	−0.47
	p	0.02	0.00	0.01	0.01	0.04

Table 4 Correlation analysis on physiological correlates of autonomic variability among conditions and SUS_speech (only significant results are reported)

		LF%[MB]	HF%[MB]	LFn.u.[MB]	HFn.u.[MB]
SUS-speech	r	−0.55	0.61	−0.60	0.60
	p	0.01	0.00	0.00	0.00

ratings could be explained by more positive attitude toward the robotic platform and its control through speech and gesture commands.

Finally, we aimed to further investigate whether usability perception, assessed specifically for multimodal interaction, could somehow be related to the physic logical responses. Actually, no significant findings resulted by inserting the SUS gesture as factor between subjects in analysis of variance. Conversely, an interesting pattern emerged from analysis of variance with the SUS speech. Analysis reported a significant interaction SUS_speech X Condition for HF% ($F_{(4,32)} = 3.73$; $p = 0.034$), LF% ($F_{(4,32)} = 3.48$; $p = 0.043$), and for normalized values of LF, ($F_{(4,32)} = 3.62$; $p = 0.038$), and HFn.u. ($F_{(4,32)} = 3.64$; $p = 0.034$), as well. Post hoc contrast for each ANOVA showed a significant effect of SUS speech in modulating the difference between the *Baseline* and *Multimodality* conditions.

Through the correlation analysis it has been possible to deeply investigate the above-described findings (see Table 4). A pattern pretty much similar to the one emerged for the association with the CSUQ emerged from this analysis. These results could be interpreted as a confirmation of a relation between the physiological activation during the interaction with the robot and the usability experienced by the users. And this is true, just when the users have to directly interact whit the robotic platform as an agent being part of a dyadic interaction, since significant results emerge only in relation with the *Multimodality* condition.

Psychophysiological correlates of affective status

Significant interactions of PA emerged with HF% ($F_{(4,32)} = 3.85$; $p = 0.031$), with LFn.u. ($F_{(4,32)} = 3.72$; $p = 0.035$), and HFn.u. ($F_{(4,32)} = 3.75$; $p = 0.034$). Everywhere, follow up contrasts showed that the comparison between *Baseline* and *Multimodality* conditions, and between *Multimodality* and *@home* conditions were significant for Positive Affect. Correlation analysis have been made between the PA

Table 5 Correlation analysis on physiological correlates of autonomic variability among conditions and positive affect (only significant results are reported)

		HF%[HM]	LFn.u.[HM]	HFn.u.[HM]	LFHF[HM]
PA	r	−0.52	0.51	−0.51	0.49
	p	0.02	0.02	0.02	0.03

and the physiological indexes in terms of differences between conditions (*HB, MB, HM*). As showed in Table 5, significant associations emerged between the affective status and the physiological response, somehow mirroring the results from analysis of variance. It seems that the variation on autonomic activity in terms of different activation between the two conditions, is associated to the emotional status of users. Specifically, increased positive feelings are associated to higher activity of sympathetic system (and consequent lower activity of parasympathetic one) suggesting higher degree of positive emotional involvement in the @*home* condition. This finding could be explained by speculating that the services of the @*home* are meant to behave as a means for supporting human-to-human interaction. Possibly, higher affective involvement due to the fact that the user is actually interacting with another person, not properly with the robot. Conversely, during the *Multimodality* condition, the user has to interact directly with GIRAFF, by providing a number of commands. Indeed, the user and the robotic platform are the two actors of the interaction in this specific situation. Moreover, an association between the positive mood reported by PANAS and the variation of autonomic activity in the *Multimodality* condition resulted significant. Taking into account that the physiological activation pattern on our sample presents slightly lower autonomic activation during this experimental condition, it seems that an increase on positive mood is associated with lower difference between basal values and values measured during the interaction with GIRAFF. It turns that a lower difference could be due to an increase on sympathetic activity—and decreased parasympathetic—in the experimental condition.

Indeed, we could speculate for an association between positive attitude toward the multimodal interaction with GIRAFF and increased autonomic activity.

4 Discussions

Results from this experiment demonstrate that users perceived in a positive way the "enhanced" GIRAFF, both with regards to its services and to its multimodal interaction features. In fact, self-ratings suggested a positive impact on users who experienced an overall positive mood during the interaction which turned out to be barely workload demanding. The experience with GIRAFF was perceived neither as stressful, annoying nor frustrating considering the low values emerged for negative affect rating. Analysis on physiological responses somehow supported the self-rating results, and allowed a deeper understanding on individual attitude towards the robot. Two psychological dimensions showed to be related to the physiological activation during the interaction, namely usability and positive mood. In fact, only when inserting these variables as covariates in the analysis of variance, significant results emerged with regard their influence on physiological activation related to the interaction with GIRAFF.

With regard to usability, the perception to interact with an effective and satisfactory robotic platform was determinant mostly when the interaction entailed the user to give commands to it. More specifically, autonomic system moved toward sympathetic activation in relation to higher usability ratings. This was true especially when the users had to directly interact whit the robotic platform as an agent being part of a dyadic interaction, since significant results emerged only when considering the Multimodality condition.

Also positive affect presented an influence on the autonomic activation related to multimodal interaction, in terms of an association between positive attitude toward the multimodal interaction with GIRAFF and the autonomic balance that juts out into sympathetic activation. It is not surprising that usability and positive mood showed the same pattern when relating them to physiological activation. First of all, these were the only two dimensions that presented a positive correlation between each other. Moreover, it is also pretty intuitive to consider that good degrees of usability can contribute in making the experience as a positive one, eliciting positive feeling on users, and this is further supported by high usability and positive affect scores of the related questionnaires. In order to better explain the influence of these subjective dimensions on the physiological activation, we can rely on findings from psychophysiological research. A number of studies on emotional stimuli processing brings evidence on HRV being correlated with valence of stimuli. Specifically, it is well known that heart rate acceleration occurs in response to pleasant stimuli, while unpleasant stimuli are accompanied by heart-rate slowing [7–16]. Considering that heart rate is affected by the autonomic nervous system, and specifically, it is increased by sympathetic activation and decreased under parasympathetic influence also our results can be discussed under this view. Further support to our hypothesis comes from ratings of others self-rating measures. We can exclude a sympathetic activation in our experimental conditions due to excessive amount of workload since results on NASA-TXL reported low degree of workload experienced by participants during the experimental tasks, and we can indeed speculate that physiological response are ascribable to positive attitude toward the robotic platform.

Under these premises, we argued about the correlation between affective status and usability perception correlation with the autonomic activation, in terms of increased sympathetic activity and decreased parasympathetic activity during the interaction with GIRAFF. Though the self-report and physiological measures are expected to converge, the physiological measures provide an added benefit since they make it possible to deeply investigate the interaction with the platform. In fact, when splitting the scenario envisaged by the experimental protocol between mere motion control of the robot and the usage of services provided by it, further interesting findings emerged. Though the physiological responses to the multimodal interaction can be somehow related both to usability perception and positive feelings resulting from the interaction, it seems that higher activation during the usage of the @home services could be rather associated to higher positive feelings experienced during the interaction with the services provided by GIRAFF, while the role of usability seems to be minimized. Actually, during the Multimodality condition users where asked to control the robot through vocal and gestures commands in order to make it to move within the environment. When analyzing this situation, it clearly comes out that the user and the robot are the two actors taking part to the dyadic interaction. The users is communicating to GIRAFF, which is the agent supposed to respond to the user's requests. On the other hand, during the @home condition, GIRAFF becomes a tool that allows the users to interact with another person. Possibly, higher autonomic activation related to higher positive mood during the usage of GIRAFF services with respect to the multimodal interaction, can be explained by the presence (virtual) of another person as communication partner in the interaction. Somehow, these last results can be explained by relying on evidences that support a different human approach depending on the amount of human-like features of their technological counterparts during an interaction. It seems that this behavior is partly due to people's specific mental model about system behavior and appearance. If a system looks and behaves much like a human being (e.g., a humanoid robot emits a human's voice), users mental model of the system's behavior may approach their mental model of humans, and consequently behave like they are interacting with a human being, suggesting that mental models actually moderate people responses to interactive systems [17, 18]. Nevertheless, with regard to ours findings, it is not really matter of anthropomorphization, but rather matter of who the user believes to be his/her counterpart. In our experiment, a different approach seems to be adopted according to whether the users were interacting with GIRAFF, or with another human being, even if this interaction was mediated through the robot.

Acknowledgements The authors work has been initially motivated by the GIRAFFPLUS project (FP7 ICT GA.288173). They are currently supported by the AAL JP under the MAESTRO project ("Sustainable reference framework for evaluating quantified self equipment and services for seniors"—AAL-2014-146).

References

1. Kulic D, Croft E (2005) Anxiety detection during human-robot interaction. In: Proceedings of the IEEE international conference on intelligent robots and system, pp 616–621
2. Kulic D, Croft E (2007) Affective state estimation for human-robot interaction. IEEE Trans Rob 23:991–1000
3. Swangnetr M, Kaber D (2013) Emotional state classification in patient-robot interaction using wavelet analysis and statistics-based feature selection. IEEE Trans Human-Mach Syst 43:63–75
4. Zhang T, Kaber D, Zhu B, Swangnetr M, Mosaly P, Hodge L (2010) Service robot feature design effects on user perceptions and emotional responses. Intel Serv Robot 3:73–88

5. Chen D, Vertegaal R (2004) Using mental load for managing interruptions in physiologically attentive user interfaces. In Proceedings of the conference on human factors in computing systems, pp 1513–1516
6. Lin T, Omata M, Hu W, Imamiya A (2005) Do physiological data relate to traditional usability indexes? In: Proceedings of the 17th Australia conference on computer-human interaction, pp 1–10
7. Anttonen J, Surakka V (2005) Emotions and heart rate while sitting on a chair. In: proceedings of the SIGCHI conference on human factors in computing systems, pp 491–499
8. Bradley M, Lang P (2000) Affective reactions to acoustic stimuli. Psychophysiology 37:204–215
9. Brouwer A, van Wouwe N, Mhl C, van Erp J, Toet A (2013) Perceiving blocks of emotional pictures and sounds: effects on physiological variables. Front Hum Neurosci 7:295
10. Codispoti M, De Cesarei A (2007) Arousal and attention: picture size and emotional reactions. Psychophysiology 44:680–686
11. Fitzgibbons L, Simons R (1992) Affective response to color-slide stimuli in subjects with physic al anhedonia: a three-systems analysis. Psychophysiology 29(6):613–620
12. Greenwald M, Cook E, Lang P (1989) Affective judgment and psychophysiological response: dimensional covariation in the evaluation of pictorial stimuli. J Psychophysiol 3:51–64
13. Hare R, Wood K, Britain S, Shadman J (1970) Autonomic responses to affective visual stimuli. Psychophysiology 7:408–417
14. Lang P, Greenwald M, Bradley M, Hamm A (1993) Looking at pictures: affective, facial, visceral, and behavioral reactions. Psychophysiology 30(3):261–273
15. Libby W, Lacey B, Lacey J (1973) Pupillary and cardiac activity during visual attention. Psychophysiology 10:210–294
16. Winton W, Putnam L, Krauss R (1984) Facial and autonomic manifestations of the dimensional structure of emotion. J Exp Soc Psychol 20:195–216
17. Lee S, Lau I, Kiesler S, Chiu C (2005) Human mental models of humanoid robots. In: Proceedings of the 2005 IEEE international conference on robotics and automation, pp 2767–2772
18. Shechtman N, Horowitz L (2003) Media inequality in conversation: how people behave differently when interacting with computers and people. In Proceedings of the CHI 2003 conference on human factors in computing systems
19. Lewis J (1995) Ibm computer usability satisfaction questionnaires: psychometric evaluation and instructions for use. Int J Human-Comput Interact 7(1):57–78
20. Brooke J (1996) Usability evaluation in industry. SUS: a quick and dirty usability scale, Taylor and Francis
21. Hart S, Staveland L (1988) Human mental workload. Development of NASA-TLX (Task Load Index): results of empirical and theoretical research. North Holland Press, Amsterdam
22. Watson D, Clark L, Tellegen A (1988) Development and validation of brief measures of positive and negative affect: the panas scales. J Pers Soc Psychol 54:1063–1070

Evaluating SpeakyAcutattile: A System Based on Spoken Language for Ambient Assisted Living

F. Fracasso, G. Cortellessa, A. Cesta, F. Giacomelli and N. Manes

Abstract The current work presents the SPEAKYACUTATTILE system, a computer based platform designed to enable its users to access a number of ICT services such as house management, health status monitoring or recreational services. It is deeply grounded on voice interaction and represents a Spoken Language System (SLS) meant to be a sort of intelligent assistant with which the users can vocally interact. The paper dwells on an experimental assessment of the system. Linear regression analysis have been carried out in order to assess the influence of system performance—in terms of dialogue efficiency metrics and dialogue quality metrics—on the perceived satisfaction of users. Results show that longer dialogues are preferred in order to positively influence the users satisfaction, suggesting the importance for people to have time for getting confident with new ICT solutions. Moreover, from the experimental analysis, it clearly emerges how system intervention should be reduced, suggesting how a good balance between user and system turns represents an important aspect for a fluid interaction. The same can be speculated for dialogues with no met requests that also tended to be associated with lower satisfaction scores. These last results support the importance for a vocal assistant to be effective in its purpose in order to be perceived as useful and satisfying.

F. Fracasso (✉) · G. Cortellessa · A. Cesta
CNR—Italian National Research Council, ISTC, Rome, Italy
e-mail: francesca.fracasso@istc.cnr.it

G. Cortellessa
e-mail: gabriella.cortellessa@istc.cnr.it

A. Cesta
e-mail: amedeo.cesta@istc.cnr.it

F. Giacomelli · N. Manes
Mediavoice S.r.l., Rome, Italy
e-mail: giacomelli@mediavoice.it

N. Manes
e-mail: manes@mediavoice.it

© Springer International Publishing AG 2017
F. Cavallo et al. (eds.), *Ambient Assisted Living*, Lecture Notes
in Electrical Engineering 426, DOI 10.1007/978-3-319-54283-6_26

Keywords Spoken language system · Ambient assisted living system · User evaluation · User satisfaction

1 Introduction

Research in Ambient Assisted Living technology (AAL) is attracting more and more interest among ICT scientists. The present work is inserted within this context and aims to introduce SPEAKYACUTATTILE, an Italian project dedicated to support the daily life of vulnerable people, with specific regard to the elderly. SPEAKYACUTATTILE is a computer based platform designed to provide the users with a simple instrument for accessing a number of services such as house management, health status monitoring or recreational purpose. The system is grounded on voice interaction and represents a Spoken Language System (SLS) meant to be a sort of intelligent assistant with which the users can vocally interact. Spoken Language Systems by definition are systems that rely primarily or exclusively on audio for interaction, this includes speech and sound [1], and nowadays they are being used more often for a wide range of applications.

Since the eighties, different systems have been developed for several applications. In working environment, some administrative information systems have been developed (APHODEX—Acoustic-PHOnetic Decoding EXpert system, [2, 3]), such as office databases (SPICOS II—Siemens-Philips-IPO-Continuous Speech Understanding and Dialogue System [4]) or document retrieval systems (i.e. Hearsay-II [5]), and speech-to-speech real-time translation systems for the domain of conference registration (DmDialog [6]). Other applications covered different areas on travel planning (HWIM—Hear What I Mean, [5, 7]), specifically in trains travel information retrieving (Ernest [8]; VODIS II [9]), flight reservation and inquiries (SUNDIAL [10]) or air traffic inquiry systems (MINDS—Multi-Modal Interactive Dialog System [11]), and hotel reservations, like HAM-ANS—Hamburg Application-Oriented Natural Language System [12, 13], as well. More recently, ICT for Ambient Assisted Living paradigms is taking advantage of this interaction modality, since it appears to be a natural and valuable way in order to overcome difficulties due to, i.e., age-related impairment. In fact, despite some results from an automatic speech recognition (ASR) performance study where the ASR performance was lower for older persons and for female [14], experiments in an assistive environment using voice recognition pointed out that the speech interface is the easiest way for the user to interact with the computer based service system [15]. Application in assistive field has been covering several areas such as intelligent environments, in-car applications, personal assistants, smart homes, and interaction with robots and assistants for disabled and elderly people [16]. These solutions have to be able to understand and produce spoken language in various applied fields, pursuing the goal to make the interaction more and more effective by tailoring on specific users features. Since speech is claimed to be one the most natural modes of interaction, the numbers of speech-enabled applications are rapidly increasing and much effort has been put into considering the special requirements of assistive environments. Among others, some efforts have been carried out in order to study, implement, and evaluate the speech interface of a multimodal interactive guidance system based on the most common elderly-centered characteristics during inter-action within assistive environments [17]. Moreover, studies on prosody, articula-tion and speech quality have been made in order to exploit this communication channel with the purpose of detecting accident-prone fatigue states from speech features [18]. The success of the SLS, and consequently their positive impact on AAL, depends on whether the user is able to accomplish the task successfully using the system and how the task is actually accomplished. For this reason, an extremely critical step in the development of a spoken language system is not only the designing of the interface and devising dialogue strategies but also evaluating how the system performs. Performance of the system includes some metrics such inappropriate utterance ratio, concept accuracy, number of turns, elapsed time and other such factors which make the whole process of comparing dialogue strategies across system and tasks difficult. A current challenge is represented by an increasing demand for standardized bench-marks to test and compare performance and usability of such of interaction modalities beyond metrics such speech recog-nition accuracy, adequate language modeling and appropriate semantic represen-tation for efficient interaction with back-end knowledge sources [19]. In this direction, Walker and her colleagues put some efforts while developing a method for evaluating spoken dialogue systems [20]. These researchers developed PARADISE (PARAdigm for Dialogue System Evaluation), an evaluation frame-work that is useful to compare performances of different dialogues strategies, and system designed for different tasks as well, in order to evaluate the performance. PARADISE considers user satisfaction ratings as an indicator of usability. Usability is, in turns, calculated as a measure composed by two factors: task success and dialogue costs using a decision-theoretic framework with the main aim to maximize users satisfaction by maximizing task success and minimizing costs. This frame-work uses methods from decision theory to combine a discordant set of perfor-mance metrics. Subjective satisfaction is placed at the center of this model, and it is supposed to be influenced by objective features of the system, measurable through dialogue quality metrics and efficiency dialogue metrics.

The present work aims to introduce the SPEAKYACUTATTILE assistive platform and the validation of the first prototype. With this purpose, section two is devoted the presentation of technical features of the platform, while section three describes the experimentation carried out with users. The last section is devoted to outline some conclusions and future development on the SPEAKYACUTATTILE system.

2   The SpeakyAcutattile Platform

SPEAKYACUTATTILE has been conceived as an intelligent assistant centered on the use of vocal interaction in order to use a set of digital services. The underline idea moves from the goal to make an interface enabling access to digital contents to all kind of people, despite their specificities. The overall platform is showed in Fig. 1. The new enabling platform consists of hardware and software components. It enables the construction and use of new digital content and services as well as allowing new modes of access to existing ones. The platform provides access from both in-house/office and on the move. It is composed of several hardware and software modules based on a client/server architecture. The client side is based of a PC Box running an avatar with speech recognition technology and is accessible by voice through a special and innovative multifunction wireless device (Speaky Acutattile), which is the heart of the new platform. It acts as a spoken interface through a remote controller with incorporated microphone, connected to the computer through an USB. This device is provided with a push-to-talk button and allows the users to give vocal commands to the PC-box in a walkie-talkie manner The PC Box is also connected to an advanced sensors system for home automation, which allows people to manage and control their house. The SPEAKYACUTATTILE platform includes also a system for monitoring person posture. The system is supposed to monitor the user at home, and by detecting the posture it may indicate a critical situation in which the person loses consciousness or falls. Finally, the system includes biometric sensors for measuring vital parameters for Telemedicine and Telecare. In the server side architecture there is a full contact center for both caregivers and technical support operators monitoring all the connected PC Boxes. It is a call center with a first level voice portal automated system and a second level with the human operator. The service center also serves as a center for data processing, Content Management System (CMS).

As depicted in Fig. 2, from the client side a number of modules are integrated in order to provide different services to the users. More in detail the following applications are accessible from the main menu of the GUI.

- *Domotics* that allows the person a complete control of the house through vocal commands (appliances, utilities, communications, security, privacy, etc.) in orchestration with environmental sensors and actuators;
- *E-learning* that is a support to educational teaching;
- *Face Recognition*, that allows the authentication to the services in order to preserve security and privacy of the person;
- *Postural monitoring*, that combined with environmental sensors is able to detect falls or critical situations;
- *Agenda*, through which the person can fix appointments and set reminders;
- *Multimedia Library*, that allow the access through speech channel to the library in order to listen to music, and see videos or photos;

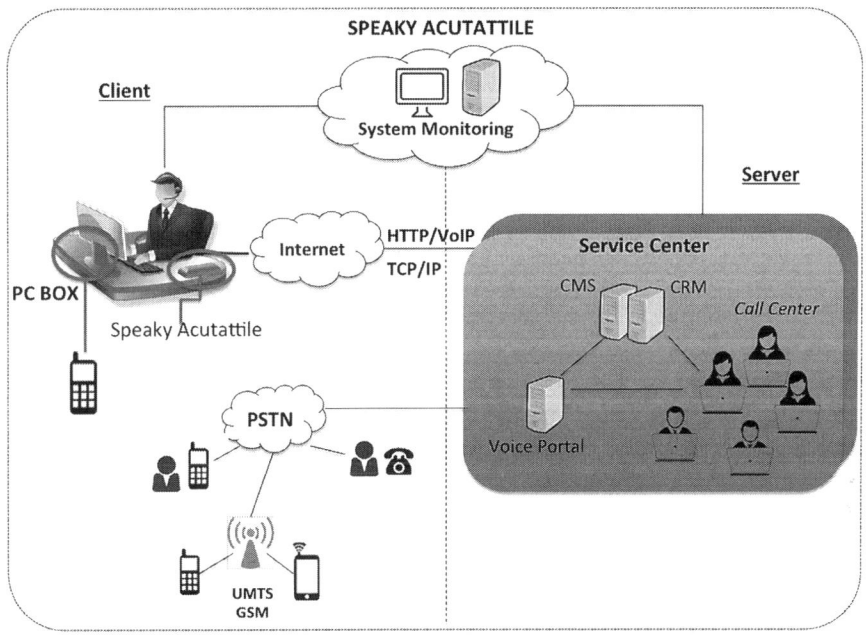

Fig. 1 The overall SPEAKYACUTATTILE platform

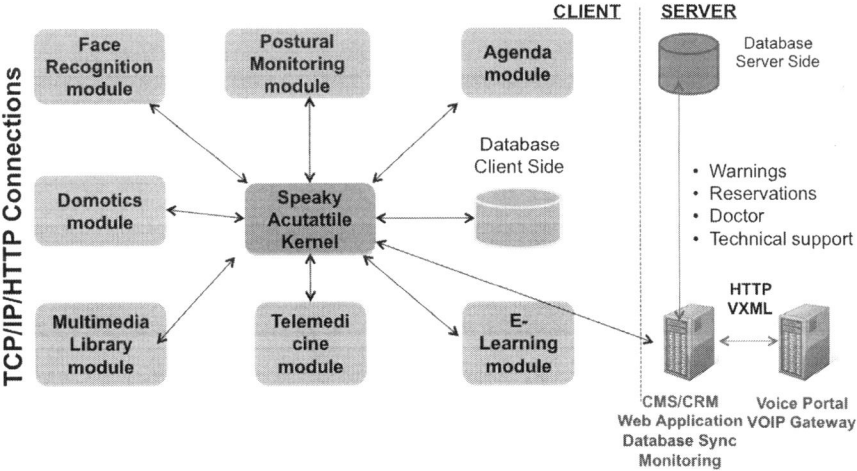

Fig. 2 The general architecture of the SpeakyAcutattile system

- *Target search.* Through the Acutattile device (see later) it is possible to explore the desktop of the PC. Thanks to it the user is provided with a feedback when an object (i.e. an icon) is reached. Both an audio feedback (a description of the object) and a tactile one (vibration) are provided to the user;
- *Telemedicine*, through which the user is allowed to make some physiological measurements (i.e. blood pressure, oximetry) and send them to the service center.

At server side, information is stored in a database and a Service Center allows a remote monitoring of some parameters detected by SPEAKYACUTATTILE. Specifically, information from Postural monitoring, Telemedicine and Agenda can be checked by a caregiver.

Finally, others components of the system deserve to be mentioned, just to provide a complete overall framework, despite they have not been subjected to evaluation. A particular mechatronic device (Acutattile), a sort of proactive mouse, that represents a further means to communicate with the platform. It acts both in a passive way—like an usual mouse do—and proactive way—by accompanying the users to perform certain movement within some modules (i.e. E-Learning module). Additionally, a network of environmental sensors and actuators are connected to SPEAKYACUTATTILE in order to allow the control of the environment, and an innovative system for postural monitoring for fall detection is part of the system as well. Finally, there are some biometric sensors useful for health status monitoring, in order to provide telemedicine and tele-assistance services. As introduced at the end of the previous section, the present work aims to present the results of experiments carried out in order to assess the speech interface. For this reason, the rest of the article will focus only on those modules, which require speech interaction.

3   Method

3.1   Participants

Thirty-five persons (19 women and 16 men), mean age 46.22 years old (SD = 18.93), took part in the experiment aimed to assess the SPEAKYACUTATTILE platform. Participants were asked to provide information regarding their attitude toward technology. As the reader can see in Fig. 3, the majority of them reported to have a pretty good idea regarding technology and its usefulness in everyday life. Moreover the majority of them reported good capability on computer usage, even if only 13 persons of the sample stated to have experienced speech dialogue system (i.e. Siri, Cortana) in their life.

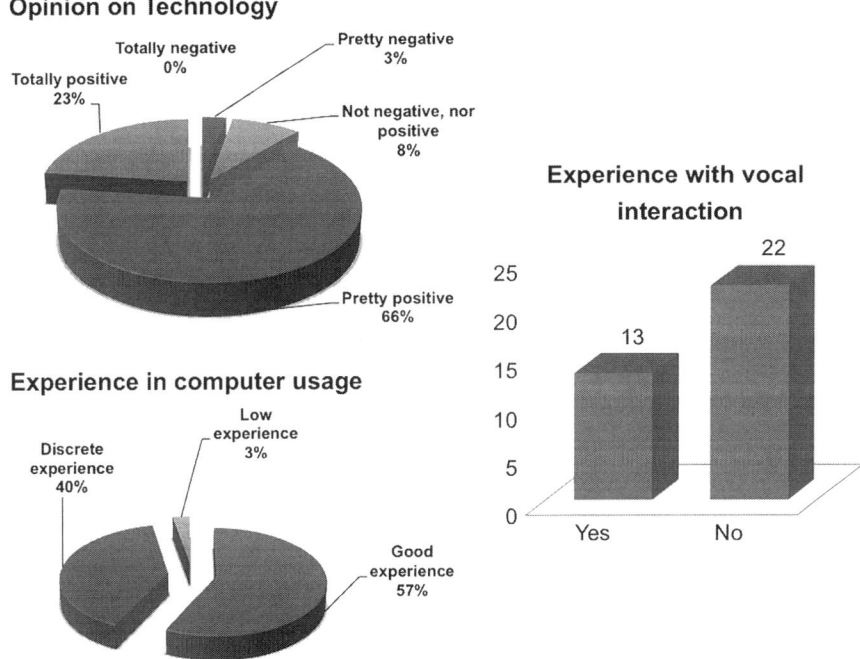

Fig. 3 Descriptive statistics on users experience and opinion with technology

3.2 Materials and Metrics

Subjects have been asked to fill in an ad hoc questionnaire for each module of the platform and a final questionnaire (SASSI [21]) regarding the whole interaction with the system. Moreover, some performance metrics (e.g., length of the interaction, frequency of system's errors) have been gathered from the log file of the system after each interaction. The following subsections are devoted to better describe the instruments used during the evaluation sessions.

3.2.1 Ad Hoc Questionnaire on Task Satisfaction

We built an ad hoc questionnaire based on the one proposed by [19] in order to gather feedback on user satisfaction for each single module. The questionnaire has been developed in order to investigate the following areas:

- *TTS Performance*—It has been easy to understand the system during the interaction.
- *Task Ease*—During this interaction it has been easy to find the information I was looking for.

Table 1 Cronbach's Alpha
for each questionnaire

Questionnaires	Cronbach's Alpha
Face recognition	0.77
Telemedicine	0.72
Domotic	0.74
Multimedia library	0.79
Agenda	0.81

- *Interaction Pace* – I think that the pace of interaction with the system was appropriate.
- *User Expertise*—During this interaction I knew what to do and what to say at each point.
- *System Response*—It often happened that the system was slow to reply to me.
- *Expected Behavior*—The system worked the way I expected it to.
- *Future Use*—I would use this system for (different according to the specific module) in the future.

In order to assess the reliability of this ad hoc instrument, the Cronbach's Alpha has been computed for all the versions of the questionnaires developed for each module of the platform. Table 1 shows the obtained values, suggesting good reliability property for each questionnaire on single module satisfaction.

3.2.2 Subjective Assessment of Speech System Interfaces (SASSI)

Subjective Assessment of Speech System Interfaces (SASSI) consists of 34 statements about the tested system, which are to be rated with level of agreement on a 5-point Likert scale. This self-report instrument has been developed by Hone and Graham [21] with the purpose to build an instrument devoted to the assessment of satisfaction on speech dialogue system. It measures six factors of users perception of speech systems:

- *System response accuracy* (e.g. "the system is reliable", "the system makes few errors");
- *Likeability* (e.g. "the system is useful", "I felt in control of the interaction with the system");
- *Cognitive demand* (e.g."I felt tense using the system", "a high level of concentration is required when using the system");
- *Annoyance* (e.g. "the interaction with the system is irritating", "the system is flexible");
- *Habitability* (e.g. "I always knew what to say to the system", "the interaction with the system felt natural");
- *Speed* (e.g. "the interaction with the system is fast", "there were not too many steps needed to perform a task");

3.2.3   Performance Metrics

Among the metrics within the PARADISE framework we took into account those which better fitted with the SPEAKYACUTATTILE platform:

- Dialogue Efficiency Metrics
  - elapsed time, system turns, user turns, total turns
- Dialogue Quality Metrics
  - errors, noinput, reprompt, help (raw)
  - errors%, noinput%, reprompt%, help% (normalized).

The **dialogue efficiency** metrics were calculated from the dialogue recordings and system logs. The length of the recording was used to calculate the elapsed time in seconds (ET) from the beginning to the end of the interaction, indeed it has been calculated for the whole interaction. Measures for the number of **System Turns**, and the number of **User Turns**, were calculated on the basis of the system logging everything the platform said and everything it heard from the user. The total amount of Turns (**Total Turns**) has been computed as well. The **dialogue quality** measures were derived from the recordings and the system logs. Some of them were automatically logged by the system like the number of times the users had to repeat a command to the system (**reprompt**), whenever it was due to an error of recognition by the system or to a timeout. The **errors** of speech recognition by the system were also computed and the times the users pushed the button just to make the system stop talking (**noinput**). User behaviors that the system perceived as a possible situation affecting the dialogue quality were also logged: these included the number of times the system played one of its specific help messages because it believed that the user had asked for *Help* (**helps**). Finally, as in [19], we normalized the dialogue quality metrics by dividing the raw counts by the total number of utterances in the dialogue and this resulted in **errors%**, **noinput%**, **reprompt%**, **help%** metrics.

   This solution has been chosen because all the efficiency metrics seems unlikely to generalize [22].

3.3   *Experimental Procedure*

Participants came to the lab and were asked to compile a consent form, and subsequently they were instructed about the experimental protocol. They were supposed to perform some specific tasks for each module of the platform, since the experimental session focused on specific modules, namely the Face Recognition, the Media Library, the Telemedicine Guide, the Domotics module and finally the Agenda one (see Fig. 4 for additional insight on the experimental setup, and Table 2 for further information on instructions provided to the participants).

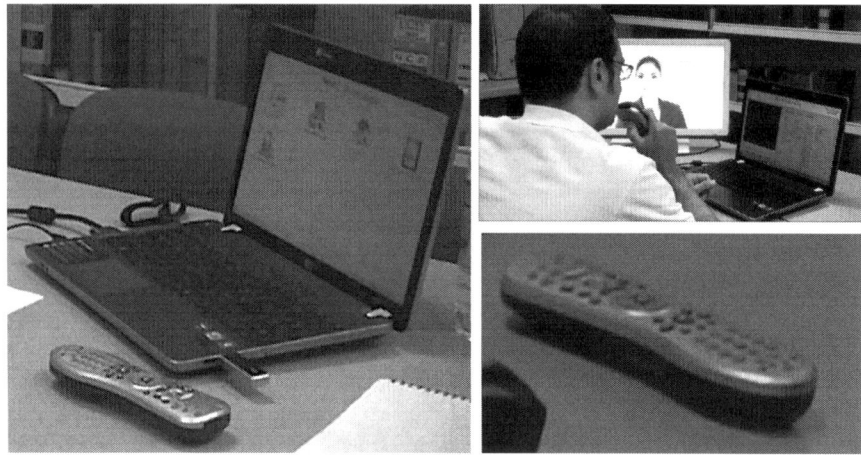

Fig. 4 The SPEAKYACUTATTILE devices. On the *left*, the remote controller connected to the pc via USB is displayed, while on the *right* it is possible to see the Speaky Avatar

Table 2 General instructions provided to the participants for each task

Task	Instruction
Face recognition	This is the first task you are asked to perform. Since you need to be registered within the system before you start using it, you have to create your account through the face recognition module. Indeed, please, create your account and register to the system
Multimedia library	Please, enter the media library module and ask the system to listen to an artist. Then, chose a particular song and adjust the volume as you prefer. Finally, check the photographs and look at the video called "countryside"
Telemedicine guide	Please, enter the tele-medicine module. You are supposed to measure your blood pressure. Follow the instruction, take the measurement, and send the data to the service center
Domotic	Please, enter the domotic module. Switch on the light, open the window, raise the shutter and turn on the air conditioner. Now, Switch off the light, close the window, lower the shutter and turn off the air conditioner
Agenda	Enter the Agenda module and check if there are any appointments for today. Now, set up a medical examination for next week

Except for the task face recognition which always was the very first one, the order of the other tasks was randomized among participants

Right after having performed each single task they have been asked to compile the ad hoc questionnaire on usability and satisfaction referring to the single task just performed. At the end of the whole experimental session, participants have been asked to fill in the SASSI questionnaire.

3.4 Statistical Analysis

The objective of the experimentation was to investigate how perceived satisfaction could be affected by performance metrics gathered by the system. For this purpose the following linear stepwise regressions have been performed. In order to investigate the satisfaction experienced by the users while interacting with the single modules, a linear regression has been carried out per each module, where the dependent variable was represented by the results from the ad hoc questionnaire on satisfaction, and the dialogue efficiency metrics and quality metrics, regarding the single task, have been inserted into the model as independent variables. In order to investigate the overall perceived satisfaction, a further linear regression have been performed with SASSI as dependent variable and the overall efficiency and quality metrics as independent variables. In a subsequent step the introduction of each dimension of SASSI as dependent variable has been considered in order to define whether the gathered metrics affected specific aspects of perceived satisfaction. Moreover, a final regression analysis has been carried out with the main aim to investigate the weight of each module on the overall perceived satisfaction. For this purpose, the SASSI score has been inserted into the model as dependent variable, while the scores on the ad hoc questionnaires per each task where inserted as independent variables.

4 Results and Discussion

In Fig. 5 the results from questionnaires on satisfaction assessment are presented. Specifically, on the left the feedback on the overall experience is depicted, both for the overall SASSI score and for each dimension of the questionnaire. On a rating scale from 1 to 5, it can be evinced how the overall experience has been judged pretty satisfactory (M = 3.42, SD = 0.23). More in detail, participants reported good degree of *Likeability* (M = 4.03, SD = 0.69), with discrete feelings of *Annoyance* (M = 2.44, SD = 0.93) and they judge the system effortless (*Cognitive Demand*: M = 4.06, SD = 0.57). Moreover, they found no particular problems with

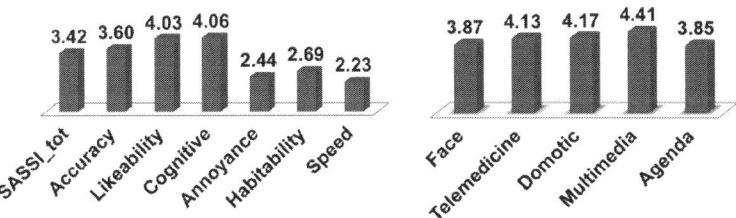

Fig. 5 Mean scores from satisfaction questionnaires. From SASSI (on the *left*) and from each module (on the *right*)

the system reactivity to their commands (*Speed*: M = 2.23, SD = 0.73), and the system behavior seemed to sufficiently match user's conceptual model on it (*Habitability*: M = 2.69, SD = 0.78).

With regard the usability and satisfaction feelings according to each module (graph on the right in Fig. 5), participants reported definitely positive judgments for every module with slight differences among them. The Multimedia Library seems to be the most appreciated module (M = 4.41, SD = 0.69), followed by the one for vocal control of the house (Domotics, M = 4.17, SD = 0.79), and the Telemedicine Guide (M = 4.13, SD = 0.79). Finally, the two modules with the lowest score were the ones devoted to the authentication to the services of SpeakyAcutattile (Face Recognition, M = 3.87, SD = 0.8), and the Agenda (M = 3.85, SD = 0.91).

In Table 3 there are the mean scores obtained by computing the performance metrics from log files and from video recordings. The table displays dialogue efficiency and dialogue quality metrics for interaction of each task according to single modules, and for the whole interaction.

4.1   Overall Satisfaction

One of the main objectives of the present study was to investigate the influence of system performance on the overall satisfaction perceived by the users during the interaction with SPEAKYACUTATTILE. The model tested through the first linear regression analysis showed that the inserted factors explained 38% of the variance in the overall satisfaction (SASSI).

More specifically, looking at Table 4, it becomes clear how the rate of system turns can affect the overall satisfaction during the interaction with the platform. Indeed, a negative association emerged, suggesting how an acceptable interaction has to be characterized by a limited intervention by the agent. This is supported also by the significant negative association with the factor *noinput*. Since this metric accounts for those times when the user pushes the button in order to stop the platform talking, it can be evinced that an increased amount of *noinput* brings to lower perception of satisfaction and usability supposedly due to excessive redundancy of system speech. Moreover, it emerged that the length of the interaction has a positive correlation with the SASSI. Namely, the more the user interacts with the platform, the higher the experienced satisfaction is resulting by the interaction itself.

These results could be reasonably interpreted as the beginning of a sort of familiarizing process where the user get confident while interacting with SPEAKYACUTATTILE increasing his/her feelings of satisfaction and confidence through time. Despite the finding that longer dialogues were associated with higher user satisfaction disagrees with the results of many previous PARADISE-style evaluation studies (i.e. [23]), our results are in line with those of [24] who also find a positive influence of dialogue length. Users could possibly need more time in order to get confident with the system and this turns in more positive feelings expressed for longer interactions that allow the users to familiarize with it. More in detail, when taking into account the subscales of the SASSI questionnaire

Table 3 Mean values (standard deviation within brackets) of performance metrics

Performance metrics	Face recognition	Multimedia library	Domotics	Telemedicine guides	Agenda	Overall interaction
TIME (sec)	185.52 (127.41)	119.35 (72.1)	156.35 (74.45)	243.55 (149.91)	156.84 (107.11)	861.61 (294.52)
USER_TURNS	6.43 (3.93)	9.91 (2.75)	10.80 (2.08)	7.46 (4.21)	12.71 (5.87)	47.23 (9.51)
SYS_TURNS	8.49 (4.00)	8.57 (1.99)	10.63 (1.78)	8.20 (3.93)	12.26 (5.33)	48.14 (8.96)
TOT_TURNS	14.49 (7.54)	18.49 (4.33)	21.43 (3.49)	15.66 (7.80)	24.97 (11.08)	95.03 (16.95)
ERRORS	0.69 (1.32)	0.86 (1.19)	0.51 (0.82)	0.46 (0.70)	1.06 (1.35)	3.57 (2.73)
NOINPUT	0.37 (0.94)	0.66 (1)	0 (0)	1.23 (2)	0.26 (0.51)	2.51 (3.93)
REPROMPT	0.83 (1.15)	1.06 (1.45)	1.49 (1.29)	0.57 (1.20)	1.31 (1.41)	5.26 (3.02)
HELP	0.06 (0.24)	0.03 (0.17)	0 (0)	0.20 (0.53)	0.20 (0.41)	0.42 (0.82)
ERRORS%	–	–	–	–	–	0.04 (0.03)
NOINPUT%	–	–	–	–	–	0.03 (0.03)
REPROPMPT%	–	–	–	–	–	0.06 (0.03)
HELP%	–	–	–	–	–	0.001 (0.04)

Table 4 Linear regression results for SASSI and its subscales

Model	AdjR^2	Factors	t	p	Beta	VIF
SASSI	0.38	Time	2.50	0.018	0.40	1.45
		Sys_turns	−3.40	0.001	−0.53	1.36
		Errors%	1.56	0.128	0.22	1.09
		Noinput%	−2.88	0.007	−0.39	1.01
Accuracy	–	–	–	–	–	–
Likeability	0.40	Tot_turns	−1.69	0.101	−0.23	1.13
		Noinput	−3.91	0.000	−0.53	1.07
		Errors%	2.56	0.015	0.35	1.07
Cognitive demand	0.13	Reprompt	−2.59	0.012	−0.45	1.19
		Errors%	1.65	0.109	0.28	1.19
Annoyance	–	–	–	–	–	–
Habitability	–	–	–	–	–	–
Speed	0.22	Time	−1.97	0.05	−0.35	1.45
		Reprompt%	−2.40	0.022	−1.13	9.90

Significant with p-value < 0.05

(Table 4), not all the models resulted significant. Specifically, no significance emerged with regard to Accuracy, Annoyance and Habitability. Nevertheless some interesting results emerged for the other subscales. Likeability seems to be affected by *noinputs* in negative way. This could mean that redundancy in interaction, and consequently the needs to stop the system, risks to undermine the perceived pleasantness and usefulness of the system.

With respect to the perceived amount of effort needed to interact with the system and the feelings resulting from this effort (Cognitive Demand), a negative influence by reprompts emerged. This means that the efforts spent in repeating several time the same commands to the platform—with no receiving answer or receiving a wrong one—can result in too much cognitive load for the users. Speed is the last dimension investigated as dependent variable in a regression linear model, and it has been found to be affected by some performance metrics. Specifically, the model showed how the percentage of repeated commands (reprompt%) and the time required to complete the task (time) influenced negatively the perceived responsiveness of the system to the users commands.

A further step envisaged within the analysis design consisted in deeper investigation of which one of the single modules could better contribute to the overall perception of usability and satisfaction during the interaction (see Table 5). The results revealed that the satisfaction experienced during the interaction with the single modules contributed for 49% to the variance of the overall satisfaction. Two modules resulted to influence the overall experience in a significant manner, the interaction with the Telemedicine Guide and the Agenda. More specifically, the

Table 5 Linear regression analysis results for SASSI and single module satisfaction

Model	AdjR^2	Factors	t	p	Beta	VIF
SASSI	0.49	Face recognition	1.77	0.08	0.25	1.34
		Telemedicine	3.00	0.005	0.56	2.34
		Domotics	−1.50	0.144	−0.27	2.27
		Agenda	3.02	0.005	0.39	1.14

P-value < 0.05 significant

Table 6 Linear regression analysis results for single modules

Model	AdjR^2	Factors	t	p	Beta	VIF
Face recognition	0.19	Time	−1.56	0.12	−0.24	1.01
		Noinput	−2.52	0.01	−0.39	1.01
Domotics	0.13	Reprompt	−2.50	0.01	−0.39	1.00
Multimedia library	0.18	Noinput	−2.95	0.005	−0.45	1.00
Agenda	0.30	Errors	−3.12	0.003	−0.45	1.03
		Help	−1.92	0.06	−0.28	1.03

P-value < 0.05 significant

contribution of the satisfaction experienced while performing these specific tasks seemed to influence in an effective way the overall experience contributing to define it as satisfactory and defining the platform as usable and useful.

It is possible to speculate on these results by recurring to qualitative comments made by the users while participating at the experimental sessions. Indeed, they particularly appreciate the Telemedicine module because of its usefulness in monitoring the health status of the persons, and because of its property devoted to foster the relation with a caregiver in order to make him aware of possible warning on the person's health status. These results can be read under the lens of well-known models of technology acceptance (TAM [25], UTAUT [26]). In fact, according to these models, the perceived usefulness represents one among the determinants of technology acceptability.

4.2 Single Module Satisfaction

Finally we were interested in understanding whether any performance metrics could somehow affect the experienced satisfaction on single modules. Actually, the coefficient of determinations did not show valuable results on the proposed models (Table 6). Moreover, many metrics have been removed through the stepwise selection and the model, where the scores from Telemedicine satisfaction were inserted as dependent variable, did not result significant at all. This could be due to a methodological issue: probably a low amount of observations per each metrics within subjects could affect the results. This issue was conversely overcome when taking into account the whole interaction.

5 Conclusions

The present work described SPEAKYACUTATTILE, an innovative assistive computer-based platform devoted to support the daily life of people. Healthy people have assessed the prototype in order to test the technology readiness, and this represented a preliminary step before introducing the solution to frail people. In fact, this solution has been conceived as an enrichment for home environment in everybody daily life, and specifically for frail people. SPEAKYACUTATTILE is primarily meant to represent a means to break down those barriers which arise when frailty comes over. Results from the evaluation bring valuable contributes to better delineate which features could be ascribable to a satisfying Spoken Language System for Ambient Assisted Living. It emerged how longer dialogues are preferred in order to positively influence the users satisfaction, suggesting the importance to let people the time to get confident with new solutions. Moreover, it emerged how system intervention should be reduced, suggesting how a good balance between user and system turns represents a further critical aspect of those systems. The same can be speculated for dialogues with no met requests that also tended to be associated with lower satisfaction scores. These last results support the importance for a vocal assistant to be effective in its purpose in order to be perceived as useful and satisfying. Overall, this experience represented a step forward bringing additional insights on SLS as valuable solutions in everyday life of people, even not taking into account possible impairment. After all, the value of such speech-based solutions in people everyday life was suggested by the wide diffusion of instruments like vocal assistants on smart phones. This work will drive the industrialization process of the SPEAKYACUTATTILE assistive platform, which will be launched on the global market in 2019. The patented product SPEAKYACUTATTILE may be a highly innovative product worldwide. Nevertheless, this work represented a preliminary step, because still further investigations on SPEAKYACUTATTILE are required now by involving frail people. The goal for further investigations is to involve blind users in order to refine the platform according to specific needs and to assess its usability within the Universal Design framework. In fact, additional efforts are still necessary in order to validate speech interfaces as meaningful means in AAL paradigms.

Acknowledgements Speaky Acutattile is partially supported by MISE under decr.conc. 00007MI01 27/05/2011.

References

1. Kamm C, Walker M (1997) Design and evaluation of spoken dialogue systems. In: IEEE workshop on automatic speech recognition and understanding, pp 14–17
2. Carbonell N, Pierrel J (1988) Recent advances in speech understanding and dialog systems. NATO ASI series F: computer and systems sciences, vol 46. Task-oriented dialogue processing in human-computer voice communication, p 491–495. Springer
3. Haton J (1988) Recent advances in speech understanding and dialog systems. NATO ASI series F: computer and systems sciences, vol 46. Knowledge-based approaches in acoustic-phonetic decoding, pp 51–70. Springer
4. Niedermair GT, Streit M, Tropf H (1990) Linguistic processing related to speech understanding in SPICOS II. Speech Commun 9:565–585
5. Ermon LD, Lesser VR (1990) The hearsay-ii speech understanding system: a tutorial. In: Waibel A, Lee K-F (eds) Readings in speech recognition. Morgan Kaufmann Publishers Inc., San Francisco, CA, USA, pp 235–245
6. Kitano H (1990) Dmdialog: a speech-to-speech dialogue translation system. Mach Transl 5 (4):301–338
7. Wood W (1990) Language processing for speech understanding. In: Waibel A, Lee K-F (eds) Readings in speech recognition. Morgan Kaufmann Publishers Inc., San Francisco, CA, USA, pp 519–533
8. Sagerer G, Kummert F (1988) Knowledge based systems for speech understanding. Springer, p 421–458
9. Young S, Russell N, Thornton J (1991) The use of syntax and multiple alternatives in the vodis voice operated database inquiry system. Comput Speech Lang 5(1):65–80
10. McGlashan S, Fraser N, Gilbert N, Bilange E, Heisterkamp P, Youd N (1992) Dialogue management for telephone information systems. In: Proceedings of the third conference on applied natural language processing, p 245–246. Association for Computational Linguistics
11. Young S, Hauptmann AG, Ward WH, Smith ET, Werner P (1989) High level knowledge sources in usable speech recognition systems. Commun ACM 32(2):183–194
12. Hoeppner W, Morik K, Marburger H (1986) Talking it over: the natural language dialog system ham-ans. In: Bolc L, Jarke M (eds) Cooperative interfaces to information systems. Springer, New York, NY, USA, pp 189–258
13. Mctear M (1987) The articulate computer. Blackwell Publishers Inc, Cambridge, MA, USA
14. Goetze S, Moritz N, Appell J-E, Meis M, Bartsch C, Bitzer J (2010) Acoustic user interfaces for ambient-assisted living technologies. Inform Health Soc Care 35(3–4):125–143
15. Becker E, Le Z, Park K, Lin Y, Makedon F (2009) Event-based experiments in an assistive environment using wireless sensor networks and voice recognition. In: Proceedings of the 2nd international conference on PErvasive technologies related to assistive environments, p 17. ACM
16. López-Cózar R, Callejas Z, Griol D, Quesada JF (2014) Review of spoken dialogue systems. Loquens 1(2):e012
17. Jian C, Schafmeister F, Rachuy C, Sasse N, Shi H, Schmidt H, von Steinbüchel N (2012) Evaluating a spoken language interface of a multimodal interactive guidance system for elderly persons. In: HEALTHINF 2012—proceedings of the international conference on health informatics, Vilamoura, Algarve, Portugal, 1–4 Feb 2012, pp 87–96
18. Krajewski J, Wieland R, Batliner A (2008) An acoustic framework for detecting fatigue in speech based human-computer-interaction. In: Proceedings of the 11th international conference on computers helping people with special needs, pp 54–61. Springer
19. Walker M, Kamm C, Litman D (2000) Towards developing general models of usability with paradise. Nat Lang Eng 6(3&4):363–377
20. Walker MA, Litman DJ, Kamm CA, Abella A (1997) Paradise: a framework for evaluating spoken dialogue agents. In: Proceedings of the eighth conference on European chapter of the

association for computational linguistics, p 271–280. Association for Computational Linguistics

21. Hone KS, Graham R (2000) Towards a tool for the subjective assessment of speech system interfaces (sassi). Nat Lang Eng 6(3&4):287–303

22. Litman DJ, Walker MA, Kearns MS (1999) Automatic detection of poor speech recognition at the dialogue level. In: Proceedings of the 37th annual meeting of the association for computational linguistics on computational linguistics, pp 309–316. Association for Computational Linguistics

23. Litman DJ, Pan S (2002) Designing and evaluating an adaptive spoken dialogue system. User Model User-Adap Inter 12(2–3):111–137

24. Foster ME, Giuliani M, Knoll A (2009) Comparing objective and subjective measures of usability in a human-robot dialogue system. In: Proceedings of the joint conference of the 47th annual meeting of the ACL and the 4th international joint conference on natural language processing of the AFNLP, vol 2. pp 879–887. Association for Computational Linguistics

25. Davis F (1989) Perceived usefulness, perceived ease of use, and user acceptance of information technology. Manage Inf Syst Q 319–340

26. Venkatesh V, Morris M, Davis G, Davis F (2003) User acceptance of information technology: toward a unified view. Manage Inf Syst Q 425–478

Quantify Yourself: Are Older Adults Ready?

Paolo Massa, Adele Mazzali, Jessica Zampini
and Massimo Zancanaro

Abstract Quantify Yourself is a recent trend by which people continuously measure walked steps, heart rate, sleep, stress and other personal indicators in order to monitor their wellbeing or life in general. Enabled by sensors currently embedded in affordable tools such as wearable devices and smartphones, Quantify Yourself has the potential for empowering each person towards an increased self-knowledge. This recent phenomenon is engaging mainly young and tech savvy people. In this paper, we explore if and how older adults track indicators related to their health and wellbeing. By means of 20 open interviews with elderly people carried out in the context of their houses, we focus on the practices and the artefacts they use. Older adults are an interesting portion of population in this regard because their health condition is usually an issue for them as individual and for the society as well and at the same time they are likely to be less prone to adopt new technologies. Some important themes are emerging from this study that might be useful to design new technology that better fits this population. In particular, the differences between the practices employed for medical and wellness indicators and between measurement and tracking; the importance of memory as the main tracking device; the sharing of artefacts between partners as well as the subjective perception of involvement during measurement with different artefacts.

Keywords Active aging · Elderly · Quantify yourself

P. Massa (✉) · M. Zancanaro
Fondazione Bruno Kessler, Via Sommarive, 18, Povo (TN), Italy
e-mail: massa@fbk.eu

M. Zancanaro
e-mail: zancana@fbk.eu

A. Mazzali · J. Zampini
Universita' di Trento, Via Calepina, 14, Trento, Italy
e-mail: adele.mazzali@hotmail.it

J. Zampini
e-mail: jessica.zampini@live.it

© Springer International Publishing AG 2017
F. Cavallo et al. (eds.), *Ambient Assisted Living*, Lecture Notes
in Electrical Engineering 426, DOI 10.1007/978-3-319-54283-6_27

377

1 Introduction

The relationship between patient and doctor has evolved little over the centuries [1]. The patient was expected to comply silently with the decisions taken by the doctor who had no obligation to provide information to the patient. This highly asymmetrical relationship, the paternalistic model, resisted up to around 30 years ago, when the relationship has moved towards greater patient control and reduced physician dominance, basically a model in which the patient is more active and autonomous but still information and knowledge is mainly in the hand of the doctor which might want or not to share it and explain it to the patient [1].

Yet, in the very few last years, we are witnessing what might be a big change in the relationship doctor-patient. Recent technologies such as different types of sensors have become smaller and hence embeddable in mobile devices such as smartphones and wearable devices and that allows anyone to continuously capture enormous amounts of information about personal life and health. This huge amount of information is going directly to the patient and not to the doctor thus possibly balancing the power between doctor and patients with the latter become more involved in understanding their own life. This empowerment of the patient might for example lead to self-diagnoses and reduced perceived needs for health professionals [2], especially as the technological trend is expected to continue and to make every human indicator automatically and continuously tracked [3]. Smartphones and wearable devices are already widespread allowing continuously tracking of indicators such as physical activities (walked steps, burnt calories), heart rate, respiration, blood pressure, sleep, diet, stress and more [2]. New revolutionary technologies are almost ready to the market, such as for example, "ingestible" technologies that collect physiological data from inside the body: smart pills detecting eaten foods, calories, responses to medications, melatonin or alcohol levels; smart miniaturized camera which once swallowed perform colonoscopies or endoscopies and communicate this data outside the body [3]. Furthermore, apps, computer programs and web sites allow to manually insert health information that are currently not automatically trackable by sensors, such as mood for instance [2].

This wealth of personal information has already attracted the interest of small and large companies: see for example ResearchKit proposed by Apple as an open source software framework by which everyone may share personal health information with the aim to advance medical research [4]. This recent phenomenon has been called in different ways, such as quantify yourself and self-tracking and, especially in the academic context, personal informatics or personal analytics [5].

Although some technologies are already widespread, self-tracking/quantify yourself is still a niche phenomenon involving a small portion of population, typically young and tech-savvy people [6]. In this paper, we focus on older adults because a quantify-yourself approach may benefit a lot this particular population although the technology acceptance may be difficult.

2   Related Work

In 2013, Pew Internet Center published a report titled "Tracking for Health" [7] whose headline was that "69% of U.S. adults track a health indicator like weight, diet, exercise routine, or symptom". They conducted telephone interviews with around 3000 adults aged 18 and older asking 30 different closed-ended questions related to health indicators tracking but also health status and use of technology. They asked how people keep track of changes about health indicators and included memory as last option in their closed-ended question ("Or do you keep track just in your head?"). Indeed, memory turned out to be the most used tool (49%) followed by paper, such as notebook or journal (34%) and only few people did use medical devices (8%), such as a glucose meter, or apps on mobile devices (7%) or computer programs, such as spreadsheet (5%). Other interesting findings are about the effects of tracking health indicators: 46% of people who tracked some indicators said tracking has changed their overall approach to health, 40% of people said it has led them to ask a doctor new questions or to get a second opinion from another doctor, hence pointing at possible changes in the relationship doctor-patient. As could be expected, people living with chronic conditions, such as high blood pressure or diabetes, were found to be significantly more likely to track a health indicator or symptom. Indeed, only 19% of U.S. adults reporting no chronic condition said they track health indicators or symptoms, whereas 40% among those reporting one chronic condition and 62% among those with two or more.

Few recent academic papers focused on the Quantify Yourself phenomenon, analyzing people who are already heavily involved in the practice and typically they are younger adults. For example, in 2010, Li et al. [5] reported results from a survey with 68 people and 11 follow-up interviews. All participants were already collecting personal information, both automatically and manually, and reflecting on it. Among information collected automatically, the most collected one were bank statements (54 out of 68), email history (52) and credit card bills (38) and interestingly there are no health related information among the top 10 automatically collected ones. Manually collected information include calendar events (27), status updates (22), work activities (22), blog posts (21) and then some indicators which are health-related: weight (21), exercise (20) and even mood (17), see Table 1 of [5]. Blood sugar level is reported to be collected only by 2 of the 68 people and it is important to highlight that participants were recruited from personal informatics sites and Quantify Yourself blogs so that for instance they were relatively young (median age range from 26 to 30) and technologically very savvy. The main contribution of this paper is a stage-based model of personal informatics composed of five stages: preparation, collection, integration, reflection, and action. Preparation occurs before people start collecting personal information and concerns itself with motivations for collecting. Collection happens when the information is really collected and is characterized by the tools used and the frequencies of collection. The integration stage is devoted to prepare and combine the different information collected. Reflection deals with looking at the collected information and exploring it.

The final stage, action, is when people decide what to do with their newfound understanding of themselves. For each stage, authors also list barriers encountered by the interviewed quantify yourselfers.

In 2011, Li et al. [2] published another paper which focuses only on the reflection phase, assuming the collection of information is already happening. In fact, authors interviewed 15 people who already self-tracked and reflected on personal data. They found that questions people ask themselves can be grouped in 6 categories: status, history, goals, discrepancies, context and factors. They also propose that the reflection stage is composed of 2 sub-phases: discovery and maintenance. Lastly, they suggest features which personal informatics tools should have to support reflection.

Finally, Choe et al. [6] focuses on extreme users of Quantify Yourself, described as "life hackers, data analysts, computer scientists, early adopters, health enthusiasts, productivity gurus, and patients". The authors analyze 52 video recordings of talks stored on the quantifiedself.com blog. In these videos extreme users, who already track personal information and often created their own technological tools for tracking and reflecting on them, explain what they did and what they have learned during the process. The goal of the paper is hence to learn pitfalls and mistakes from these extreme users.

All the papers above focused on extreme users of Quantify Yourself which have peculiar characteristics while in this paper we are interested in investigating if and how tracking of health indicators happens for older adults, a portion of population that typically is not among early adopters of new technological trends. We are aware of only one paper with this same focus: the authors interviewed 20 adults aged 51 to 94 using contextual enquiry as methodology [8]. They found that, along different artifacts for tracking personal health information, use of memory is anyway the largest and this confirms the Pew report [7]. Memory is described by participants as either a tool or a privacy strategy. They also list reasons for non-tracking such as problems with technology and routine interruption. The other main finding is related to a specific artefact, the calendar, in which older adults track doctor related information such as appointments and for which different privacy control strategies were used depending on the context: calendars in public areas such as the living room contained minimal details while in private areas such as bedrooms more detailed information were tracked. Based on this, authors suggest that new digital calendars should incorporate a feature that "allows information presented to change based on location".

3   Interview Study of Health Tracking in Older Adults

Our study involved 20 older adults living in North East Italy (Verona, Mantova and Vicenza provinces). They were recruited starting from two relatives of the authors and using a snowball sampling which consists in asking the participants to involve other acquaintances and neighbors. We included only adults with 60 or more years and living independently. The age ranged from 61 to 87 with a mean age of 74. Females were 13 out of 20.

Similarly to the Pew report [7] (and differently from all the papers discussed above) we chose to not adopt as an inclusion criterion whether the participants already tracked some indicators or not. We did that because we were interested also in patterns of non-tracking and motivations behind it.

From a methodological point of view, we used contextual inquiry [9] because we believe the importance of the context is crucial in letting emerge real practices and motivations for tracking of health indicators. For this reason, all interviews occurred in the houses of the participants and were semi-structured and complemented by observations of context and artefacts. Moreover, when some tracking was described by the older adults, we asked them to perform the tracking itself and explain it (perform and think aloud) possibly using the real artefacts. All participants lived in their houses, sometimes with a partner, sometimes alone.

The health status is expected to influence the need for and attitudes towards health indicators tracking so we describe it here briefly. All 20 participants have at least one health condition (as in [8]): 16 have health issues related with their blood pressure, 9 heart issues and 5 diabetes, 5 reported high cholesterol levels, 2 osteoporosis and 2 reported breathing difficulties.

Another important aspect is related to technology: among our 20 participants, only one was able to use apps on smartphones and to browse the web with a computer. That is very different from the 20 older adults interviewed in [8] where 17 had computer or laptop experience and 11 of them owned their own computer.

Regarding the protocol to guide the semi-structured interviews, we considered the indicators that emerged in previous works discussed above but we decided to exclude those not related to health or wellness (for instance Li et al. [5] reports how the most collected indicators are related to finance).

For each indicator, we set out to investigate: motivation for tracking that indicator (both for starting and for keeping doing it regularly) or for non-tracking it; how the tracking actually happens, when and how frequently, where, the consequences of tracking, and the possible sharing of the information tracked.

According to the tenets of contextual inquiry, we also focused on the specific artefacts used and the practices involved. These aspects were investigated asking the participants to perform and think aloud the tracking as it occurs normally in their houses and by using the real artefacts. Following the suggestion of previous studies [7, 8], we included memory as a tool for tracking.

All interviews were recorded and later transcribed. During the interviews, we asked older adults permission to take photographs of artefacts. The interviews lasted from 10 to 70 min with a mean of 52. The transcriptions were coded using thematic analysis [10].

4   Results

In this section we report results of the analysis of interview transcripts.

4.1   Two Types of Indicators: Health and Wellness

Eleven (11) different health indicators were tracked at least once by the 20 older adults we interviewed: blood pressure (90%), weight (75%), physical activity (65%), sleep patterns (55%), heart rate (50%), medications (40%), mood (35%), blood sugar level (30%), cholesterol (25%), blood oxygen saturation (5%) and eaten food (5%). We did not investigate doctor appointments since we considered them as being an event reminder, even if connected with health, rather than an indicator to be tracked.

We found that indicators could be grouped into 2 main categories: medical indicators and wellness indicators. Medical indicators were blood pressure, heart rate, blood sugar level, blood oxygen saturation, cholesterol and taken medications. Wellness indicators were physical activity, eaten food (diet), weight, sleep patterns and mood.

The differences between the two categories are mainly due to motivation for tracking and tools used for tracking.

Typically, medical indicators were required to be tracked by a medical professional because they were necessary to monitor a chronic condition which, if not controlled, might result in serious health problems. On the other hand, wellness indicators were not immediately tied to important chronic conditions so there was no external pressure for tracking them and the motivation was hence only intrinsic.

With regard to the tools used, medical indicators were usually characterized by technological artefacts, medical devices able to measure the indicator itself, for example the sphygmomanometer, for measuring blood pressure and heart rate, or the glucometer, for measuring glucose (sugar) in the blood.

Wellness indicators, on the other hand, were usually not characterized by the use of a technological artefact (with the exception of weight, of course). Indeed, for wellness indicators our participants just use their memory for measuring so there was a high level of ambiguity in analyzing the interviews on whether the indicator was tracked or not. For example, for sleep patterns, we regarded the indicator as tracked if the participant was reporting some kind of reflection about the quality of their sleep almost every day: we had 11 out of 20 older adults tracking sleep patterns as wellness indicator. Mood was considered tracked only if the participant was actively reflecting about their mood, at least some times in a week (7 older adults reported this practice). Diet was even more ambiguous: all participants had a degree of awareness of which foods they ate but only one was actively reflecting about the properties of the foods eaten and the possible impact on his health.

4.2 Measurement and Tracking: Two Different Sub-phases

From the analysis of the transcripts of the 20 interviews, it emerges that older adults were engaged in two different phases in tracking the indicators: the measurement and the tracking itself.

Measurement is the phase in which a numerical information (data) is obtained, while tracking is the phase in which something is done with this information: for example, some of our participants measure the blood pressure and heart rate with the sphygmomanometer and then track the numerical values (max, min and pulse) with a pen on a piece of paper (see Fig. 1).

It is worth noting that usually these technological medical devices used for measuring also support the phase of tracking by allowing an automatic recording of the data. Yet, none of the 20 older adults we interviewed used this feature and preferred to rely either on their memory or on pen and paper. We will further discuss this aspect below.

When there are no artefacts for measurement, the process is in general more ambiguous: for example, someone can "measure" their mood by reflecting on it, simply by asking themselves if they are happy or sad and trying to think about the reasons and then "track" their mood using an app for smartphone or pen and paper or just using their memory to remind themselves about their past mood. None of the 20 older adults actively use technological artefacts for tracking. However, when the mind is involved as a tool, either for measurement or tracking, the processes are

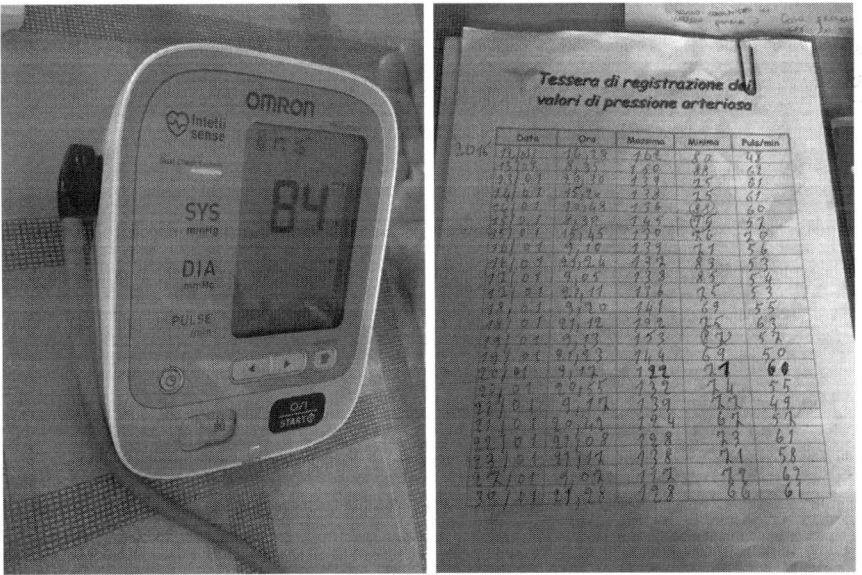

Fig. 1 Artefacts used for measurement (sphygmomanometer, *left*) and for tracking (sheets of paper). The health indicator is blood pressure and heart rate

mental and internal to the mind of the older adults and hence more difficult to unambiguously characterize. On the other hand, when there is an artefact involved, as for most of the medical indicators, it is easier to ask to think about the practice with perform and think-aloud methodology and hence to get a clearer picture of the practice.

Nevertheless, we believe it is extremely useful to keep the two phase of measurement and tracking separated and this division is not proposed in previous papers such as [2, 5, 6, 8]. We believe these two phases can be considered as a specification of the stage "collection" of the stage-based model for personal informatics [5] which suggests to divide the Quantify Yourself practice in five stages: preparation, collection, integration, reflection, action. Just as the authors of [5] in a following paper [2] suggested to divide the stage "reflection" into two phases: discovery and maintenance, we have some evidence about the division of the stage "collection" in two phases: measurement and tracking.

4.3 Tools for Measuring and Tracking: Artefacts and Mind

As already introduced, different artefacts characterize the two phases, measurement and tracking, and the two types of indicators, medical and wellness.

Medical indicators typically have dedicated artefacts for measurement, medical devices specifically designed for that indicators which the older adults own and keep in their houses and use frequently, in general at least daily. Those include the sphygmomanometer, for measuring blood pressure and heart rate, that is used by 18 of the 20 older adults we interviewed. As noted above, 6 of our participants had diabetes and so they used the glucometer for measuring glucose in the blood (see Fig. 2). Other artefacts used are the pulse oximeter, used by one person for measuring the oxygen saturation of the blood because of a chronic condition related to breathing issues (see Fig. 2).

Interestingly, nobody used computer programs or smartphone apps for tracking indicators. The reason for this is that the 20 older adults we interviewed reported an almost non existent use of technology: as already reported, only one is able to use apps on smartphone. This result is very different from what emerged in the related researches [2, 5, 6] but we somehow expected that because on those works authors analyzed extreme users of quantify yourself while we focused on older adults with very low technological skills. Indeed, our findings are in line with the 2013 Pew study [7] whose results, grouped also for different age ranges, show that, for the 830 adults aged 65 or more they interviewed by telephone, 12% of them use a medical device for tracking, only 2% use computer programs, 1% use smartphone apps while paper-based tools are used by 41% and mind from 44% of the older adults. A similar effect was also noted in the 20 interviews to older adults analyzed by Miller and colleagues [8].

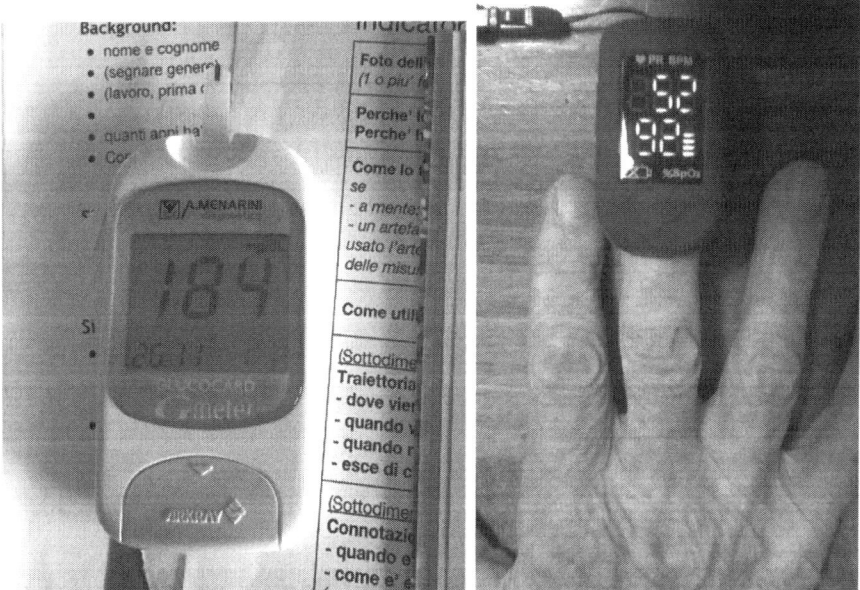

Fig. 2 glucometer (*left*) and pulse oximeter (*right*)

For what concerns wellness indicators, we observed the lack of technological devices used for the measurement (with the exception of the weighing machine for weight): this means self-reflection and memory are usually used for measurement and also memory is usually used for tracking. Thirteen (13) participants reported that they do some physical activity but none of them use an artefact for tracking it even if wearable devices for tracking steps and calories burnt are easily available on the market. Sleep patterns were measured and tracked without artefacts by 11 of our participants, mood by 7 and 1 for diet.

Actually, the situation is different for weight since there is a common artefact used for measuring it and widely available: the weighing machine. Fifteen (15) older adults reported that they measure weight and 13 of them used the weighing machine, either one they own in their houses or one they can use in a community center. Still, 2 older adults reported they "measure" their weight using their clothes which is an artefact already present in their life and that, if properly augmented with technology, might be more acceptable to older adults than other technologies.

In conclusion, medical indicators are characterized by the use of physical artefacts for measurement and tracked mainly with paper-based tools while wellness indicators are measured mainly with self-reflection and memory and tracked mainly by memory as well.

4.4   Sharing: Of Artefacts, Not of Tracked Data

In our interview protocol, we decided to investigate older adults also for what concerns their sharing of the tracked data. Indeed, the Pew Report [7] found that 761 (25%) out of 3014 interviewed people shared the tracked information with someone, typically the medical professional (52%) and the partner (22%).

Indeed, some of the older adults we interviewed reported that they share the information with the doctor by bringing the block-note or diary with them when they visit him or her.

However, we found it is much more common to share the measurement artefact itself: in fact 14 out of 20 older adults live with the partner and often the partner has similar chronic conditions which require monitoring the same medical indicator. So, they actually share the same artefact for measurement.

In fact, 10 older adults reported how they share the same artefact for measurement, typically the sphygmomanometer. Interestingly, in all these cases but one, there is one senior which take care of the process for both partners, i.e. he or she measures the blood pressure for both and also keep track of the measured information for both. In this way, they also share the results, compare them and somehow monitor each other. It is interesting to note that often the medical device has a feature for keeping two separated profiles and recording the measurements in a separate way: all of them are aware of the feature but none of them use it and prefer to use one profile because they are not confident with technology and this feature is too complex for them.

4.5   Perception of Active Involvement
During Measurement and Tracking

We also investigated if tracking health indicators had consequences. This again was inspired by the Pew study [7] which reported how 46% of trackers said tracking has changed their overall approach to health, 40% of trackers said it has led them to ask a doctor new questions or to get a second opinion from another doctor.

Yet, among our 20 participants, only 2 reported similar consequences: one decides the amount of medications by herself and also ask advice to a different doctor. Another one tried to predict when and how the doctor proposes changes in medications and, considering himself successful in doing this, he felt as good as the doctor.

The Pew report [7] found larger consequences of health indicator tracking but the reason behind this difference might be that the Pew interviews were done as close-ended questions, yes or no answers to the question "*In which of the following ways, if any, has tracking this health indicator affected your own health care routine (…)? Has it changed your overall approach to maintaining your health (…)*" and respondents might have been more inclined to answer positively to this closed-ended questions by telephone than to our open-ended questions asked in their houses.

Indeed, another interesting element emerged: their perception of active involvement, physical and mental, during the measurement phase. In particular, 3 older adults elicited how they felt passive and not involved when they use their digital sphygmomanometer. They felt that it is too much automatic and they do not have to do anything. They also reported their belief that the measurement is not as accurate as with analogical sphygmomanometers especially since they see that their doctor uses the analogical sphygmomanometer and not the digital one. These participant not only lamented this fact but also suggested to design future digital artefacts for tracking health indicators in a way that does not exclude too much the tracker, especially if they are designed for older adults which might prefer to remain in control of the process and physically participate in it.

4.6 Barriers to Tracking

We classified four kinds of barriers to tracking with artefacts that emerged from the analysis of the interview transcripts.

The first obstacle is related to confidence in use of technology. As we already discussed, the 20 participants do not routinely use technology such as smartphones or computers. This means that, differently from hackers and extreme quantifiers analyzed in [2, 5, 6], our participants were not able to consider and possibly use the many apps for smartphone already available for tracking physical activity, sleep patterns, mood and other indicators [4].

A second barrier, especially for wellness indicators, is related to the perceived importance of these indicators: since doctors do not usually require to monitor them, they are perceived as not too important and hence measurement and tracking is very light, and only with the mind.

The third barrier is related to the fact measurement and tracking have not become part of their daily routines: our participants reported they have very regular and repetitive days with consolidate routines and the specific measurements were not part of these routines. In general, it seems it is only the doctor who is able to induce a change in these routines when he or she requires the older adults to start tracking a medical indicator which is related to a critical chronic condition. Two similar aspects emerged also from [8]: that tracking interrupts daily routine and that tracking is time intensive.

Finally, emotions can act as a barrier for tracking health indicators. Older adults are worried of becoming obsessed with the measurement tools and health indicators and to keep measuring them too often. Similarly, we found a negative feeling looking at the measurement, some sort of dissatisfaction. In a similar way in [8] one of the obstacles was "want to avoid thinking about their health condition".

5 Conclusion

While a portion of the population, young, tech-savvy adults, are already using smartphones and wearable devices to automatically track walked steps, heart rate, sleep quality and more, in this paper we explore if and how older adults track health indicators and they are likely to be ready to get the new wave of personal devices and sensors. Older adults, who might benefit immensely from self-tracking and an increased self-knowledge of themselves, usually do not use these tools.

With our field study, we aimed at understanding the practices around measurement and tracking of health and wellness indicators when artefacts are involved and when they are not. We carried out interviews with 20 people aged 60 and more using semi-structured interviews and we used contextual enquiry as methodological viewpoint. We found that there are differences in terms of motivation for tracking and artefacts used between medical and wellness indicators: typically, medical indicators such as blood pressure, heart rate and blood sugar level are required to be tracked by a doctor and measured with medical devices while wellness indicators such as sleep or mood were measured with the mind and the motivation for tracking them originated from the older adults and not someone else.

We also found evidence of the need to keep separated the two phases of measurement and tracking: measurement is when a numerical data is obtained while tracking is the following phase in which something is done with this information. They are characterized by different artefacts and practices and we believe they constitute a specification of "collection" which is one of the 5 stages of the model for personal informatics which comprises preparation, collection, integration, reflection and action.

Artefacts were presented mainly for medical indicators: medical devices for measuring them and paper-based artefacts (block-notes and journals) for tracking them. The presence of technology was very reduced among the 20 older adults we interviewed and none of them used computer programs or smartphone apps for tracking them. Wellness indicators were measured and tracked mainly with the mind.

Some older adults reported that digital devices were making them feel excluded from the measurement process because they had nothing to do. As a consequence of this, they also believed their measurements were not as precise as with analogical devices which require physical participation in the process of measurement.

The information tracked about indicators was in general little and consequently there was not too much sharing of it with other people such as the doctor. However, there were interesting practices of sharing measurement artefacts among co-living partners and also almost always one of the two partners was in charge of measurement and tracking of health indicators for the other partner.

We also identified 4 barriers to tracking health indicators as they emerged from the analysis of the interviews. First, the lack of confidence with technology; second, the perception that some health indicators, especially wellness ones, are not important and so there is a lack of motivation for tracking them; third, tracking is not part of a routine. Fourth, emotions, such as fear of becoming obsessed with an indicator or to be disappointed in seeing a disliked measurement, might also refrain older adults from measuring and tracking medical and wellness indicators.

We believe that these results can help in designing better tools and practices for tracking health indicators which might be easier to be adopted and enjoyed also by older adults.

Acknowledgements This research has been funded by project ActiveAgeing@Home (Ministero dell'Istruzione, dell'Università e della Ricerca, Italy).

References

1. Kaba R, Sooriakumaran P (2007) The evolution of the doctor-patient relationship. Int J Surg 5 (1):57–65
2. Li I, Anind KD, Jodi F (2011) Understanding my data, myself: supporting self-reflection with ubicomp technologies. In: Proceedings of the 13th international conference on Ubiquitous computing. ACM
3. Ingestibles, Wearables and Embeddables. Federal Communications Commission. Web. https://www.fcc.gov/general/ingestibles-wearables-and-embeddables
4. Research Kit. Apple. Web. http://www.apple.com/researchkit/
5. Li I, Anind D, Jodi F (2010) A stage-based model of personal informatics systems. In: Proceedings of the SIGCHI conference on human factors in computing systems. ACM
6. Choe EK et al (2014) Understanding quantified-selfers' practices in collecting and exploring personal data. In: Proceedings of the 32nd annual ACM conference on Human factors in computing systems. ACM
7. Fox S, Maeve D (2013) Tracking for health. Pew Research Center's Internet & American Life Project. http://pewinternet.org/Reports/2013/Tracking-forHealth.aspx
8. Miller, S, Bilge M, John L (2013) Artifact usage, context, and privacy management in logging and tracking personal health information in older adults. In: Proceedings of the human factors and ergonomics society annual meeting, vol 57, no 1. SAGE Publications, USA
9. Beyer H, Karen H (1997) Contextual design: defining customer-centered systems. Elsevier, The Netherlands
10. Boyatzis RE (1998) Transforming qualitative information: thematic analysis and code development. Sage publishing, USA

Telemedicine for Dementia-Affected Patients: The AAL-ACCESS Project Experience

Gianfranco Raimondi, Paolo Casacci, Giuseppe Sancesario, Beatrice Scordamaglia, Gaia Melchiorri and Massimo Pistoia

Abstract Alzheimer's disease now affects about 5% of people over 60 years and in Italy, it means about 500,000 patients. It is the most common form of dementia, a state caused by an alteration of the brain function that implies a serious difficulty to conduct normal daily activities. This work describes the experience gained with development and experimentation of an ICT system to remotely support the care of the person with cognitive impairment within the AAL ACCESS Project.

Keywords Telemedicine · Alzheimer · Remote control · HRV

1 Introduction

The elderly and their family carers face many barriers in their daily life, as do the professionals providing care services. The sharing of information is a crucial issue, especially when medical information is needed to adapt drug prescription to the patient's specific condition. The communication and interaction between an elder person and relatives, home carers, nurses, and other professionals is typically unreliable and not coordinated. Therefore, the information about how the situation

G. Raimondi
"Sapienza" University of Rome, P.le Aldo Moro, 8, 00185 Rome, Italy

P. Casacci (✉) · M. Pistoia
Liferesult s.r.l., Via Stefano de Stefano n. 23, Foggia (FG) 71121, Italy
e-mail: paolo.casacci@liferesult.it

M. Pistoia
e-mail: massimo.pistoia@liferesult.it

G. Sancesario · B. Scordamaglia · G. Melchiorri
Tor Vergata University of Rome, Via Orazio Raimondo,18, 00173 Rome, Italy
e-mail: beatricescorda@gmail.com

G. Melchiorri
e-mail: gaiamelchiorri79@gmail.com

© Springer International Publishing AG 2017   391
F. Cavallo et al. (eds.), *Ambient Assisted Living*, Lecture Notes
in Electrical Engineering 426, DOI 10.1007/978-3-319-54283-6_28

evolves is not effectively shared between those stakeholders and prevents proper adaptation of intervention to the actual evolution.

The ACCESS project designed and implemented a communication system for sharing data between elderly people and "their" stakeholders, especially family carers, through electronic devices. The project aimed to implement all necessary coordination and electronic communication between the different actors involved in home care. One of the objectives was to implement an easy and permanent communication system to remotely monitor the old person's state of health, in order to assess the effectiveness of therapies and medications.

The use of technology as a support and medical attention to different types of diseases is now a common feature in several research projects conducted at European and national level. Diseases such as Alzheimer's or stroke, considered among the leading causes of disability, are at the center of these projects [7].

In the integrated management of the disease, the patient and his family are the center of a network which includes specialized outpatient services, day centers, home care services, the nursing homes, the long-term care and the hospital.

The integrated management is made easier by the use of electronic health records, which allow the sharing of patient information from all those involved. The adoption of this approach seems to be the most appropriate care, since it can allow a slowing in the progression of the disease and improved quality of life for the patient and his family.

The innovation of this proposal lied on the development of an integrated system allowing storage and transmission of large volumes of information and data, generated not only by the senior (user) and the family carers or professionals but also by automatic devices.

The project was developed in three countries: Italy, France and Belgium, each one in a specific way according to the demand and context, providing an adaptable panel of services. In Italy the project was declined in the direction of clinical monitoring of vital parameters and patients' mood and state of health, to assess efficacy of Alzheimer treatment. The work was carried on by the group of Neurology at the Tor Vergata University (Rome), with the contribution of La Sapienza University Group of Cardiology, along with technology partner Liferesult.

In this concern we worked on the ability to remotely monitor patients with dementia in their own homes, with the support of a caregiver and especially of high-tech devices with data transmission to a reference center. Our approach required the monitoring of several parameters considering the patient as a whole, i.e. taking into account not only the cardiovascular circadian rhythms, but also the respiratory activity and movement, thus providing a more complete and comprehensive appreciation of the person in his normal everyday activities.

The chosen devices to be employed in the work were a wearable device (detector of heart parameters), a tablet to collect data at the patient's premises, and a cloud server to compute data.

2 Materials and Methods

The ACCESS project has accounted for the technological partner Liferesult, already normally engaged in the study of information technology solutions for life-sciences, a strong push to study the matter of clinical monitoring of vital signs. In particular, a considerable amount of effort was spent on the use of an advanced biomedical sensor, able to record with considerable precision data on cardiac functions and patient mobility while presenting very reduced dimensions.

The research carried out in the project began with the study of sensor data transmission, which takes place via Bluetooth communication protocol. The inherently limited range of the signal, less than 10 m, required the development of a local software layer, installed on a tablet PC also equipped with Bluetooth functionality. This additional layer would allow the interconnection of two devices and would allow data transmission from the sensor to the tablet on one side, while on the other would allow sending software strings for appropriate sensor configuration.

The vital parameter detection device used was MR&D's Pulse Sensor™, based on ST Microelectronics BodyGateway™ chipset. It is a wearable, battery operated device intended for use as a part of a multiparameter analysis system. It uses a sensorized component adhesive (plaster), placed on the body of the assisted person. It can record symptomatic and asymptomatic events and is suitable for ambulatory monitoring of non-lethal cardiac arrhythmias. The device permits to record heart rate, respiratory rate and, through a specific algorithm, the level of activity of the person, providing the management system of continuous or periodic messages of information to/from the server according to specific settings defined by operators. Available data and parameters depend on the selected operative mode. In fact the device can be configured to operate in two different modes:

- Streaming Mode: is when the device is powered ON and sampling the data as specified in the configuration settings, sending them directly to the associated device with periodicity specified by the last configuration commands received from the associated device.
- Monitoring mode: is when the device is powered ON, gathering and storing in the internal memory data at the frequency specified in the configuration settings, and sending the data as requested by the associated device.

Sampling frequencies for each monitored parameter can be read in the table below (Table 1).

From the device we can obtain a record for 5-min each hour in which the ECG (signal and R-R interval), breath frequency, position and activity level are reported; then in the day we can potentially observe 24 records and we have the possibility to have not only the ECG abnormalities (arrhythmias or conduction's defects) but also the neurovegetative assessment during the normal activity.

The next step in the project was the creation of software modules constituting an application installed on a tablet, to store the downloaded data locally before its transmission to the central server. This latter is the architectural element of the

Table 1 Sampling frequencies in the Pulse™ device

Signals and parameters	Streaming mode	Monitoring mode
ECG raw	128/256 Hz	128/256 Hz
Heart rate	1 each 10–15–30–60 s	1 each 10–15–30–60 s
Heart rate reliability	1 each 10 s	1 each 10 s
R-R variability	1 each 10 s	1 each 10 s
XYZ raw	50.0 Hz	–
Activity level	1 each 5–10–15–30–60 s	1 each 5–10–15–30–60 s
BIOIMP-Z0 raw	32 Hz	–
BIOIMP-DZ raw	32 Hz	–
Respiration rate	1 each 15–30–60 s	1 each 15–30–60 s
Battery level	1 each 10–15–30–60 s	1 each 10–15–30–60 s

system on which doctors log on to see patient data and operate analysis and evaluation of the recorded information. In order to allow an easier management of patients at home, Liferesult has chosen, in agreement with the medical team of the Regional Centre of Alzheimer's Policlinico Tor Vergata, an asynchronous mode for data transmission. The tablet keeps waiting for the connection of a monitoring device; when one paired device falls within the Bluetooth detection range, the tablet start the download process of all data in the device. If the transfer is successful, the device's internal memory is cleared to leave more space for new data and the tablet returns a visual confirmation of the successful acquisition of data in the user interface window (Graphical User Interface, GUI). Then the tablet, by means of a 3G mobile data connection, provides to transfer the patient data on the central server, exploiting a data exchange methodology based on Web Services. In the tablet app, available to the caregiver of the patient, an additional feature of daily "diary" is implemented: the family member or the person who is treating the patient may signal the occurrence of physical problems or alteration of the normal behavior through a feature available in the application. In this way, information on any adverse reactions to medications, mood changes, or changes in the circadian rhythm, may be brought promptly and effectively to knowledge of the treating specialist.

The medical team, if desired, can set an "agenda" of daily activities to be performed or to be monitored at the patient's home. A specific functionality of the application notifies to the caregiver, with visual and sound reminders, the need to verify the assumption of medicines and fluids, or the need to monitor certain patient behaviors during the day. This feature can be configured easily and is fully customizable by the doctor, depending on the patient's specific needs and situation. Refer to Fig. 1 for a screenshot of the tablet application.

The central server, that collects and makes available all data of patients in punctual and aggregate form, by showing graphs and trend curves, has been realized through the Omniacare platform. Omniacare is a software product endowed with very broad characteristics of configurability, scalability and robustness.

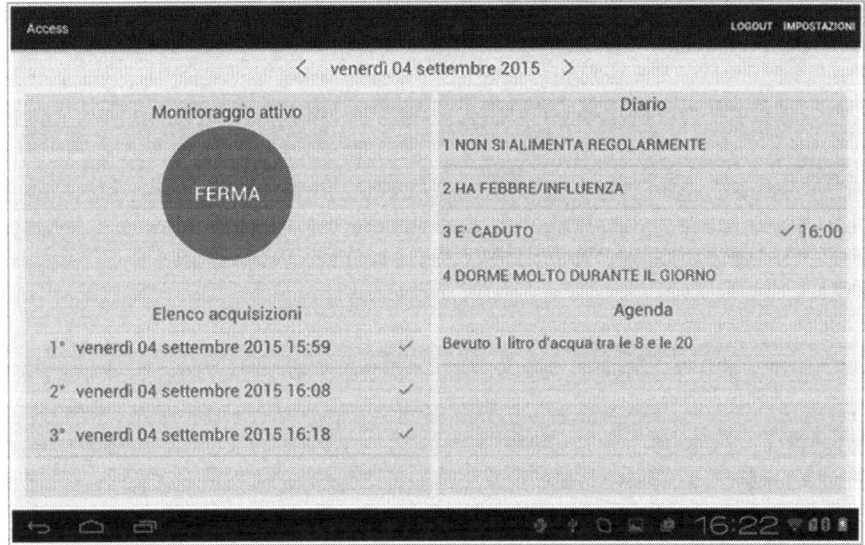

Fig. 1 Tablet application

A specific verticalization for the ACCESS project was realized, comprising a series of features:

– Patient management (personal data, medical history, medical records, current therapies).
– Charts of monitoring data (ECG curve, R-R interval, level of physical activity, heart rate, respiratory rate).
– Comparative analysis of data and curves of vital signs.
– Therapy management.
– Agenda Setting and patient diary.

Omniacare offers a comprehensive list of comparative charts, including ECG curves on equivalent grid graph paper, where the x axis is scaled on 1 mm = 40 ms (25 mm/s). The platform is accessible via any Internet connection, using the most common browsers (Internet Explorer, Mozilla Firefox, Google Chrome ...). The doctor, with appropriate credentials and permissions, can access information about his patients anywhere and prepare comparative analyses, based on the curves of recorded parameters. This allows the evaluation of the disease evolution, with particular regard to the patient's response to drug therapy, in order to adapt the type and dosage of medication to the situation of the individual patient, based on objective factors and thus improving the quality of care (Figs. 2, 3, 4, 5, 6, 7 and 8).

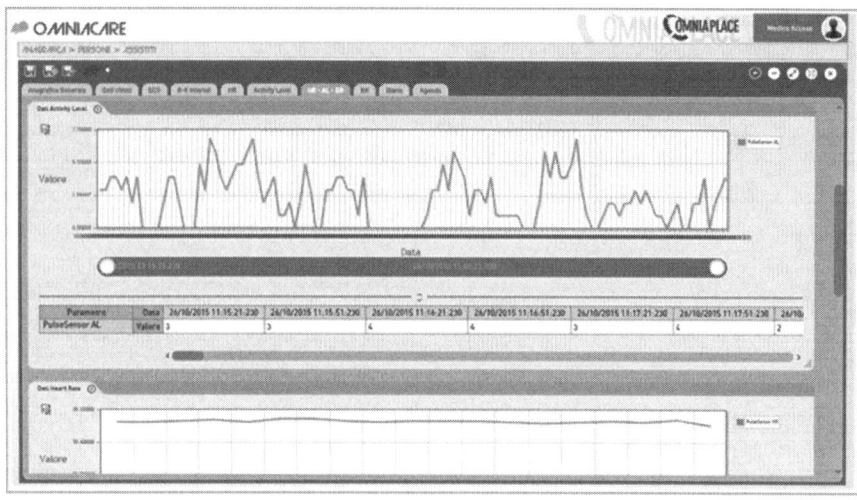

Fig. 2 Central server

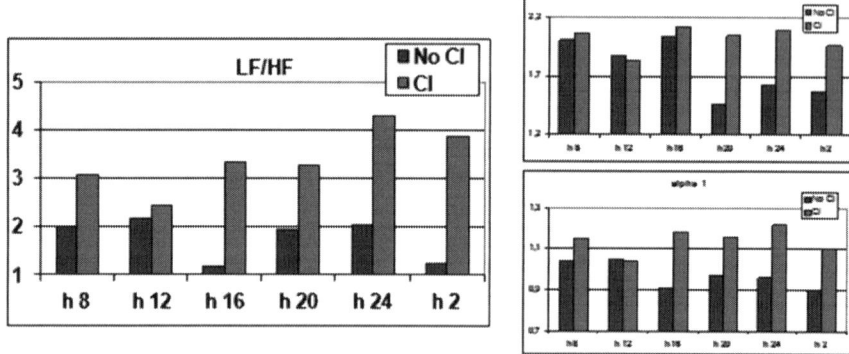

Fig. 3 Graphical HRV analysis of the enrolled patients

3 Clinical Aspects

Particular attention is required when prescribing psychotropic medications in patients affected by Alzheimer, because sometimes they may induce serious, although preventable, iatrogenic effects [8]. The cholinergic activity of acetyl cholinesterase inhibitors and the anticholinergic properties of the antipsychotics agents are both related to the vagal modulation that can be observed from the surveys of the electrocardiogram (ECG) [6, 11]. We hypothesized that the early ECG recording with remote control can be predictive of not only the side effects of treatment with neuroleptics and with acetyl cholinesterase inhibitors, but also the

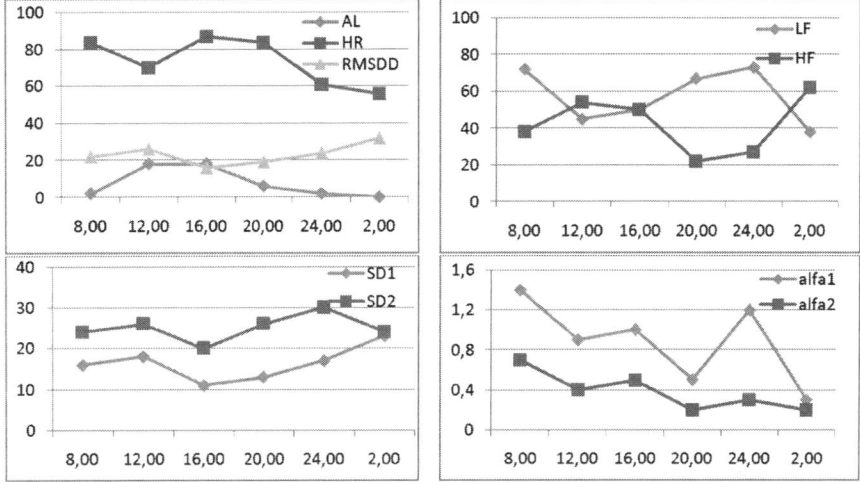

Fig. 4 Patient with pseudo normal neurovegetative assessment

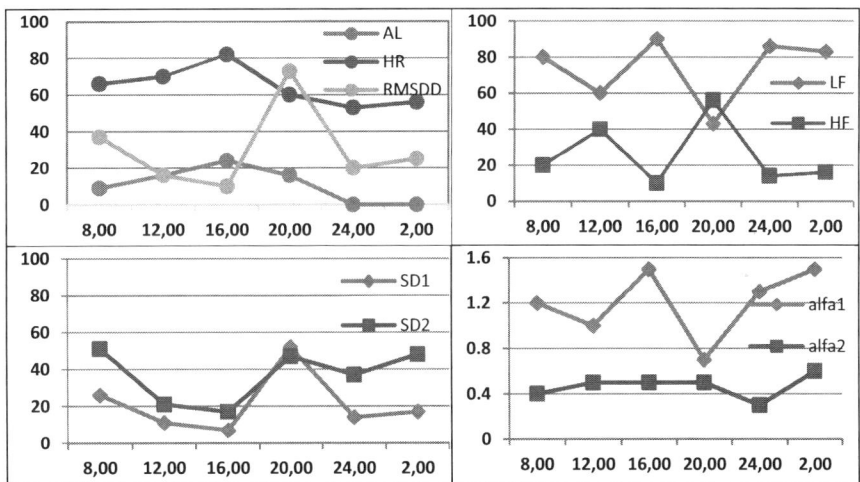

Fig. 5 Patient with sympathetic hyperactivity

neurovegetative cardiovascular daily assessment [10, 14]. Then the clinical aim of this project was to evaluate the ability to monitor the daily autonomic assessment in patients with dementia by means of the HRV analysis of ECG signal [2].

The Pulse sensor employed in the ACCESS Project permits to record heart rate, respiratory rate and, through a specific algorithm, the level of activity of the person, providing the management system of continuous or periodic messages of information to/from the server according to the specific settings defined by operators.

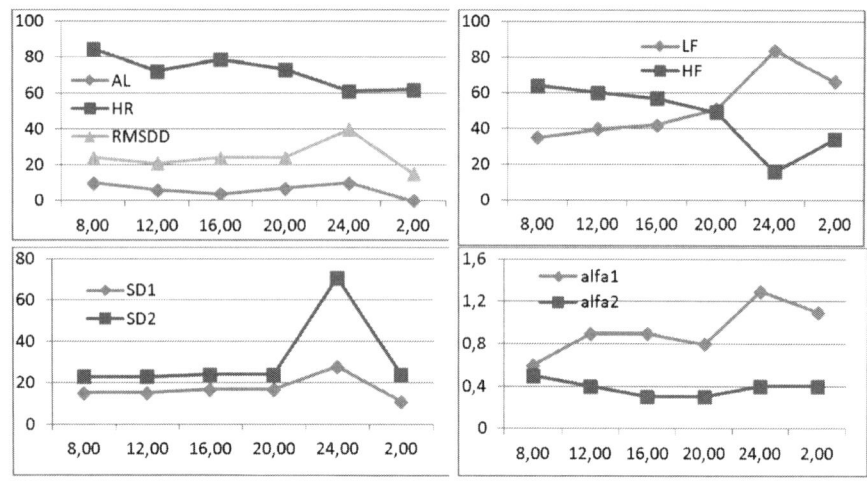

Fig. 6 Patient with sympathetic hyperactivity only during the evening and the night

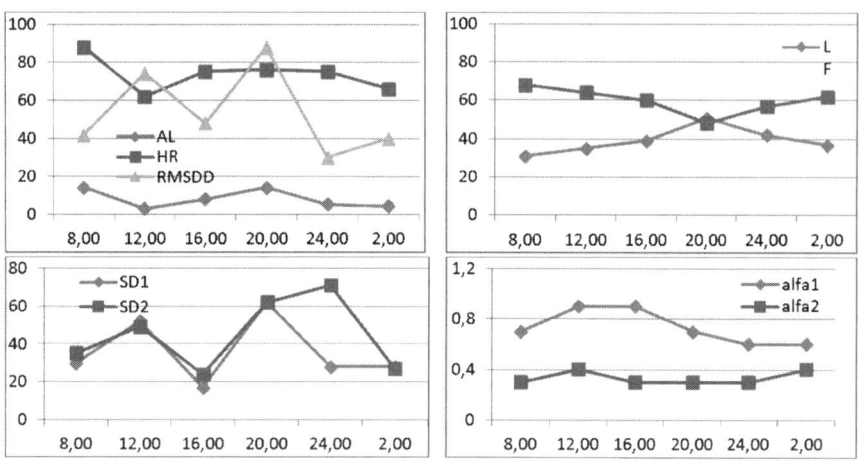

Fig. 7 Patient with parasympathetic hyperactivity during all the day

From the records we can extrapolate by means of KUBIOS-HRV software the HRV analysis, both linear and nonlinear. Linear methods include traditional statistical analysis (SDNN, RMSSD) and the analysis of the HRV through the frequency domain [1] calculating the LF, HF and LF/HF Ratio components. Nonlinear methods include the Poincarè plot (SD1 and SD2 indexes) and the Detrended Fluctuation Analysis (DFA-α1 and α2 indexes) [16, 17, 19].

Heart rate variability (HRV) is a powerful non-invasive method for analyzing the function of the autonomic nervous system [18]. It is useful to understand the interplay between the sympathetic and parasympathetic autonomic nervous system,

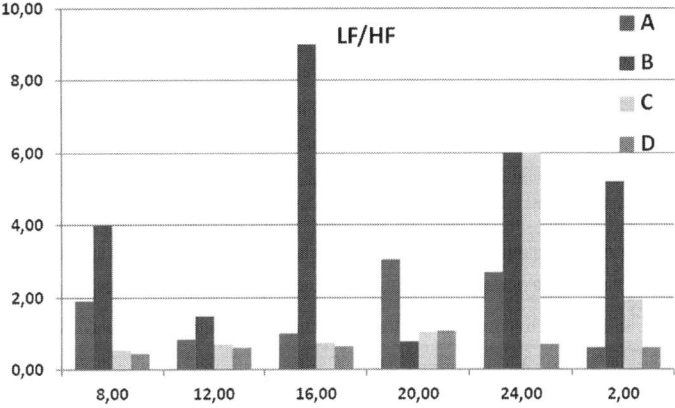

Fig. 8 LF/HF ratio in the 4 patients

which serves to speed up and slow down the heart rate, respectively. HRV, the variation of the time period between consecutive heart beats, is thought to reflect the heart's adaptability to the changing physiological conditions. It is dependent predominantly on the extrinsic regulation of the heart rate. Assessment of HRV provides quantitative information about the modulation of heart rate (HR) by sympathetic nervous system (SNS) and parasympathetic nervous system (PNS). Interactions of SNS and PNS using HRV signal have been well studied and their importance established with a number of cardiac diseases including myocardial infarction, patients with congestive heart failure [20], patients at risk of sudden cardiac death and patients with hypertension. There are two main approaches to the analysis of HRV: time-domain and frequency-domain analysis.

Time-domain indices, i.e., Mean, standard deviation (SD), standard deviation of normal RR intervals (SDNN), standard deviation of averaged normal RR intervals (SDANN) are derived from simple statistical calculations based on interbeat intervals (RR intervals). These indices are sensitive to transients and trends in the sample of heartbeats, and as such provide estimates of overall and beat-to-beat variability [4].

Frequency-domain analysis, which is based on the power spectral density of the heart rate time series, highlights the issue of the underlying rhythms of the mechanisms controlling heart rate (HR) and identified three major spectral peaks (high frequency (HF: 0.15–0.4 Hz), low frequency (LF: 0.04–0.15 Hz) and very low frequency (VLF: below 0.04 Hz) in the adult HR spectrum. These measurements can be derived from short-term (i.e. 5 to 30 min) or long-term ECG recordings (i.e. 24 h). HRV has been used as a non-invasive marker of the activity of the autonomic nervous system for over two decades [12, 13]. The necessary guidelines for comparing different studies of HRV have been established by the Task force of ESC and NPSE. It has been suggested that the time-domain methods are ideal for the analysis of long-term HRV signal.

As concerns nonlinear analysis, namely Poincarè plots [5, 15], a two-dimensional vector analysis was used to quantify the shape of the plots. In this quantitative method, short-term (SD1) and long-term (SD2) R-R interval variability and the ellipse area of the plot are quantified separately. SD2 is considered to reflect vagal modulation of the sinus node. As concerns Detrended fluctuation analysis (DFA), this technique is used to quantify the fractal scaling properties of short- and intermediate-term R-R interval time series. The HR correlations were defined separately for short-term (<11 beats, $\alpha1$) and longer-term (>11 beats, $\alpha2$) R-R interval data. Reduction of the $\alpha1$ index is a predictor of mortality in patients with ischemic cardiac diseases or heart failure [9].

We studied 139 patients, affected by Alzheimer disease according to the diagnostic criteria as reported in our previous works [3, 7]. 58 Patients were enrolled but only 33 patients (16 F and 17 M, 74.5 ± 8.4 years) completed the study. Dropouts were due to lack of caregivers or errors committed by caregivers during data acquisition. Patients who effectively participated were monitored for a week.

Rather than evaluating 24 periods in the day, in our opinion it was better to analyze the following periods:

- Morning (8.00 and 12.00 a.m.) in which the sympathetic activity is high.
- Afternoon (16.00 and 20.00 p.m.) in which there is an initial decrease of the sympathetic activity and after an increase in the evening.
- Night (24.00 and 2.00 a.m.), in these periods the parasympathetic activity progressively increases).

With this analysis, it is possible to better explore the daily cardiovascular neurovegetative pattern of the patients.

4 Results

In all the patients enrolled the ECG conduction was not influenced by neurological therapy, but in each period considered the indexes of the sympathetic activity, both linear in the time and the frequency domain and non linear, showed a marked increase also during the night period, in which the rest condition was confirmed by the low indexes of the activity level and then there should be an increase in vagal tone instead.

Data are expressed as Mean ± SD (Table 2)

Table 2 HRV analysis of the enrolled patients; both linear and non-linear parameters show an increase of the vagal tone in the evening and night

Hour	R-R ms	LF/HF	SD1/SD2	$\alpha1$
08.00	875.6 ± 159.4	2.4 ± 1.9	1.9 ± 0.6	1.1 ± 0.3
12.00	839.9 ± 143.8	2.4 ± 2.2	1.9 ± 3.9	1.0 ± 0.3
16.00	825.2 ± 128.7	2.4 ± 2.0	1.8 ± 0.7	1.1 ± 0.1
20.00	830.8 ± 135.3	2.8 ± 2.4	1.9 ± 0.8	1.1 ± 0.3
24.00	952.9 ± 140.5	3.3 ± 2.6	2.1 ± 0.8	1.1 ± 0.3
02.00	972.1 ± 130.2	2.8 ± 3.4	1.8 ± 0.7	1.0 ± 0.3

Table 3 HRV analysis of the patients treated with acetyl cholinesterase inhibitors

Hour	R-R ms	LF/HF	SD1/SD2	α1
08.00	894.2 ± 180.2	3.1 ± 2.1	2.1 ± 0.7	1.2 ± 0.3
12.00	863.9 ± 142.7	2.4 ± 2.2	1.9 ± 0.7	1.1 ± 0.3
16.00	840.7 ± 135.9	3.3 ± 2.6	2.1 ± 0.7	1.2 ± 0.1
20.00	843.5 ± 132.6	3.2 ± 2.4	2.0 ± 0.8	1.2 ± 0.3
24.00	971.2 ± 159.6	4.3 ± 3.1	2.1 ± 0.8	1.2 ± 0.3
02.00	1001.6 ± 119.7	3.8 ± 4.7	2.0 ± 0.8	1.1 ± 0.4

A greater increase of vagal tone can be observed during the evening and night

But if we consider only the patients (19-9 F) with acetyl cholinesterase inhibitors we found a surprisingly greater increase in sympathetic activity in all period considered especially during the night periods despite no difference in HR (Table 3).

These preliminary data show that the system can analyze also the effects of different therapies on the neurovegetative cardiovascular control.

The principal result of this study is the possibility to evaluate from remote not only the ECG signals but also, in post-analysis but in real-time, the behavior of the neurovegetative assessment of the cardiovascular system during the day. It is also to couple this aspect with the activity level, the breath frequency and the heart rate. Indeed, the system performs a real-time recording of physiological signals:

- 1-lead ECG Electrocardiogram,
- Bio-impedance
- Activity through 3–axis Accelerometer.

The signals are processed online to determine several physiological indexes (RR Heart rate and Heart rate Variability, Respiration Rate, Activity Level and Body Posture). From the central server it is possible to measure the ECG parameters, especially the impulse formation and conduction, very important in patients under therapy with acetyl cholinesterase inhibitors; these drugs, as known, both interfere with the formation of the electrical impulse and with the impulse conduction (QT prolongation) [6, 11].

Hereafter we show 4 patients who represent the various neurovegetative behaviors. The figures below show the potentiality of this system, as we can observe the activity level, the HR and the behavior of the principal indexes of HRV, expression of the sympathetic and parasympathetic activity during a day, analyzed by means of linear and non linear analysis in different patients. Namely, we indicate as AL, Activity level; HR, Heart Rate; RMSDD, index of HRV in the time domain; Lf and HF spectral components in the frequency domain; SD1 and SD2 (Poincarè Plot) and α1 and α2 (DFA) indexes of HRV analyzed by means of non linear analysis:

If we consider the LF/HF ratio, expression of the sympato-vagal balance, in the previous 4 patients we can observe the four different neurovegetative assessments. The patient A presents an almost normal pattern (sympathetic hyperactivity in the morning and in the evening); the patient B shows a prevalence of sympathetic modulation while patient D shows a prevalence of parasympathetic modulation. In the patient C the sympathetic hyperactivity is present only during the evening and the night.

5 Discussion

Telemedicine applications play an increasingly important role in health care. They offer indispensable tools for home healthcare, remote patient monitoring, and disease management, not only for rural health and battlefield care, but also for nursing home, assisted living facilities, and maritime and aviation settings.

In addition, multiple comorbid conditions among older patients require frequent physician office and emergency room visits, at times leading to hospitalization. In recent years, mobile health systems utilizing hand-held devices (e.g., smart phones or tablet) have been developed, which could be used for health-related interventions. Studies have demonstrated that technological innovation is vital for prosperous economies, and greater technological innovation leads to improved public health indicators. Moreover an optimal model for telemedicine use in the international care setting has not been established.

Our objective was to devise a new home system for cardiovascular and motor control of the patients with dementia. In fact in this study, although of a pilot nature, we used the Pulse Sensor™ which is a wearable electronic, battery operated device that is worn on the chest for the acquisition, recording and transmission of physiological parameters to external devices which can analyze or forward the data to additional storage elements or system. Alongside, we employed Liferesult's tablet PC application and the Omniacare software platform for information display and data analysis.

The overall system permits to monitor not only the normal parameters (ECG, respiratory rate or activity level) but also to have a daily behavior assessment of the neurovegetative cardiovascular pattern related to activity level and respiratory rate. The 4 patients presented in this study show 4 different sympato-vagal system patterns, and then it is possible to modify or to adapt the therapy in a personalized way in real time. For example, the patient B shows an increase of the sympathetic activity during all day and, because the high sympathetic activity correlates with an increase of the cardiovascular risk, it is important to carefully monitor this patient.

In conclusion, the proposed system can help the physician and the caregiver in the control of particular patients. The wireless connection allows various device application and several monitoring arrangements ranging from real-time monitoring to long-term recording of biological signals. Implementation of this model may facilitate both accessibility and availability of personalized monitor and therapy. Further studies would validate it in the clinical and healthcare environment.

Acknowledgements The authors gratefully acknowledge the financial support from the Italian Ministry of University and Research through the project "ACCESS—Information Technology for Assisting Carers at Home" (Fund for Research Enablement "FAR: Fondo per le Agevolazioni alla Ricerca", prog. 280/281–2012 call AAL-JP European Programme).

Further Reading

1. Akselrod S, Gordon D, Ubel FA, Shannon DC, Berger AC (1981) Cohen RJ-power spectrum analysis of heart rate fluctuation: a quantitative probe of beat-to-beat cardiovascular control. Science 10;213(4504):220–222.
2. Allan LM, Kerr SR, Ballard CG, Allen J, Murray A, McLaren AT, Kenny RA (2005) Autonomic function assessed by heart rate variability is normal in Alzheimer's disease and vascular dementia. Dement Geriatr Cogn Disord 19(2–3):140–144
3. Amadoro G, Corsetti V, Lubrano A, Melchiorri G, Bernardini S, Calissano P, Sancesario G (2014) Cerebrospinal fluid levels of a 20–22 kDa NH2 fragment of human tau provide a novel neuronal injury biomarker in Alzheimer's disease and other dementias. J Alzheimers Dis. 42(1):211–226
4. Balocchi R, Cantini F, Varanini M, Raimondi G, Legramante JM, Macerata A (2006) Revisiting the potential of time-domain indexes in short-term HRV analysis. Biomed Tech 51:190–193
5. Brennan M, Palaniswami M and Kamen P (2001) Do existing measures of poincare plot geometry reflect nonlinear features of heart rate variability? IEEE Trans Biomed Eng 48:1342–1347
6. Coppola L, Mastrolorenzo L, Coppola A, De Biase M, Adamo G, Forte R, Fiorente F, Orlando R, Caturano M, Cioffi A, Riccardi A (2013) QT dispersion in mild cognitive impairment: a possible tool for predicting the risk of progression to dementia? Int J Geriatr Psychiatry 28(6):632–639
7. Ferrazzoli D, Sancesario G (2013) Development and significance of the frailty concept in the elderly: a possible modern view. CNS Neurol Disord Drug Targets. 12(4):529–531
8. Howes LG (2014) Cardiovascular effects of drugs used to treat Alzheimer's disease. Drug Saf 37(6):391–395
9. Huikuri HV, Mäkikallio TH, Peng CK, Goldberger AL, Hintze U, Moller M (2000) Fractal correlation properties of R-R interval dynamics and mortality in patients with depressed left ventricular function after an acute myocardial infarction-circulation.
10. Kasanuki K, Iseki E, Fujishiro H, Ando S, Sugiyama H, Kitazawa M, Chiba Y, Sato K, Arai H (2015) Impaired heart rate variability in patients with dementia with Lewy bodies: efficacy of electrocardiogram as a supporting diagnostic marker. Parkinsonism Relat Disord. 21(7):749–754
11. Leitch A, McGinness P, Wallbridge D (2007) Calculate the QT interval in patients taking drugs for dementia. BMJ 15:335(7619):557
12. Malliani A, Pagani M. Lombardi F. Cerreti S (1991) Cardiovascular neural regulation explored in the frequency domain. Circulation 84:1482–1492
13. Martinmaki K, Rusko H, Saalasti S, Kettunen (2006) Ability of short-time Fourier transform method to detect transient changes in vagal effects on Hearts: a pharmacological bloking study. AM J Physiol Heart Circ Physiol 290:H2582–H2589
14. Mellingsæter MR, Wyller TB, Ranhoff AH, Bogdanovic N, Wyller VB (2015) Reduced sympathetic response to head-up tilt in subjects with mild cognitive impairment or mild Alzheimer's dementia. Dement Geriatr Cogn Dis Extra 13;5(1):107–115
15. Mourot L, Bouhaddi M, Perrey S, Cappelle S, Henriet MT, Wolf JP, Rouillon JD, Regnard J (2004) Decrease in heart variability with overtraining: assessment by the Poincaré plot analysis. Clin Physiol Funct Imaging 24:10–8
16. Peng CK, Havlin S, Stanley H, Goldberger A (1994) Quantification of scaling exponents and crossover phenomena in nonstationary heartbeat time series. Chaos 5:82–87
17. Raimondi G, Legramante JM, Scordamaglia B, Masci I, Montanari G, Pampena R, Skroza N, Potenza MC (2014) Linear and non-linear R-R interval variability analysis in the neurovegetative cardiovascular assessment in Psoriasis and Obesity. Appl Inf Syst Eng Biosci 61–69

18. Sayers BM (1973) Analysis of heart rate variability. Ergonomics 16:17–32
19. Scordamaglia B, Masci I, Sindona F, Cuozzo R, Ciaramella A, Raimondi G (2016) Non-linear analysis of the heart rate variability during passive Tilt test. Intern Emerg Med 10:163
20. Woo MA, Stevenson WG, Moser DK, Trelease RB, Harper RH (1992) Patterns of beat-to-beat heart rate variability in advanced heart failure. Am Heart J 123:704–710

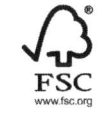

Druck:
Customized Business Services GmbH
im Auftrag der KNV-Gruppe
Ferdinand-Jühlke-Str. 7
99095 Erfurt